P aul Bedson has university qualifications in philosophy and counselling and has integrated these western sciences with a deep understanding of traditional Chinese medicine, oriental philosophy and meditation. He has studied natural medicine in India, South-East Asia, the Philippines and the United States, and has practised as an acupuncturist, body worker, counsellor, meditation instructor and teacher of natural therapies for 17 years.

Paul worked as a resident seminar facilitator, counsellor and natural therapist at the Camp Eden Health Retreat in the Gold Coast hinterland for 14 years. He now works as a counsellor, group psychotherapist and meditation instructor for the Gawler Foundation in Victoria. Each year he teaches hundreds of cancer patients and others the healing power of meditation, a positive spirit and an open heart.

the COMPLETE FAMILY GUIDE *to* NATURAL HEALING

Paul Bedson BA, BAcu, BCouns

HB
HINKLER
BOOKS

Cover Design: Hinkler Design Studio

 Published in 2005 by Hinkler Books Pty Ltd
17–23 Redwood Drive
Dingley VIC 3172 Australia
www.hinklerbooks.com

ISBN 1 7412 1597 8
Printed and bound in China

*I dedicate this book to the healing powers of self-respect and self-love.
I urge all readers to make a commitment to heal themselves.*

Many thanks to Jena, for her support and assistance in creating *The Complete Family Guide to Natural Healing*, and to my son, Jordan, for his unspoken inspiration.

CONTENTS

INTRODUCTION

The Complete Family Guide to Natural Healing is a home reference book for achieving natural health and well-being. I have attempted to provide the reader with an understanding of the major body systems as well as offering options for the prevention and treatment of a wide range of common health complaints.

Knowledge is a powerful tool and in many ways the general public has been disempowered by allowing the knowledge of health and healing to be monopolised by a relatively small number of professionals. *The Complete Family Guide to Natural Healing* is an attempt to circulate information throughout our community and to encourage more individuals to become involved in their own process of health and healing. Disease is such an important learning and awareness opportunity; it can be missed if we relinquish the responsibility for our own healing. In my own life I have found that making a commitment to my health, by listening to my body's voice and respecting its wisdom, has been essential for my healing journey.

The information in *The Complete Family Guide to Natural Healing* has been arranged in a way to facilitate access both for prevention and possible treatments for disease. Chapters One to Ten are set out in terms of the ten major body systems: respiratory, integumentary, nervous, circulatory, digestive, reproductive, hormonal, musculo-skeletal, lymphatic and urinary. Each chapter has an introduction which describes the main functions of that particular body system and recommends nutrients, herbs, essential oils, foods and juices which generally strengthen the organ functions of that system.

If you are aware (based on your personal history of weakness and/or disease) which of your body systems are prone to problems then these specific systems can be fortified by using the general information from the introduction to the relevant chapter.

If you regularly suffer from a certain common complaint then, by referencing that complaint, you can access specific advice for preventing its recurrence. Maintenance of your health, by a commitment to strengthening your inherited or acquired weaknesses, is far preferable to treating illness after it has taken root.

If, however, you are suffering acute symptoms of a particular complaint *The Complete Family Guide to Natural Healing* can be used as a source of treatment options which include: nutrition, herbs, homeopathy, aroma-therapy and dietary and lifestyle recommendations. Common complaints are described in terms of their potential causes and likely symptoms.

Orthodox medicine

The Complete Family Guide to Natural Healing offers options for complementary treatments which can often be used in conjunction with your current medical treatment. The options offered in this book are *not* intended as replacements for direct, personal, medical advice from your doctor or natural therapist. Orthodox medicine can be particularly helpful for a precise diagnosis. Although I encourage self-responsibility in terms of your health, that health also deserves the utmost in professional support.

TREATMENT OPTIONS

Nutritional treatment

Vitamins and minerals can provide valuable nutrition for the body. They supply nutrients which may be lacking from dietary sources. Many common complaints can be treated effectively by improving the diet and/or by taking nutritional supplements. In today's developed countries many people still have an inadequate dietary intake of a range of vitamins and minerals. Stressful lifestyles, environmental pollution and ill health further increase our need for nutrients. Due to preservatives and artificial additives much of our food is lacking in nutrients. Preventing and treating disease through nutrition has been used throughout the world for centuries. The dosages recommended in this book for nutritional supple-ments are therapeutic dosages which are generally higher than the recommended daily allowance. (Recommended daily allowances [RDA] sustain the wellbeing of a fairly healthy individual, whereas therapeutic doses restore health where there is poor health or disease.) When increasing the dosage of supplements, do so gradually and monitor for any reactions. Some individuals may have allergic reactions to certain supplements or the form in which they are administered. Use hypo-allergenic supplements wherever available and check with your health care professional for the appropriateness of the supplement. Always take supplements with a full glass of water and change or rotate brands every 12 months if taking them over a prolonged period of time.

In this book the recommended dosages are for adults, unless otherwise specified. A child weighing 25 to 40 kilograms should be given three-quarters of the adult dose; a child under 25 kilograms should be given half the adult dose; and a child under six years of age should be given specifically designed children's formulas. In the appendix of this book there are lists of dietary sources of vitamins and minerals so you can choose to adjust your diet as well as (or instead of) taking supplements.

Herbal treatment

The use of herbal medicines is an ancient healing legacy. Herbs have been used in numerous countries and cultures for thousands of years. Today herbs and their derivatives are used both by natural therapists and 'orthodox' pharmaceutical chemists. However, natural therapists generally believe that plants in their natural states are preferable to pharmaceutical drugs. The natural plant is a whole organism which is in perfect balance; as such it offers a buffering action (minimising the possibility of undesirable side effects) and also offers a synergistic action (blending subtle qualities of the plant to enhance its effect).

Pharmaceutical science is beginning to prove what herbalists have known for thousands of years: herbs are made up of mutually dependent complex chemicals which work best when used in their organic state. Pharmaceutical chemists have only recently discovered secondary plant products such as alkaloids and glycosides which greatly enhance the primary action of many herbs. In other words, the whole plant is more than just the sum of its active chemical ingredients. For example, aspirin, which is derived from herbs like Meadowsweet and Black Willow, can upset the stomach if taken in excess. On the other hand, Meadowsweet, the whole herb, is used to settle the stomach and reduce excess acidity.

INTERNAL USE
Herbal remedies can be taken as teas (infusions), tinctures or tablets/ capsules. All of these forms are readily available from your herbalist, naturopath, health food store and many chemists, or you can make your own.

- Herbal teas and infusions
To make a herbal tea or infusion use one teaspoon of the dried herb (or mixture of herbs) for each cup of tea required. Place the herbs into a teapot or cup, cover with hot water and leave to steep for ten to 15 minutes. Most herbal teas should be drunk three times a day. Herbal teas can be taken hot or cold, and many are available as tea bags. Any aromatic herbs should be infused in a teapot which has a self-sealed lid to stop the vital oils from being lost through evaporation.

- Tinctures
These are much more concentrated than herbal teas so the dosage is smaller; five–15 drops, taken three times a day. Tinctures can be taken straight or added to a little hot or cold water.

- Tablets and capsules
Tablets and capsules are now available for most single herbs and also for some herbal mixtures. This form of herbal treatment is quicker, more portable and helps to minimise the unpleasant taste of some herbs. Follow the instructions on the container for the correct dosage. Generally children under 25 kilograms should be given half the adult dosage; children over 25 kilograms can take three-quarters the adult dosage.

EXTERNAL USE

For external application herbal remedies can be used as lotions, ointments, gels, douches, compresses and poultices.

- Douches
Herbal infusions or teas can be used as douches (if prescribed). Douches are particularly used for local infections of the vagina. Pour the cooled infusion into a douche bag (available from chemist) and insert the applicator into the vagina. This is easiest done in the bathtub or on the toilet as the liquid will run out of the vagina.

- Lotions
To make a herbal lotion, heat 50 ml of almond oil and add 20–30 drops of the herbal tincture. Simmer on a low heat for a few minutes.

- Gels and ointments
Herbal gels and ointments are available from health food stores and chemists.

- Herbal pillows
To make a herbal pillow, place a handful of each of the recommended dried herbs inside a pillowcase, or sprinkle ten–15 drops of the essential oil on a piece of cloth and place it inside the pillowcase. Sleep on the pillow at night to inhale the fumes.

- Compresses
A compress is a cloth soaked in a warm or cooled herbal infusion (or a tincture added to water) which is

applied directly to an injured area or to a skin condition. Sometimes the heat of the compress is desirable for the treatment so the compress should be changed when it cools down.

- Poultices
  Poultices are similar to compresses, only the solid herbal material is applied directly to the skin or between thin gauze. Dried herbs can be bruised, boiled or added to apple cider vinegar to make something like a paste. This is then either placed behind a thin gauze and placed on the skin, or applied directly to the affected area.

IMPORTANT NOTE
Some people may be allergic to or have negative reactions to certain herbal products. Herbal medicines must be used sensitively as some have ex-tremely strong actions. Although herbs are generally a very safe treat-ment, consultation with a herbalist or naturopath is recommended, especially if the herbs are to be taken over a prolonged period of time.

Homeopathic treatment

Homeopathic medicine has been in use for over 200 years. It is a safe treatment for many common ailments. Homeopathy was founded by Dr Samuel Hahnemann, an eighteenth century German physician and chemist. Hahnemann rediscovered a treatment principle proposed by the 'father of medicine' Hippocrates (c. 460–357 BC); the principle of 'like curing like'. Hahnemann created a system of remedies designed to enhance the body's innate self-restorative powers. He experimented with a wide range of natural remedies derived from animal, vegetable and mineral substances and used his remedies in a manner which is in some ways similar to vaccination. The principle of homeopathy is that a substance that causes symptoms of illness can also cure similar symptoms.

Some homeopathic remedies are as exotic as snake's venom; others as common as onions. All of them are diluted (in preparing them) to such an extent that no possible side effect can be attributed to them. The dilution is to such a degree that only the vibration (or the energetics) of the original substance can be found in the homeopathic remedy. This factor makes homeopathic remedies very safe even for children and pregnant women.

Homeopathics are most effective when all symptoms of the disease are taken into account and the remedy is specific to the individual. Consulting a homeopath is generally more effective than self-diagnosis, although a home first aid kit for common complaints can be very effective.

Homeopathic remedies can be obtained in the form of small pills, tablets, granules, powders or as a tasteless, colorless liquid. The most common dosage is seven–12 drops taken directly under the tongue (for best absorption) or in a small amount of water. The potency of the homeopathic is generally 6C for acute problems and 30C for less acute problems.

Aromatherapy treatment

Aromatherapy uses the medicinal properties of essential plant oils to treat health complaints. It was used in ancient times by the Egyptians, Phoenicians, Romans and Greeks.

Aromatherapy works on both mind and body simultaneously in a gentle and nurturing manner. About 60 essential oils are currently being used for their curative qualities. Oils have various healing properties: antiseptic, antispasmodic, aphrodisiac, calming, warming, anti-inflammatory, balancing, digestive, antidepressant, stimulating, diuretic, clarifying the mind and relaxing the muscles.

Aromatherapy oils are mostly used as massage oils, bath oils, compresses or burnt in an oil burner for inhalation. Some oils can be taken internally.

- Massage oils
  Essential oils should not generally be used straight onto the skin. Mix essential oils with a base oil (ratio of one drop of essential oil per 2 ml of base oil) before using as a massage oil. Recommended base oils include 100 percent pure, cold-pressed fine vegetable oil such as: avocado, hazelnut, wheat germ, grapeseed, olive, safflower and almond. Then add five percent Wheat Germ oil to your mix and store in a dark glass bottle in a cool place.

- Bath oils
  Simply add five–ten drops of essential oil to a hot bath. The essential oils will be absorbed through the skin as well as inhaled.

- Oil burners and inhalation
  Add five–ten drops of essential oil to the bowl of an oil burner and fill the rest of the bowl with water. Light the candle under the bowl and enjoy the aromatic effects. Other methods of inhalation include the traditional bowl of hot water with five–ten drops of essential oil, or a few drops of the essential oil on a handkerchief or pillow.

- Compresses
  This method is used where a specific part of the body needs to be treated directly. Soak a clean cloth in warm water and add five–ten drops of essential oil. Squeeze out excess water and apply to the desired area and then wrap with a warm, damp towel.

IMPORTANT NOTE
Consult a qualified aromatherapist or herbalist before using essential oils if you suffer from: high blood pressure, epileptic seizures, if you are pregnant, or if you have sensitive skin which is prone to allergic reactions.

CHAPTER ONE

THE RESPIRATORY SYSTEM

Maintenance of the lungs, throat and breathing

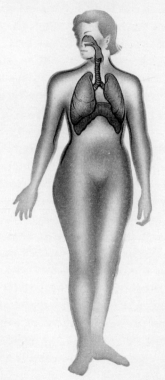

What does it consist of?

The upper respiratory system consists of the nose and the throat. The lower respiratory system consists of the larynx (voice box), the trachea (wind pipe), the bronchial tubes (bronchi) and the lungs. It is important, from a preventative medicine standpoint, to view this network of organs and passageways as a whole system.

Diseases that begin as a minor infection in the upper respiratory system, such as the common cold and hay fever, can then develop into more serious diseases of the lower respiratory system such as pneumonia and bronchitis. By becoming sensitive to the early signs of a respiratory system disorder and by taking responsibility for healing them at this stage, we can often prevent more serious diseases.

What does it do?

The cells which make up every tissue, structure and organ of our bodies continually burn up oxygen in metabolic reactions. These metabolic reactions create energy from nutrient molecules (which come from our food) providing the raw materials for the growth, development and repair of our bodies.

The respiratory system supplies fresh oxygen to the blood so that it can be transported to every cell of the body. At the same time, these metabolic reactions release carbon dioxide as a waste product. Since an excessive amount of carbon dioxide produces acidity—which is harmful to cellular functions—this excess must be eliminated through the respiratory system as we exhale. Our bodies cannot store oxygen, so we need to breathe to replenish our supply of oxygen and eliminate carbon dioxide. The air passes through the nasal passages, where it is warmed, filtered and moistened. This filtering process continues as air flows down through the throat, voice box, wind pipe and bronchial tubes to the lungs. The linings of these air passageways are covered with a specialised membrane which produces mucus. Mucus is necessary to moisten the air and to trap dust particles. These air passages are also lined with tiny hairs, called cilia, which move the mucus and dust bundles along the throat where they can be eliminated by swallowing or spitting. If there is no mucus, this can cause inflammation and a sore, dry throat. If there is an excess of sticky mucus, this can cause congestion and prevent the normal functioning of the air passageways.

What goes wrong with it?

The respiratory system is affected by the quality and content of the air we breathe. The most common problems of this system are related to viral infections, allergies and chemical or mechanical irritants in the form of pollution or smoking. Viral infections such as the common cold are mostly self-limiting (meaning they run their own course). We experience a runny nose, cough, headache, temperature, muscular pain and a sore throat for a few days, but if our immune system is strong we recover without the need for further treatment. However, if our body's natural defences are weak as a result of fatigue or mental and physical stress, then we may not have the energy or the immunity to heal ourselves naturally. If we do not take responsibility for assisting our bodies to heal this initial phase of disease, the virus might spread or cause a secondary infection such as tonsillitis, bronchitis or pneumonia. Most of the patterns of disease of the respiratory system can be grouped into three categories:

(i)   inflammation and dryness;
(ii) congestion from excess mucus;
(iii) spasms of the bronchial muscles.

The wholistic treatments for the respiratory system are used to either prevent weaknesses of the above three categories, or to heal such imbalances once they have appeared.

Orthodox medicine often blames bacteria and viruses as being the causes of respiratory problems, but these organisms can only take hold and multiply in the body if they are given the right conditions in which to thrive. The respiratory system has its own natural defences against disease, namely: lymphatic tissue (e.g. tonsils, lymph nodes), the production of mucus, and the function of cilia. But these defences can be affected by stress, smoking and a poor diet. Stress weakens our immune system, smoking irritates and congests our air passageways, and a poor diet can create an excess of mucus causing congestion. Respiratory disorders involving an excessive formation of mucus (such as catarrh and asthma) can be treated preventively by limiting the consumption of such mucus-forming foods as:

- dairy products, including goat's milk (a little yoghurt may be tolerated);
- refined foods, especially sugar and white flour;
- grains, especially grains high in gluten such as wheat, oats, rye and barley;
- starchy root vegetables such as potatoes, swedes, turnips and parsnips;
- eggs;
- chocolate;
- sweet fruits.

Herbal treatment

There are many herbs that benefit the respiratory system and they fall into three groups.

RESPIRATORY STIMULANTS
These herbs encourage the loosening and expulsion of mucus (i.e. expectoration): Bittersweet, Cowslip, Comfrey, Chickweed, Catnip, Daisy, Senega, Soapwort, Squill and Thuja.

RESPIRATORY RELAXANTS
These herbs relax lung tissue and can ease the flow of mucus and thus encourage expectoration: Angelica, Aniseed, Bitter Almond, Coltsfoot, Elecampane, Eucalyptus, Ephedra, Flaxseed, Hyssop, Greater Plantain, Thyme, Wild Cherry Bark and Wild Lettuce.

RESPIRATORY DEMULCENTS
These herbs relieve and soften irritated or inflamed mucus membranes by lubricating and protecting them: Comfrey Root, Coltsfoot, Flaxseed, Licorice, Irish Moss, Marshmallow Leaf, Mulberry and Mullein.

Traditional Oriental approach

In Oriental medicine the lungs are called the 'Master of Chi' (energy); therefore one of the early signs of a weakness of lung chi is tiredness.

Other signs are:

- shortness of breath (i.e. breathlessness on exertion);
- weak voice;
- physical and mental exhaustion;
- dry skin and/or hair;
- cough;
- slouched shoulders, collapsed chest;
- pale complexion;
- either no sweating or excessive sweating;
- susceptibility to coughs and colds.

The lung meridian (energy pathway) governs:

- the moisture of the skin and hair;
- the opening and closing of the pores of the skin for perspiration;
- the body's defences against the penetration of wind, cold and infections;
- energy levels;
- functioning of the nose, throat and the volume of the voice.

On an emotional level the lung meridian governs grief. Grief is a healthy emotion which enables us to complete situations and let them go. Too much (indulgence) or too little grief (denial) gives rise to a disharmony of lung chi. Pain, sadness or trauma from our childhood, if not completely grieved and released, can cause a weakness or stagnation of our lung chi.

Too much grief can take the form of excessive worry or sorrow which can stagnate the fullness of the breath and create shallow breathing. A victim role and a 'poor-me' attitude can also stagnate lung chi. The slouched shoulders and sunken chest posture of the victim will also restrict the movement of lung chi.

Emotional symptoms of lung chi imbalance are:

- an excess or overindulgence of grief, or prolonged sorrow;
- becoming excessively attached to things and people (i.e. being possessive and unable to let go);
- fatalism, despair and pessimism;
- apathy, a lack of energy and lack of inspiration;
- withdrawal, introversion and a soft voice.

The condition of your skin and hair, energy level, voice and immune system can all be improved by strengthening your lung chi. Lung chi can be increased by: appropriate intensity of exercise, breathing exercises, acupressure and shiatsu massage, stretching, tai chi, acupuncture and Chinese herbs (as prescribed by a practitioner of Chinese herbalism).

Dietary and lifestyle recommendations

- Drink six to eight glasses of fluids a day: herbal teas, juices or mineral water.
- Chicken soup can work wonders if sipped, as it increases the flow of nasal mucus.
- Drink potato peeling broth two or three times daily.

- Yoghurt will build immunity to prevent coughs and colds.
- Have a mustard foot bath. Mix one teaspoon of mustard powder into a paste with water and then add it to a hot foot bath.
- Mucus-forming foods (see page 3) should be avoided.
- Rug up and rest, conserve your energy to fight the infection.

FOODS

Foods which benefit the respiratory system include:

- garlic, parsley, onions, carrots, apricots, sprouts, melons, watercress, tahini, wheat germ, corn, green beans;
- almonds, raw nuts, seeds, pepitas;
- grated beetroot and apple salad;
- grated carrot with chopped oranges;
- grated carrot with finely chopped fennel root;
- sources of vitamin C with bioflavonoids;
- lemon juice;
- celery and grapefruit juice, carrot juice, fresh vegetable juices.

ASTHMA

Description

Asthma is a temporary narrowing of the tubes through which air flows into and out of the lungs. During an attack, spasms in the muscles surrounding the air tubes constrict the outward passage of air making it difficult for the lungs to deflate properly. The spasms are not the cause of the attack, but merely the result of chronic hypersensitivity and inflammation of the muscle wall of the airways to certain stimuli.

Symptoms

The main symptom is a wheeze that is sometimes followed by violent coughing to expel mucus from the lungs. A number of sufferers describe a tightness in the chest area and a tiredness or lethargy caused by the decrease in lung function and the extra effort required to breathe. Varying degrees of breathing difficulties are experienced depending on the severity of the attack.

Causes

It would be a mistake to think that asthma begins and ends with the lungs. It is important to look at the health of the entire body, particularly the immune system. Common triggers for asthma attacks vary widely, but include chemicals such as: tobacco smoke; drugs; food additives such as MSG; foods such as dairy products, nuts, chocolate and colas; as well as allergens such as dust mites, moulds, pollens, cats and dogs. Other triggers include anxiety, stress, exercise, changes in temperature and respiratory infections such as bronchitis.

Nutritional treatment

Nutritional supplements that may be beneficial in the treatment of asthma are listed in the following table—see page xii for information on how to use these supplements.

Herbal treatment

Herbs used to treat the symptoms of asthma are listed below. For infor-mation on how to use these herbs see pages xiii–xv.

EXPECTORANT

An infusion made from the following herbs will help to eliminate mucus: Aniseed, Blood Root, Coltsfoot, Comfrey root, Licorice, Senega, Elecampane and Lobelia.

Nutritional supplements for asthma

SUPPLEMENT	DOSAGE	COMMENT
Vitamin A	15,000 iu daily (if pregnant no more than 15,000 iu daily)	Lungs and the respiratory system require vitamin A to maintain and heal tissues
Beta-carotene	10,000 iu daily	An anti-oxidant
Vitamin B complex	50 mg four times daily	Stimulates the immune system
Vitamin B6	50 mg three times daily	Aids in the absorption of B12
Vitamin B12	100 mg twice daily between meals	Decreases inflammation in lungs during an attack
Vitamin E	600 iu and up daily	Potent anti-oxidant
Vitamin C with bioflavonoids	1500 mg three times daily	Helps fight inflammation and keeps down infection
Kelp	1000–1500 mg daily	A balanced source of a wide range of minerals
Magnesium	750 mg daily	May help stop the acute asthmatic episode by increasing the vital capacity of the lungs. Has a dilating effect on the bronchial muscles
Multivitamin and mineral complex with Selenium	200 mg daily	Necessary to enhance the immune system
Bee pollen	Up to one teaspoon daily	Soothes the mucus membranes
Coenzyme Q10	100 mg daily	Necessary in the utilisation of vitamins and minerals

To dilate bronchioles use: Licorice root, Slippery Elm, Ephedra.

SPASM-REDUCING HERBS
These include: Grindelia, Lobelia, Sundew, Wild Cherry, Aniseed, Oregano, Garlic, Thyme and Angelica root.

TENSION-REDUCING HERBS
Anxiety and tension are often associated with an attack. Try the following herbs: Hops, Skullcap and Valerian.

ANTI-INFLAMMATORY HERBS
Ginko biloba has been used effectively to treat asthmatic symptoms. It is a potent anti-inflammatory, as is ginger.

OTHER USEFUL HERBS
An infusion made from the leaves of Coltsfoot can be beneficial in soothing any irritation in the lungs.

Homeopathic treatment

Treatments that may be prescribed by a homeopath for asthma include:

- Antimonium tartaricum;
- Bryonia;
- Drosera;
- Spongia.

See page xv for information on how to use these homeopathics.

Aromatherapy treatment

Add the following essential oils to an oil burner for relief from the symptoms of asthma:

- Eucalyptus (also good massaged into the chest and back);
- Sandalwood (also good massaged into the chest and back);
- Frankincense;
- Myrrh;
- Roman Chamomile.

See page xvi for information on how to use these essential oils.

Dietary and lifestyle recommendations

- Avoid mucus-forming foods such as dairy products, refined foods, grains, most starchy root vegetables, eggs, chocolate and sweet fruits. Eat a diet consisting of lots of fruit and vegetables which are high in vitamin C such as: capsicum, blackcurrants, parsley, broccoli, brussels sprouts, cauliflower, strawberries, lemons, oranges, spinach, grapefruit, asparagus, fresh beans, peas, tomato, blackberries, sweet potato, lettuce, pineapple, garlic and avocado. Eat hot foods such as chilli peppers and curries three times weekly.
- Avoid very cold drinks and ice-cream.
- Use an elimination diet to detect allergens in your diet. Common triggers include: alfalfa, corn, peanuts, soy products, eggs, beets, carrots, colas, dairy products, fish, red meat (especially pork), processed foods and refined foods (such as white flour and sugar).

For more information on diet see Chapter Eleven. If fish is not an allergic trigger, eating fish three times weekly may also be helpful.

- Manage stress by learning a breathing, relaxation or meditation technique such as yoga, tai chi or qigong.
- Exercise is helpful to keep your breathing pattern efficient, but sustained, strenuous exercise can also trigger an acute attack in some individuals. Try swimming or tennis. Singing can also be beneficial.
- Avoid smokers and dusty environments. Try a negative ioniser which draws dust and other particles from the air; it may be especially helpful in getting a better night's sleep.
- Have a mustard foot bath (see page 5).
- Chinese massage, shiatsu, acupuncture and Chinese herbs have all been found to benefit asthma sufferers. Consult a qualified practitioner for specific treatment advice.

BRONCHITIS

Description

Bronchitis is an inflammatory condition of the main air tubes (bronchi) that carry air to the lungs. The inflammation causes a blockage of the airways resulting in coughing and a build up of mucus due to irritation. There are two main types of bronchitis: acute bronchitis and chronic bronchitis.

Acute bronchitis often follows a respiratory tract infection such as a cold or influenza. It usually runs its course and is over in a couple of weeks, however symptoms can persist and the condition may lead to pneumonia.

Chronic bronchitis is the result of constant irritation of the bronchi. This condition can lead to cardiovascular problems, high blood pressure and fluid retention.

Symptoms

Symptoms of acute bronchitis include fever, chills, coughing, infected mucus, wheezing, chest pains, a sore throat and difficulty in breathing.

Symptoms of chronic bronchitis include chronic cough, infected mucus, shortness of breath, chest and back pain, blue lips and swollen fingertips known as clubbing.

Causes

Acute bronchitis is usually caused by a viral or bacterial infection such as a cold or influenza. Chronic bronchitis is often caused by cigarette smoke, inhaled pollutants, viral or bacterial infections, allergies, or an hereditary predisposition.

Nutritional treatment

The following nutritional supplements (see table below) may benefit those suffering from acute bronchitis. Chronic bronchitis sufferers, however, should seek medical advice first. A course of nutritional supplements may be of benefit in helping boost the immune system of chronic bronchitis sufferers in the long term. See pages xii–xiii for information on how to use these supplements.

Herbal treatment

The most commonly used herbs in the treatment of bronchitis are:

- Angelica;
- Aniseed;
- Blood Root;
- Coltsfoot;
- Elecampane;
- Hyssop;
- Mullein;
- Thyme;
- White Horehound.

These herbs work not only as expectorants to clear the mucus, but they also have demulcent properties to soothe the inflamed tissues of the airways. Fenugreek is another herb that helps reduce mucus flow.

Nutritional supplements for bronchitis		
SUPPLEMENT	DOSAGE	COMMENT
Vitamin A	20,000 iu twice daily for one month then reduce to 15,000 iu daily	For the healing and protection of lung tissue
Beta carotene	15,000 iu daily	An anti-oxidant
Vitamin B complex	100 mg three times daily	Promotes healing of lung tissue
Vitamin C with bioflavonoids	3000 to 10,000 mg daily	Boosts the immune system and reduces histamine levels
Vitamin E	400 iu and up twice daily Take with 50–100 mg vitamin C	Free radical scavenger and oxygen carrier needed for healing tissue. Also helps breathing
Zinc lozenges	One 15 mg lozenge five times daily	Needed for tissue repair
Chlorophyll or fresh wheatgrass juice	Take three times daily or as directed on the bottle	Keeps tissues free of toxins and improves circulation
Garlic	Two 500 mg tablets three times daily with meals	Works as a natural antibiotic by reducing infection

Other herbs for treating bronchitis include Echinacea, Golden Seal, Eucalyptus (taken externally), Licorice, Marshmallow and Peppermint.

Echinacea and Golden Seal extracts help to fight viruses and bacteria by boosting the immune system. At the first sign of illness place one dropperful in your mouth and hold there for ten minutes, then swallow. Do this every three hours but not for more than one week at a time. Caution: only use Golden Seal internally for one to two weeks. Do not use it if pregnant.

HERBAL TEAS
Any of the following teas will help relieve the symptoms of bronchitis:

- Damiana tea;
- Elecampane tea;
- Peppermint tea;
- Wild Cherry Bark tea.

Or you can make your own tea. Combine the dried leaves or flowers of Mullein, White Horehound, Coltsfoot and Lobelia so there are one–two teaspoons of the mixture. Place in a cup of boiling water and infuse for ten to 15 minutes. Take three times daily.

HERBAL BATH
Infuse five drops of Eucalyptus and five drops of Thyme with boiling water and let stand for 30 minutes. Then pour the infusion into a hot bath and soak for 15 minutes.

For more information on how to use herbs see pages xiii–xv.

Homeopathic treatment

Treatment that may be prescribed by a homeopath for bronchitis includes:

- Arsenicum album;
- Belladonna;
- Bryonia;
- Lycopodium;
- Mercurius solubilis;
- Phosphorus;
- Pulsatilla.

See a qualified homeopath for an effective, specific remedy. For more information on how to use homeopathics see page xv.

Aromatherapy treatment

The essential oils that help relieve the symptoms of bronchitis include:

- Myrrh (healing, anti-inflammatory, respiratory, tonic);
- Cypress (circulatory, respiratory, decongestive, head clearing, antispasmodic);
- Eucalyptus (head clearing, respiratory, decongestive, anti-inflammatory, antispasmodic);
- Lavender (respiratory, antibacterial, decongestive, muscle relaxant);
- Peppermint (respiratory, anti-inflammatory, balancing, calmative);
- Thyme (circulatory, respiratory, nervine, relaxant).

There are a variety of ways that you can use these essential oils. See page xvi for more information on how to use them.

- Add a few drops of essential oil to the water of an oil burner for a soothing and healing fragrance.
- A vaporiser can also be helpful in some cases. A few drops of Eucalyptus oil or Lemon oil can be added to the water.
- Cypress oil is often found in commercial preparation for the treatment of colds, flu and bronchitis. A few drops on a handkerchief can help relieve nasal congestion.
- A herbal pillow can be made by putting a handful of dried Cypress, Eucalyptus and Thyme inside a pillowcase, or by putting a few drops of oil on a piece of cloth inside the pillowcase. This will aid congestion and help clear the head.

Dietary and lifestyle recommendations

- A well-balanced diet high in vitamins A and C is recommended. Include garlic and onions in your diet; garlic is a natural antibiotic and both garlic and onions inhibit inflammation.
- Avoid mucus-forming foods such as dairy products, refined foods, fried and fatty foods, red meat, sugar, sweet fruits, white flour, grains, starchy root vegetables, eggs and chocolate.

- Drink plenty of fluids: pure water, herbal teas and soups (especially chicken soup, which fights congestion and thins the mucus). Hot, spicy foods are recommended at least three times a week. Add garlic and hot red peppers to the chicken soup and other dishes.
- Avoid cigarettes and cigarette smoke.
- Avoid caffeinated products like coffee, tea and colas as they make you urinate and thereby lose more fluids than you gain (and become dehydrated).
- Add moisture to the air. Use a vaporiser or steam inhalations to loosen up mucus which is thick and difficult to cough up.
- Don't rely on over-the-counter cough medicines and expectorants. These medicines suppress coughing and coughing is essential for eliminating mucus. Better and cheaper results come from drinking lots of fluids.

IT'S IMPORTANT TO SEE YOUR DOCTOR IF:
- your cough is persistent or very severe;
- you are coughing up blood;
- you are short of breath and have a profuse cough;
- you have a very high fever (over 38.5°C) or a fever that lasts more than three days;
- you feel very tired and lethargic.

CROUP

Description

Croup affects children between the ages of three months and five years. It usually occurs at night because when children sleep their breathing becomes shallower and the muscles in the neck, which assist breathing, don't function as well as usual.

Treatment is directed towards any underlying infections and any swelling or obstruction to the throat should be removed. Any anxiety or emotional agitation will further narrow the air passages so the child should be nurtured and calmed. The vast majority of children recover within a few days. Croup usually follows a cold, bronchitis or an allergy attack.

Symptoms

The symptoms of croup include a sharp cough (which sounds like a seal barking), difficulty breathing in, and excessive movement of the chest with the laboured breathing. The inflammation of the throat is only slightly painful and there may be a mild fever. The cough (called strider) is high-pitched and sharp and wheezing often accompanies the breathing.

Causes

Croup is usually caused by a viral infection which results in inflammation of the windpipe and voice box.

Nutritional treatment

The nutritional supplements that may be beneficial to children suffering croup are listed in the table below. See pages xii–xiii for information on how to use these supplements.

Herbal treatment

The following herbs are especially recommended in the treatment of croup:

- Blood Root (an expectorant which also relaxes the bronchial muscles);
- Echinacea (for the infection and the fever);
- Elecampane (an expectorant which also soothes inflammation);
- Thyme (an expectorant which fights the infection);
- Golden Seal (a powerful tonic for the mucus membranes). Only use for one to two weeks and don't use if pregnant;
- Comfrey (an expectorant which also soothes and reduces irritation);
- Eucalyptus (fights the infection, works well as an inhalant in a vaporiser).

You can also find relief from the symptoms of croup in these herbal remedies.

- Apply hot onion or ginger packs over the chest and the upper back, between the shoulder blades. Make these packs by slicing onion or ginger and placing the slices

Nutritional supplements for croup

SUPPLEMENT	DOSAGE	COMMENT
Vitamin A	2000 iu daily	For healing the inflamed mucus membranes. Give liquid form for young children
Vitamin C	Under four years: 100 mg four times daily Over four years: 500 mg four times daily	Boosts the immune system and controls infection
Vitamin E	Under four years: 10–20 mg daily Over four years: 20–50 mg daily	Speeds up healing of mucus membranes. Use liquid form
Zinc lozenges	As directed on label	Boost the immune system and assist the healing of damaged tissue
Cod liver oil	One tablespoon twice daily in juice	Can be substituted for Vitamin A

between damp, warm cloths. Keep reheating cloths.

- Put one teaspoon of Blood Root into a cup of cold water, bring to the boil and then leave until it's just warm. Drink this Blood Root tea three times daily.
- Ginger herb baths also give relief from the symptoms of croup. Add four ginger tea bags or four tablespoons of chopped raw ginger to a hot bath.
- Make a Eucalyptus and Thyme hot bath. Add five–ten drops of both Eucalyptus and Thyme oils to a hot bath.

For more information on how to use herbs see pages xiii–xv.

Homeopathic treatment

The types of homeopathic treatment used for croup varies according to the specific symptoms that accompany the croup. If there is:

- a loose cough use Aconite or Hepar sulphuris;
- wheezing use Hepar sulphuris;
- rattling sounds use Hepar sulphuris;
- a greenish phlegm use Sulphur;
- croup only on waking use Calcarea sulphurica;
- recurrent croup use Hepar sulphuris;
- croup with barking cough use Aconite, Bellis perennis, Drosera, Spongia, Hepar sulphuris or Kali muriaticum;
- a bluish face use Antimonium tartaricum;

- a cold sweat use Antimonium tartaricum;
- croup worse on waking or worse after sleep use Lachesis.

Consult your homeopath for a specific remedy and see page xv for information on how to use homeopathics.

Aromatherapy treatment

A vaporiser or steam inhalations with a few drops of Eucalyptus and Thyme oil (keep the child's eyes closed) helps to fight the infection and loosen the mucus.

Dietary and lifestyle recommendations

- Milk and dairy products create mucus so they should be avoided. To help break up the mucus give plenty of fluids, such as: water, juices, homemade soups and herbal teas. Water or juice before bedtime can help.
- Add humidity to the air by using a vaporiser or hot showers. This will help relieve the inflammation and stop the coughing.
- Keep the child's head raised when sleeping as this makes breathing easier.

IT'S IMPORTANT TO SEE YOUR DOCTOR IF:
- you have a high fever;
- you have difficulty in breathing;
- you have a sore throat with difficulty swallowing.

EMPHYSEMA

Description

Every breath we take adds oxygen to the blood and removes carbon dioxide. The exhalation releases carbon dioxide and stale air from the lungs. A person suffering from emphysema cannot exhale fully without great effort because the air sacs in the lungs lose their elasticity, enlarge and may rupture.

Symptoms

The most common symptoms of emphysema are: breathlessness followed by coughing during even the slightest exertion, excessive sputum (spittle mixed with mucus) and a barrel-shaped chest. Weight loss may also occur as the pressure of the diaphragm on the stomach causes discomfort when eating full meals. Complications of emphysema include recurrent attacks of bronchitis and pneumonia and an increased risk of heart disease. Although severe cases of emphysema may be very difficult to heal, treatment can minimise the symptoms and make breathing easier.

Causes

Most sufferers of emphysema are long-term cigarette smokers and their emphysema is directly related to their smoking. Other causes include air pollution and occupational exposure to industrial dust.

Nutritional supplements for emphysema

SUPPLEMENT	DOSAGE	COMMENT
Vitamin A	50,000 iu daily (if pregnant no more than 10,000 iu daily)	Needed for repair of lung tissues and to boost immune system
Vitamin C with bioflavonoids	5000 mg daily in divided doses	Aids the healing of damaged and inflamed lung tissues. Boosts the immune system
Vitamin B complex	As directed on label	For proper functioning of immune system
Vitamin E	Up to 1000 iu daily	Anti-oxidant and carrier of oxygen
Selenium	200 mg daily	A destroyer of free radicals created from air pollution
Chlorophyll	As directed on label	Facilitates ease of breathing
Garlic	Two 500 mg capsules three times daily with meals	Promotes sleep, protects nerve endings and acts as a nerve tonic
Kelp	Five tablets daily	Provides important minerals needed for healing lung tissue
Coenzyme Q10	60 mg daily	Anti-oxidant and promotes oxygen absorption by lungs
Proteolytic enzymes	As directed on label between meals	Helps cleanse the lungs
L-cysteine L-methionine	500 mg twice daily on an empty stomach	Amino acids which protect and repair lung tissue

Nutritional treatment

Nutrients may be helpful in treating emphysema. Vitamins A and C in particular help to maintain healthy tissues in the air tubes. Vitamin B, vitamin E and selenium are also important for their anti-oxidant properties. See the above table for nutritional supplements.

Herbal treatment

EXPECTORANTS
- Coltsfoot plays a role in the treatment of most respiratory disorders, as it combines a soothing expectorant with an antispasmodic action. Drink as a herbal tea three times a day.
- Elecampane is an expectorant which also soothes bronchial tissues

and acts as an antibacterial. The root of the plant is used by pouring a cup of cold water onto a teaspoon of the shredded root. Allow to stand for eight to ten hours, then heat. Take three times daily.

- Comfrey Root can also be used with Coltsfoot and Elecampane as it can soothe and protect inflamed tissue and help expectoration. Put one–three teaspoons in a cup of water, bring to the boil and simmer for ten to 15 minutes. Take three times daily.

OTHER HERBAL TREATMENT

The following herbs may also be helpful in treating emphysema: Alfalfa, Fenugreek, Horseradish, Rosemary, Ginkgo, Mullein tea and Thyme.

For information on how to use herbs see pages xiii–xv.

Aromatherapy treatment

Add the following essential oils to an oil burner for relief from the symptoms of emphysema:

- Eucalyptus;
- Pine;
- Thyme;
- Rosemary.

See page xvi for information on how to use these oils.

Dietary and lifestyle recommendations

- If eating causes abdominal discomfort due to the pressure of the diaphragm against the stomach, then eat smaller meals more often.

Eat lots of raw foods such as fresh fruits and vegetables which are high in vitamin C and beta-carotene. All anti-oxidant foods (dark green and orange vegetables) are recommended.

- In addition eat soups, skinless chicken and turkey, fish, brown rice, millet and wholegrain cereals. Chicken soup thins mucus and is good for all respiratory complaints.
- Avoid mucus-forming foods such as dairy products, fried and fatty foods, refined foods, sugar, sweet fruits, red meat, eggs, grains, starchy root vegetables, chocolate and white flour. Salt should be used sparingly.
- Eat spicy foods such as garlic, onions, tabasco sauce, chilli peppers at least three times a week.
- Avoid gas-forming foods such as cabbage and legumes as they can cause bloating which will hinder breathing.
- Develop the muscles of your shoulders and upper chest as they assist in your breathing. Either hand-held weights, push-ups or a gym weight training program may help. Remember to begin with moderate exercise.
- When breathing, concentrate on blowing out slowly through pursed lips to help keep the airways open. Also, practice belly breathing (slow, deep breathing during which you can see your belly moving in and out with the exhalation and inhalation) rather than just breathing into your upper chest.

- Give up smoking and avoid smoke, dust, animal fur, pollution, and hot, humid climates.
- Try a cleansing fast every four months using carrot, celery, spinach and all dark green fresh juices. See pages 329–30 for more details.

IT'S IMPORTANT TO SEE YOUR DOCTOR IF:
- You've caught a cold or flu as these infections can aggravate your condition and make breathing more difficult.

HAY FEVER

Description

Hay fever is an inflammation of the mucus membranes of the respiratory tract, caused by inhaling an allergen. Whatever the cause, the response to the allergen is the same: the sensitive, moist membranes that line our nose and sinuses first encounter the allergen, then histamines are released by the blood and these cause the tissues to become inflamed. The lining of the nose becomes swollen, blocking the air passages, and it secretes large amounts of clear mucus to flush away the offending allergen.

Symptoms

- sneezing
- red eyes or itchy, teary eyes
- runny nose
- itching of the nose
- bad breath
- nervous irritability
- lack of energy

Causes

The allergic symptoms of hay fever are caused by inhaling animal hair, pollen, dust, feathers, fungus, spores or some other environmental agent.

Alcoholic beverages, stressful situations, and changes of the temperature may also precipitate an attack.

Nutritional treatment

When using nutritional supplements (see following table), hay fever sufferers should always choose hypoallergenic supplements. Vitamin E (which decreases the permeability of the capillaries and, therefore, suppresses the release of histamines) is more effective when taken before the symptoms begin rather than after.

For information on how to use nutritional supplements see pages xii–xiii.

Herbal treatment

For information on how to use these herbs see pages xiii–xv.

- White Horehound, Mullein leaf, Nettle, and Wild Cherry Bark in tea, tincture or tablet form will help ward off severe allergic reactions.
- Elder is used for any catarrhal inflammation of the upper respiratory tract such as hay fever and sinusitis.

Nutritional supplements for hay fever

SUPPLEMENT	DOSAGE	COMMENT
Vitamin A	100,000 iu reduced to 25,000 iu daily within four months (if pregnant no more than 10,000 iu daily)	Essential for health of the respiratory system
Vitamin B complex	As directed on label	All B vitamins are essential for the proper functioning of the immune system
Vitamin B6	50 mg twice daily	
Vitamin B5	100 mg three times daily	
Vitamin C with bioflavonoids	2000–10,000 mg three times daily	Acts as an antihistamine
Vitamin E	400–800 iu daily	Decreases the permeability of the capillaries
Kelp	As directed on label	A rich source of minerals: potassium, sodium, magnesium, iron, and calcium
Alfalfa	Use in liquid form, one tablespoon in juice twice daily	Supplies chlorophyll and vitamin K
Zinc	50–80 mg daily	

Elder Flower herbal tea should be drunk hot three times daily.

- Ephedra also reduces allergic responses, and is useful in the treatment of hay fever. Drink as a hot herbal tea three times a day. Caution: do not choose this herb if you suffer from anxiety, glaucoma, heart disease, high blood pressure or insomnia.
- Eyebright is an excellent anti-inflammatory for the upper respiratory tract, and it also benefits symptoms of the eyes. Drink as a hot herbal tea, three times daily.
- A tea made of a combination of the above herbs (Elder Flower, Ephedra and Eyebright) can be more effective than using the herbs individually.
- Fenugreek can also help relieve the symptoms of hay fever. Drink two cups of herbal tea per day.
- Other useful herbs are: Dandelion, Licorice and Parsley. Ginger also

has powerful anti-inflammatory properties. Dandelion, Licorice and Ginger are all available as herbal teas. Parsley can be eaten raw or taken in tablet form.

Homeopathic treatment

The type of homeopathic treatment used for hay fever varies according to the specific symptoms that accompany the hay fever.

For hay fever with:

- a profuse runny nose use Arsenicum album;
- burning eyes use Arsenicum album or Euphrasia;
- irritations to eyes use Nux vomica or Euphrasia;
- an aching face use Gelsemium;
- nasal irritation use Nux vomica;
- a constant desire to sneeze use Arsenicum album;
- a runny nose, worse in morning use Gelsemium;
- a dry or burning throat use Gelsemium or Sabadilla.

Other homeopathic remedies include Allium cepa, Ragweed, Pulsatilla and Naphthaline. Consult your homeopath for a specific remedy and see page xv for information on how to use homeopathics.

Aromatherapy treatment

Add the following essential oils to an oil burner for relief from the symptoms of hay fever:

- Melissa (to soothe the inflammation and calm the allergic response);
- Chamomile (calms inflammation and allergies);
- Eucalyptus (helps cleanse and disinfect the air to make breathing easier).

For more information on how to use essential oils see page xvi.

Dietary and lifestyle recommendations

- Eat more fruits (especially bananas for their magnesium content), vegetables, grains, and raw nuts and seeds. Use onions, garlic and horseradish in cooking. Maintain a high-fibre diet.
- Increase your dietary amounts of fish oil, such as cod liver oil.
- Eating yoghurt for three months prior to the pollen season may lessen the allergic symptoms.
- Try using an air purifier, or even air-conditioning during the pollen season.
- Try yogic nasal cleansing and breathing practices (neti and pranayama). Pour warm salty water into the nose as douche (see pages 333–35 for breathing techniques).

INFLUENZA

Description

Influenza is a very contagious viral infection of the upper respiratory tract. It usually occurs in epidemics as it can be easily spread (particularly in winter) by coughing and sneezing. Influenza is difficult to differentiate from the common cold except that the flu characteristically has a much more rapid onset, often appearing and manifesting symptoms within minutes.

Symptoms

The symptoms of influenza may include some or all of the following:

- chills;
- fever;
- headache;
- runny nose;
- cough;
- anxiety;
- fatigue;
- dry throat;
- hot sensations;
- nausea and vomiting may occur;
- enlarged lymph nodes;
- muscular aches (especially shoulders, back and limbs).

Usually the illness lasts one to seven days, but if not healed it can lead to sinus infections, ear infections, bronchitis and pneumonia. The flu can be a very serious disease for elderly people.

Causes

The cause of an influenza attack is a viral infection, but predisposing factors such as diet, stress and emotional imbalances can weaken the immune system and create susceptibility to infection. Treatment is aimed at relieving the symptoms, strengthening the lungs and preventing secondary infections. All life habits which put stress on the immune system should be avoided, such as smoking, alcohol, drug use, excessive use of fats and sugar, emotional excess and physical stress.

Nutritional treatment

Nutritional supplements that may be beneficial in the treatment of influenza are included in the following table (see next page). For information on how to use these supplements see pages xii–xiii.

Herbal treatment

Herbs used in the treatment of influenza include: Echinacea, Garlic, Ginger, Golden Seal, Boneset, Peppermint, Yarrow, and Elder Flower. These herbs can be taken as teas, tablets or tinctures.

- Make a hot tea with Boneset, Elder Flower, Peppermint and Licorice. Take every two hours.
- Skullcap or Vervain may be useful to treat the depression that often accompanies the flu.
- Golden Seal is a natural antibiotic which helps to relieve congestion. Only use internally for one to two weeks and don't use if pregnant.
- Echinacea is effective for strengthening the immune system.
- Cayenne (capsicum) helps to prevent congestion and headaches by keeping the mucus flowing. Add cayenne and ginger to soups and other foods and make a hot drink of cayenne, ginger, garlic, lemon and honey.

- Fenugreek breaks up mucus and phlegm and facilitates expectoration. It also soothes inflamed tissue.
- Slippery Elm helps remove excess mucus from the body.

See pages xiii–xv for information on how to use these herbs.

Homeopathic treatment

The type of homeopathic treatment used for influenza varies according to the specific symptoms that accompany the influenza.

For influenza with:

- aching limbs use Bryonia, Gelsemium or Nux vomica;
- throbbing pain and red, dry skin use Belladonna;
- chilliness use Arsenicum album
- exhaustion and anxious feelings use Arsenicum album;
- a painful cough use Bryonia;
- irritability use Nux vomica;
- a painful throat use Bryonia;
- stubborn catarrhal symptoms, yellow mucus use Pulsatilla;

Nutritional supplements for influenza

SUPPLEMENT	DOSAGE	COMMENT
Vitamin A plus Beta-carotene	15,000 iu daily of vitamin A (if pregnant no more than 10,000 iu) 15,000 iu daily of beta-carotene	Boosts the immune system and protects the tissues lining the throat
Vitamin B complex	100 mg daily	Helps metabolise calories and assists nutritional levels
Vitamin C with bioflavonoids	5000–20,000 mg daily in divided doses	Stimulates the production of interferon, a virus killer
Zinc	Take in lozenge form as directed on label every two hours	Powerful stimulant for the immune system and nourishes the cells
Amino acid complex	As directed on label	Helps to regulate the fever and repair damaged tissue
L-lysine	500 mg daily on an empty stomach	Combats viral infections
Garlic	Two 500 mg capsules three times daily	For its antiviral and antibacterial properties
Kelp	Five-ten tablets daily	Excellent mineral source

- heaviness use Gelsemium;
- hot and cold chills up the spine use Gelsemium.

Consult your homeopath for a specific remedy and see page xv for information on how to use homeopathics.

Aromatherapy treatment

For information on how to use these essential oils see page xvi.

- Eucalyptus oil in the bath or as a steam inhalation eases congestion.
- Diluted Tea Tree or Thyme oil rubbed on the palms of the hands, the sides of the neck and the enlarged lymph nodes of the groin will help.
- Add the following essential oils to an oil burner for relief from the symptoms of influenza: Basil, Black Pepper, Ginger, Grapefruit, Lemon, Orange, Juniper, Lavender, Marjoram, Myrrh, Peppermint, Tea Tree, and Sandalwood.

Dietary and lifestyle recommendations

- Increased fluid intake is essential if a fever is present. Also keep up your nutritional levels in order to maintain and strengthen your immune system. If solid food is undesirable take stews, soups, vegetable juices and herbal teas. Energy sources like carbohydrates are important to keep the immune system strong.
- Take hot chicken or turkey soup with a dash of cayenne and plenty of garlic. Carrot is a helpful anti-oxidant food, while chillies have natural aspirin as well as being antibacterial and anti-oxidants.
- Don't exercise. Sleep, rest, meditate and breathe slowly and deeply.
- Use a humidifier or a vaporiser as they both moisten the mucus membranes in the nose and throat, so microbes are trapped and expelled.
- Boosting your immune system all year round is by far preferable to flu vaccinations as the side effects of the vaccinations may be considerably worse than the flu itself.

IT'S IMPORTANT TO SEE YOUR DOCTOR IF YOU HAVE ANY OF THE FOLLOWING SYMPTOMS:
- hoarseness;
- pains in the chest;
- difficulty breathing;
- vomiting which continues for more than a day;
- severe abdominal pain (may be a sign of appendicitis).

This is especially important for people over 65 years of age.

LARYNGITIS

Description

Acute laryngitis is a viral or bacterial infection or irritation of the larynx, the voice box or Adam's apple at the front of the throat. It often results from an untreated common cold or some other upper respiratory infection. The characteristic hoarseness results from swelling of the mucus membranes around the vocal cords. If resulting from the common cold or other upper respiratory tract infection, those illnesses must be treated at the same time.

Laryngitis may settle and resolve itself within five to ten days but recovery can be prolonged if the sufferer smokes cigarettes or uses the voice excessively.

Chronic laryngitis appears more slowly and the symptoms persist for a longer time.

Symptoms

- hoarseness of voice or loss of voice
- throat pain and cough
- fever and tiredness
- constant urge to clear the throat
- difficulty swallowing

Causes

Underlying factors in acute laryngitis include a diet low in vitamin C, congestion of the lymphatic system, stress and environmental pollution or smoking. Chronic laryngitis is caused by excessive smoking, coughing or overuse of the voice box.

Nutritional treatment

Nutritional supplements that may be beneficial in the treatment of laryngitis are included in the following table. For information on how to use nutritional supplements see pages xii–xiii.

Herbal treatment

Herbs used in the treatment of laryngitis are most effective if taken as teas or gargles. For relief from the

Nutritional supplements for laryngitis

SUPPLEMENT	DOSAGE	COMMENT
Vitamin A	25,000 iu daily (if pregnant do not exceed 10,000 iu daily) or one capsule of cod liver oil	Strengthens the immune system and heals inflamed mucus membranes
Vitamin C with bioflavonoids	5000 mg daily in divided doses	Aids the healing of inflamed mucus membranes
Zinc	50–80 mg daily	Necessary to mobilise vitamin A from liver
Garlic	Two capsules three times daily with meals	Boosts the immune system

symptoms of laryngitis, try the following.

- Sip Red Sage tea.
- Gargle with Red Sage or Thyme tea to help relieve inflammation as well as for their anti-microbial properties.
- Agrimony and Raspberry can also be used together as a gargle.
- Echinacea and Myrrh are also anti-microbial herbs, and can be used together with lymphatic tonics like Poke Root, Marigold and Golden Seal. (Only use Golden Seal for one to two weeks and don't use if pregnant.)
- Comfrey and Marshmallow tea (drunk while still warm) will also soothe a sore throat.
- Blackcurrant juice or syrup is high in vitamin C and very effective in treating sore throats. It is particularly tolerated by small children.
- Blood Root tea taken three times a day benefits laryngitis.
- A drink made of hot water, lemon, honey and grated ginger can soothe a sore and inflamed throat.

For more information on using herbs see pages xiii–xv.

Homeopathic treatment

Treatment that may be prescribed by a homeopath for laryngitis will vary according to the symptoms but may include:

- Pulsatilla or Drosera for an irritated larynx;
- Drosera, Pulsatilla or Rhus toxicodendron for a tickling throat and larynx area;
- Argentum nitricum or Rumex crispus for a lost voice;
- Argentum nitricum, Bryonia, Drosera, Natrum muriaticum, Phosphorus, or Sulphur for a hoarse voice;
- Belladonna or Silicea for a sore throat with swollen glands;
- Aconite for laryngitis with high fever;
- Phosphorus for laryngitis with a dry, tickly cough;
- Causticum for laryngitis with a dry, raw throat and violent coughing.

See page xv for information on how to use homeopathics.

Aromatherapy treatment

Try inhalations of the following oils (individually or combined) for relief from the symptoms of laryngitis:

- Clove;
- Peppermint;
- Eucalyptus;
- Sandalwood;
- Lemon.

Tea Tree oil is effective as a gargle. Place a few drops in a glass of warm water and gargle daily.

See page xvi for information on how to use essential oils.

Dietary and lifestyle recommendations

- Rest your vocal cords.
- Warm salt-water gargles can relieve a sore throat.
- Drink lots of warm water: eight to ten glasses a day. Juices, soups and liquefied foods are most appropriate while the throat is red and sore.
- Steam inhalations can restore lost moisture in your throat and thereby quicken the healing process.
- Menthol chest rubs (particularly when applied at night) may make breathing easier and facilitate rest.
- Cold water and apple cider vinegar can be applied externally as a compress to cool the throat.
- As laryngitis is associated with the throat chakra (centre), a lack of communication and creative expression may be an underlying cause of laryngitis.

IT'S IMPORTANT TO SEE YOUR DOCTOR IF:

- pain is so bad you have difficulty swallowing, as the swelling could also block your airways;
- you cough up blood;
- there is difficulty breathing or you hear severe wheezing when you breath;
- the laryngitis doesn't improve after a week of voice rest.

PNEUMONIA

Description

Pneumonia is a serious infection of the lungs which occurs when the tiny air sacs in the lungs become irritated and inflamed and filled with mucus and pus. The causes of pneumonia are primarily bacteria, viruses or fungi.

BACTERIAL PNEUMONIA

Bacterial pneumonia is extremely serious and most commonly found in very young children or the elderly. A chest X-ray is the only way to identify the condition, which can last between four and eight weeks. When bacteria exists in the lungs your resistance to further infection is lowered making you more vulnerable to secondary bacterial infection. If this occurs it is known as double pneumonia.

VIRAL PNEUMONIA

Viral pneumonia is usually less severe than bacterial pneumonia, however if not cared for properly a bacterial infection can set in.

FUNGAL PNEUMONIA

Fungal pneumonia is less common than bacterial and viral pneumonia. It tends to affect people with HIV and AIDS, certain cancers or organ transplant patients.

Symptoms

The symptoms of pneumonia include: fever, chills, chest pain, sore throat, rapid respiration, bluish colour to the nails, fatigue, and a cough that produces thick yellow/green mucus (and sometimes blood as well).

Causes

The causes of pneumonia include: chemicals, allergies, alcoholism, malnutrition, smoking, cardiovascular disease, diabetes, HIV infection, kidney failure and cancer.

Pneumonia can also be preceded by a cold or influenza.

Nutritional treatment

Nutritional supplements that may be beneficial in the treatment of pneumonia are included in the table below.

See pages xii–xiii for information on how to use nutritional supplements.

Herbal treatment

The following herbs are recommended for a number of respiratory conditions: Blood Root, Coltsfoot, Echinacea, Garlic, Ginger, Golden Seal (only use internally for one to two weeks and don't use if pregnant), Licorice, Lobelia, Thyme, White Horehound.

- Herbal pillows and poultices can provide some relief for respiratory ailments.

Nutritional supplements for pneumonia

SUPPLEMENT	DOSAGE	COMMENT
Beta-carotene	15,000 iu daily	Beneficial for the lungs and the respiratory system
Vitamin A	Up to 100,000 iu daily— use emulsion form only	Enhances immune system and promotes repair of lung tissue
Vitamin B	100 mg three times daily	Helps digestion and assists nutritional levels
Vitamin C	3,000–10,000 mg throughout the day	Helps reduce inflammation
Vitamin E	1500 iu emulsion daily	Promotes immune system
L-carnitine and L-cysteine	As directed on label	Helps protect lungs from free-radical damage
Zinc	80 mg daily	Needed for tissue repair and immune function

- For a sore throat try Sage tea with a few clove buds as a gargle.
- Also try the herbal remedies listed under Bronchitis and the Common Cold.

EXPECTORANTS

Expectorants loosen the mucus from the respiratory system. Expectorants recommended for pneumonia include: Cowslip, Bittersweet, Daisy, Senenga and Soapwort.

RESPIRATORY RELAXANTS

Respiratory relaxants help relax the lung tissue. Try Angelica, Aniseed, Coltsfoot, Flaxseed, Hyssop, Sundew and Wild Lettuce.

See pages xiii–xv for information on how to use herbs.

Homeopathic treatment

Homeopathy is recommended both during illness and after recovery to aid in building up immune resistance to further infection. In the case of pneumonia, orthodox consultation with your doctor is recommended first.

Treatment that may be prescribed by a homeopath for pneumonia includes:

- Aconite for coughs with a fever, and/or a sore throat;
- Bryonia for chest pain;
- Phosphorus for respiratory problems with tightness in the chest;
- Ferrum phosphoricum for cough during the day only;
- Kali muriaticum for barking, hard cough.

See page xv for information on how to use homeopathics.

Aromatherapy treatment

Useful oils in the treatment of pneumonia include:

- Thyme (antiseptic, circulatory, respiratory nervine, muscle relaxant. Use as a bath or massage oil);
- Sandalwood (if you are chilled a few drops in a warm bath will leave you feeling warm);
- Pine (a powerful antiseptic used for treating infections of the respiratory system. Used in poultices or as an inhalation);
- Lemon (effective in treating colds and sore throats. Immune system enhancer. Use as a bath or body oil);
- Clove (antiseptic, antispasmodic, respiratory, warming. Use in an oil burner);
- Basil, Black Pepper, Clove, Eucalyptus, Ginger, Juniper, Lavender, Lemon, Peppermint, Pine, Tea Tree (use in an oil burner for relief from the symptoms of pneumonia).

See page xvi for information on how to use essential oils.

Dietary and lifestyle recommendations

- It is important to note that a chest X-ray is the only positive way of identifying pneumonia and in most cases antibiotics are administered. Natural therapies can be used alongside traditional/orthodox medicine to help build the immune system, however see your doctor first.

- Generally a light diet is recommended and a high fluid intake is extremely important. Try fruit and vegetables juices, herbal teas, soups and broths.
- Avoid all refined and processed foods, alcohol, coffee, tobacco and dairy products.
- Bed rest is highly recommended.
- Use a vaporiser with Eucalyptus and Pine oil to help ease the breathing.
- If taking antibiotics also take acidophilus in capsule or liquid form three times daily.

SINUS PROBLEMS/ SINUSITIS

Description

Sinuses are cavities situated below, above and between the eye sockets; they are located within the bones of the face. The sinuses are connected by small holes and tubes, and they are lined with mucus membranes. The whole network of tubes and cavities is kept moist by the mucus and it slowly drains into the back of your nose and throat. The mucus linings of the sinuses secrete excess mucus when irritated, and if bacteria or viruses are present, an infection may result. Any factor which causes excess mucus secretion may result in the obstruction of mucus flow and drainage. The sinus holes become blocked and pus (from the bacteria) is formed. The mucus linings become swollen and inflamed.

Treatment may involve nutritional changes, strengthening the immune system, resolving the inflammation and assisting the drainage of the sinuses.

Symptoms

The symptoms of sinusitis include any or all of the following:

- nasal congestion;
- fever (usually low grade);
- thick pussy discharge;
- facial pain and tenderness;
- frontal headache;
- earache and/or toothache;
- redness and swelling over the sinuses;
- fatigue.

Causes

There are many things that can precipitate an attack of sinusitis. Some of the most common causes include: allergy, hay fever, viral or bacterial infections, dental infections, nasal polyps, air pollution, underwater swimming, and extreme changes of temperature and dampness.

Environmental and nutritional causes are also pre-disposing factors. Sinusitis can be caused by dairy products, toxins and pesticides from sprayed foods, and vitamin A and C deficiencies.

Nutritional treatment

Nutritional treatments that may be beneficial in the treatment of sinusitis are included in the following table.

See pages xii–xiii for information on how to use nutritional supplements.

Herbal treatment

Herbs that may help sinusitis include: Marjoram, Honeysuckle, Horseradish, Golden Seal, Peppermint, Garlic, Anise, Fenugreek, Ginger, Marshmallow and Red Clover.

• Drink two cups of Fenugreek tea per day.
• A tea of Echinacea (boosts the immune system), Golden Seal and Marshmallow (a powerfully soothing herb) taken every three to four hours may be very beneficial.

• Golden Seal can be taken as a tea or as an intranasal douche (to rinse out the nose). Only use internally for one to two weeks and don't use if pregnant.
• Hydrastis tea can also be used as a douche.
• Ginger root can be grated or crushed, warmed in water and applied to the forehead and nose as a poultice to stimulate drainage.
• Mullein, Licorice and Comfrey root reduce inflammation and soothe irritation. These herbs can be used as teas or tinctures.

See pages xiii–xv for information on how to use herbs.

Homeopathic treatment

Treatment that may be prescribed by a homeopath for sinusitis depends on the symptoms.

• For blocked and painful sinuses try Kali bichromicum, Lycopodium, Mercurius solubilis or Silicea.
• For sinusitis accompanied by weepiness, and pain above the eyes

Nutritional supplements for sinus problems/sinusitis		
SUPPLEMENT	DOSAGE	COMMENT
Vitamin A	10,000 iu daily	Maintains health of mucus membranes and boosts the immune system
Vitamin C with bioflavonoids	3000–10,000 mg daily in divided doses	Prevents further infection and facilitates repair of damaged sinus tissues
Vitamin E	400–1000 iu daily	Improves circulation and facilitates repair of damaged sinus tissues

---

Nutritional supplements for sinus problems/sinusitis

SUPPLEMENT	DOSAGE	COMMENT
Garlic	Two 500 mg capsules three times daily	Boosts the immune system
Bee pollen	Take with juice one teaspoon daily, slowly increasing to one tablespoon	Boosts the immune system and repairs damaged tissue
Flaxseed oil	As directed on label	Reduces inflammation and eases pain
Coenzyme Q10	60 mg daily	Oxygenates cells and repairs damaged tissues

---

or cheekbones take Pulsatilla.

- For sinusitis with facial tenderness take Hepar sulphuris.
- For sinusitis with stringy mucus take Kali bichromicum.

See page xv for information on how to use homeopathics.

Aromatherapy treatment

- Add the following essential oils to an oil burner for relief from the symptoms of sinusitis: Aniseed, Lavender, Lemon, Eucalyptus, Tea Tree, Orange, Pine, Bergamot, Peppermint, Chamomile, Basil and Black Pepper.
- Steam inhalations with Eucalyptus oil may be very beneficial.
- Apply Menthol or Eucalyptus packs over the sinuses.

See page xvi for more information on how to use aromatherapy oils.

Dietary and lifestyle recommendations

- Douche nasal passages with warm salty water. Yoga practitioners use a neti pot to douche, these pots can be very handy (see page 334).
- Eat a diet high in raw foods. Increase your intake of garlic, onions, and ginger. Eat some hot chilli peppers to cause nasal discharge and relieve congestion, or sniff an onion.
- Drink hot soup (chicken) or other hot drinks from a cup, the steam actually helps to unclog the nasal passages and the fluids help dilute the mucus. Hot showers, humidifiers, vaporisers and negative ionisers are all helpful in the same way.
- Avoid mucus-forming foods such as dairy products, refined, processed, tinned, bottled and frozen foods, alcohol, coffee and smoking.

- Consider going on a cleansing juice fast (see pages 329–30).
- Blowing your nose forcefully actually forces mucus back into the sinus cavities. It's better to sniff excretions to the back of the throat than to expectorate.

IT'S IMPORTANT TO SEE YOUR DOCTOR IF:
- a fever develops
- the symptoms continue for weeks without relief

COMMON COLD

Description

The common cold is an infection of the upper respiratory tract. Colds are caused by viruses, of which there are over 200, and they are transmitted by inhaling the infected droplets from air when someone sneezes or coughs. Colds are most contagious during the first few days.

Poor nutrition, tiredness and stress will all make the immune system more vulnerable to these viruses.

Ordinarily a cold will last for between five and ten days. After this the symptoms should reduce.

Symptoms

The symptoms of the common cold include:

- tiredness/lethargy;
- fever;
- muscle aches and pains;
- running nose;
- sore throat;
- sneezing;
- headaches;
- coughing.

Causes

Colds are caused by viral infections, however, a sluggish immune system, stress and poor nutrition will all increase vulnerability to a cold virus.

Nutritional treatment

Nutritional supplements that may be beneficial in the treatment of the common cold are included in the following table. See pages xii–xiii for more information on how to use these supplements.

Herbal treatment

For information on how to use the following herbs see pages xiii–xv.

- The herbs that are most effective in treating colds are Elder, Fenugreek, Horseradish, Hyssop, St John's Wort, Slippery Elm and Yarrow.

Nutritional supplements for the common cold

SUPPLEMENT	DOSAGE	COMMENT
Vitamin A	15,000 iu daily (if pregnant do not exceed 10,000 iu daily) or one capsule of cod liver oil daily	Strengthens immune system and helps heal inflamed mucus membranes
Beta-carotene	15,000 iu daily	An anti-oxidant
Vitamin C	5000–20,000 mg daily	For children use calcium ascorbate or buffered vitamin C Boosts the immune system
Vitamin B complex	50–100 mg three times daily	Boosts the immune system
Kyolic Garlic	Two 500 mg capsules three times daily	A natural antibiotic
Kelp	Five to ten tablets daily	A rich source of minerals
Calcium	As directed on label	
Zinc gluconate	As directed on label	Has anti-oxidant properties and boosts the immune system
Zinc and C lozenges	15 mg lozenge every three hours (do not exceed 100 mg daily from all supplements)	Boosts the vitamin immune system

- In the initial stages of a cold use an Echinacea and Golden Seal combination to prevent infection by boosting the immune system. Take Golden Seal and Echinacea as a tea or take one to two capsules of each twice daily. Both herbs are recommended for children and Echinacea in liquid form works well for children. (Do not use Golden Seal internally for more than one to two weeks and don't use if pregnant).
- Eat garlic for its antibacterial and antiviral properties.
- The following herbal teas are helpful for coughs and colds: Anise, Balm, Basil, Chamomile, Garlic, Horseradish, Peppermint, Licorice root, Spearmint, and Thyme. See page xiv for information on how to make herbal teas.

- Licorice-root tea soothes irritated throats and relieves coughs.
- Herbs such as Elderflower, Peppermint and Yarrow can be combined equally to make a tea. This combination has anti-catarrhal decongestive qualities. The tea should be drunk three times a day as hot as possible (see page xiv).
- Ginger, Catnip and Yarrow can be used to promote sweating. Use these herbs as hot herbal teas (see page xiv).
- A tea made with a few slices of fresh ginger is an excellent single herb remedy to counteract the early stages of a simple cold or flu.
- Rosehips are rich in vitamin C and bioflavonoids. Vitamin C can never be overestimated in the prevention and relief of colds and flu. Rosehip can be taken as a tea (see page xiv).
- Make a garlic, lemon and honey syrup. Blend a few cloves of garlic into honey and add freshly squeezed lemon juice. Taken as a syrup this mixture makes an excellent treatment for sore throats and bronchial disorders.

Homeopathic treatment

Treatment that may be prescribed by a homeopath for a cold includes Gelsemium, Hepar sulphurs, Allium cepa and Mercurius solubilis.

- Nux vomica is prescribed for colds with irritability, chilliness, watery eyes, headache and sore throat.

- Pulsatilla is prescribed for a cold with yellow mucus, lack of thirst and loss of smell.

For information on how to use homeopathics see page xv. Consult a qualified homeopath for the most effective, specific remedy for your individual case.

Aromatherapy treatment

Add the following essential oils to an oil burner or massage diluted oil directly onto the skin for relief from the symptoms of a cold: Basil, Lavender, Ravensara, Black Pepper, Lemon, Eucalyptus, Orange, Ginger, Peppermint, Grapefruit, Tea Tree, Juniper and Thyme.

- Combine Eucalyptus or Peppermint oil with boiling water and use as an inhalant to help clear nasal passages.
- Three drops of Tea Tree oil to one cup of warm water gargled three times daily helps relieve a sore throat.

For information on how to use essential oils see page xvi.

TONSILLITIS
Description

Tonsillitis is an inflammation of the tonsils, which are small glands of lymphatic tissues located at the back of the throat. These glands become very red and irritated, often with yellow or white spots of pus.

Tonsillitis is most common in children but can occur at any age. Some people have recurring bouts of tonsillitis and the condition can become chronic. This causes scar tissue to build up on the tonsils.

Symptoms

The symptoms of tonsillitis include headache, earache, fever, chills, difficulty swallowing, bad breath, sore throat and swollen lymph glands in the neck.

Causes

Tonsillitis is usually caused by streptococcus bacteria (this is where the term strep throat comes from). However it can also be caused by a virus.

Tonsils are there to trap germs and develop antibodies to fight infection. However, if the body is run down resistance to infection is lowered. Cigarette smoking, influenza, measles, and allergies and inhaled irritants can also cause tonsillitis.

Nutritional treatment

Nutritional supplements that may be beneficial in the treatment of tonsillitis are included in the following table. See pages xii–xiii for information on how to use these supplements.

Herbal treatment

Herbs that may be beneficial in the treatment of tonsillitis include:

- Catnip;
- Echinacea;
- Golden Seal;
- Slippery Elm;
- St John's Wort;
- Thyme;
- Mullein;
- Chamomile;
- Garlic;
- Ginger;
- Peppermint;
- Sage.

Gotu Kola is especially recommended for sore throats and tonsillitis.

HERBAL TEAS

Pour a cup of boiling water onto two teaspoons of the herbs listed below and leave to infuse for ten to 15 minutes; drink three times a day:

- Echinacea (can help boost the immune system and fight infection);
- Thyme (reduces fever, headaches and mucus, and is good for sore throats);
- Catnip (a traditional herb used for colds and flu, helps reduce fever);
- Chamomile (excellent for headaches, fever and pain; do not use on an ongoing basis as an allergy may result);
- Sage and/or Thyme (warm); gargle to relieve sore throat;
- Golden Seal (a powerful tonic herb especially useful for upper respiratory tract infections; do not use internally for more than one to two weeks and don't use if pregnant).

POULTICES

Mullein poultices are very soothing applied externally to the throat.

For information on how to use these herbs see pages xiii–xv.

Homeopathic treatment

Treatment that may be prescribed by a homeopath for tonsillitis varies according to the symptoms. Use:

- Belladonna for a very sore throat;
- Hepar sulphuris for splinter-like pain spreading up to your ear and swollen tonsils;
- Mercurius solubilis for swollen, ulcerated tonsils and bad breath

- Calcarea phosphorica if a common cold brings on tonsillitis;
- Baryta carbonica, Belladonna or Ignatia amara for inflamed tonsils.

For information on how to use homeopathics see page xv.

Aromatherapy treatment

The following oils can be very beneficial in helping to treat sore throats, either as a rub (by combining with a base oil such as Apricot, Avocado or Grape Seed oil) or as an inhalant using an oil burner or vaporiser. See page xvi for information on how to use these oils:

Nutritional supplements for tonsillitis

SUPPLEMENT	DOSAGE	COMMENT
Vitamin A	10,000 iu daily for three days then reduce to 5000 iu daily	Needed for the repair of tissues
Vitamin B complex	50 mg three times daily with meals	Helps reduce swelling
Vitamin C	5000–20,000 mg daily	Boosts the immune system and fights infection
Zinc lozenges	As directed on label	Aids healing
Chlorophyll	Use as a gargle	Can help to heal irritations in the mouth and throat. Has an antibiotic effect
Cod liver oil	As directed on label	Aids in tissue repair and boosts the immune system
Colloidal silver	As directed on label	Promotes healing
Vitamin E	400 iu daily	Destroys free radicals

- Clove;
- Eucalyptus;
- Lemon;
- Peppermint;
- Pine;
- Sandalwood;
- Tea Tree;
- Bergamot;
- Lavender;
- Thyme.

Dietary and lifestyle recommendations

Avoid dairy foods as these may aggravate the condition. Juices, soups and blended drinks are easier to take when the throat is inflamed and sore. A cleansing juice fast for two to five days can be very helpful.

- Use a warm salt-water gargle made up of $1/4$ teaspoon of salt in a glass of warm water, three times a daily.
- Diluted hydrogen peroxide or glycerine may also be used as a gargle.
- Do not smoke, avoid smokers, rest and drink plenty of fluids.

IT'S IMPORTANT TO SEE YOUR DOCTOR IF:
- there is no improvement after two weeks.

WHOOPING COUGH

Description

Whooping cough begins as a cold then develops into a cough which steadily worsens. The coughing becomes very severe, beginning with a spasm and ending with a 'whoop'-like sound as the patient gasps for breath between each coughing bout.

Thick stringy mucus can be coughed or vomited up. The patient can turn blue and lose consciousness from lack of oxygen. Whooping cough causes the whole of the respiratory track to become inflamed.

Whooping cough mainly affects very young children and infants and is highly contagious. It can also be potentially life threatening if not treated promptly. The symptoms can last for up to ten weeks.

Life-threatening illnesses such as whooping cough need to be treated immediately and with great care. The patient must be isolated as this illness is highly contagious. Orthodox medicine prescribes antibiotics in the first stage of whooping cough, however these are of little use once the coughing has taken hold. Oxygen and sedatives are also used in the treatment to give some relief to the patient.

Whooping cough can be avoided as there is a vaccine given to infants at two, four, six and 18 months called

Nutritional supplements for whooping cough

SUPPLEMENT	DOSAGE	COMMENT
Vitamin C	5000–20,000 mg daily in divided doses	Improves immunity and eliminates mucus
Vitamin A	15,000 iu daily (if pregnant no more than 10,000 iu daily)	Improves immunity and heals inflamed mucus membranes
Vitamins B5 and B6	50 mg daily	Benefits respiratory system and immunity
Vitamin E	10 mg daily for children under three years 20 mg daily for children between three and six 50 mg for children over six years	Assists the healing of inflamed respiratory tissue
Zinc lozenges	15 mg every three hours for three days	Boosts the immune system

triple antigen, (combined with the diphtheria and tetanus vaccines). There is a minimal risk of side effects, the most common being fever and crying.

Symptoms

Whooping cough begins with cold or flu-like symptoms, followed by a severe cough, loss of appetite, fatigue, difficulty with breathing that causes blue extremities, vomiting and thick mucus.

Causes

Whooping cough is caused by a bacteria that is transmitted through airborne droplets exhaled or coughed up by the patient. Adults can pass on the illness to children. In adults it often appears to be an ordinary cold, but it effects children much more severely.

Nutritional treatment

Nutritional supplements that may be beneficial in the treatment of whooping cough are included in the above table. See pages xii–xiii for information on how to use these supplements.

These vitamin and mineral supplements have been found to be closely linked to the proper functioning of our immune system. In illnesses such as whooping cough one must look at building up the immune system to improve the general health and well-being of the patient and to prevent the

Nutritional supplements for whooping cough

SUPPLEMENT	DOSAGE	COMMENT
Iron phosphate	*Adults suck two 50 mg pills three times daily Children over six suck one 50 mg pill twice daily*	*Specific tissue salt recommended for whooping cough*
Magnesium phosphate		*Specific tissue salt recommended for whooping cough*
L-lysine	*500 mg daily on an empty stomach*	*Assists the immune system in eliminating viruses*

further infection and ongoing complications which are often associated with this illness.

Herbal treatment

The following herbs are very helpful in treating whooping cough (see pages xiii–xv for information on how to use these herbs):

* Horseradish;
* Hyssop;
* Lavender;
* Mullein flowers;
* Sundew;
* Thyme;
* White Horehound.

Poultices and compresses are a must for whooping cough sufferers. You can use an onion compress, horseradish poultice or mustard poultice. These are very strong and can be used with severe cases. Cover the skin with a small amount of olive oil to protect the skin before applying the compress. A hot water bottle can be placed to the outside of the poultice to keep it warm. Check the skin every five to ten minutes for signs of blistering and remove the poultice if necessary. Care must be taken not to expose skin for too long to the active ingredients of the poultices as blistering of the skin can occur.

Homeopathic treatment

Treatment that may be prescribed by a homeopath for whooping cough include:

* Ipecacuanha if breathing is difficult and fast, there is wheezing, and if child goes blue in the face during coughing;
* Drosera for a ticklish throat;
* Kali carb for a hard, dry, hacking cough;
* Cuprum for coughing, exhaustion and breathlessness;
* Antimonium tartaricum for a rattling cough, nausea, vomiting, mucus and chest pain;
* Belladonna for coughing, spasms until mucus is raised, stomach pains and a dry throat.

- Bryonia for whooping cough after eating or drinking or dry cough;
- Carbo vegetabilis and Kali sulphuricum.

For more information on how to use homeopathics see page xv.

Aromatherapy treatment

Place a few drops of aromatheraphy oils in an oil burner and allow the perfume to permeate the room. The following create a soothing and healing atmosphere for the patient:

- Basil (respiratory, calming, muscle relaxant);
- Chamomile (relaxant, soothing, balancing);
- Lavender (respiratory, antibacterial, nervine);
- Eucalyptus (refreshing, respiratory, anti-spasmodic, anti-inflammatory, decongestive);
- also try the essential oils recommended for pneumonia (see page 27).

See page xvi for information on how to use essential oils.

Dietary and lifestyle recommendations

See dietary and lifestyle recommendations for the respiratory system (pages 4–5), and the common cold (page 31–33).

CHAPTER TWO

THE INTEGUMENTARY SYSTEM

Maintenance of the skin, hair and sense organs

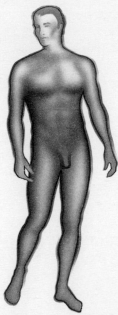

What does it consist of?

The skin, hair, and nails make up the largest of the body's organs. The skin of an adult covers about 1.69 square metres and weighs approximately 2.73 kilograms. The skin is a waterproof, protective covering for the body, with numerous very important functions. It is an organ nourished by blood and lymph vessels, and it contains the surface endings of many nerve fibres.

What does it do?

PROTECTION
The skin covers the body and protects it from physical abrasion, invasion of bacteria, dehydration, chemicals and ultraviolet radiation. Hair and nails perform similar protective functions. Some of these protective functions are performed by the skin's maintenance of a friendly community of natural bacteria, which create an environment

unfavourable to invading bacteria. Antibiotic therapy can threaten these friendly bacterial communities; so, too, can deodorants and anti-perspirants.

EXCRETION

The skin is responsible for the excretion of about a quarter of the body's waste products and in this role is related to the other excretory organs: the lungs, the kidneys, the liver and the bowels. This is why a problem in the functions of these other organs can increase the burden of elimination of the skin, often showing up as a skin disorder. Conversely, a problem with the excretory function of the skin can put more stress on these other organs. External treatments for skin problems are often ineffective as the problem may be more internally related to the other excretory organs.

Perspiration from the sweat glands is excreted through the skin, carrying small amounts of salts, chemicals and organic compounds. Perspiration also allows for regulation of body temperature.

SYNTHESIS OF VITAMIN D

Vitamin D synthesis is activated by ultraviolet rays in sunlight. Vitamin D controls the levels of calcium in the blood and regulates normal glandular activity for the body's muscles, including the heart. Vitamin D also assists the growth, maintenance and repair of all bones and teeth.

IMMUNITY

Skin cells play an important role in recognising and beginning the breakdown of foreign chemicals and microbes.

SENSATION

Skin contains the surface endings of many motor, sensory and secretory nerve fibres. These detect temperature, touch, pressure and pain. They also regulate the excretion of perspiration from the sweat glands and sebum from the oil glands.

What goes wrong with it?

The skin may be affected by a wide range of disorders and imbalances. Many of the disorders may be the outer reflection of internal problems (especially of the lungs, kidneys, liver and bowels). The skin may also be affected by physical injury, chemical damage, infections by viruses, bacteria, fungi and protozoa, as well as infestations by mites and parasites.

The skin's own sweat and oil glands may become dysfunctional, nerves may be disordered and the skin may suffer from various allergic reactions. Blood supply to the skin may be adversely affected and tumours may develop. Emotional factors, stress and anxiety are important in the development, aggravation and continuation of many of the abovementioned skin conditions.

Nutritional treatment

There are many vitamins and minerals that benefit the skin.

VITAMIN A

Vitamin A helps to form and maintain healthy function of eyes, skin, hair, teeth, gums, several types of glands and mucus membranes. It prevents drying of the skin, promotes healthy hair and strong teeth and bones. Vitamin A also prevents the formation of cells which could develop into cancerous cells. It softens and lubricates dry, rough skin.

VITAMIN C

Vitamin C has a major role in the formation of collagen, which allows for the stretching and contraction of the skin, provides strength, and aids in the healing of wounds. Vitamin C also helps to detoxify cancer-causing substances by strengthening the body's natural defence systems. Vitamin C deficiency may lead to anaemia and scurvy.

VITAMIN E

Vitamin E creams or oil, as well as ingested Vitamin E, are excellent for healing skin lesions, scar tissue and burns. It increases and releases blood platelets, which are required for tissue healing. It slows down the ageing process by improving blood circulation. Deficiency may cause easy bruising, anaemia, hair loss, dandruff and varicose veins. Vitamin E lubricates and softens dry, rough skin.

VITAMIN B2

Vitamin B2 is essential for good eyesight, healthy skin, nails and hair. Of all the B group vitamins, B2 is the one most likely to be deficient. A deficiency can lead to dermatitis, cracked lips, sore mouth, acne, oily skin, baldness and ulcers.

VITAMIN B3

Vitamin B3 deficiency can cause numerous types of skin allergies, dermatitis, ulcers, hair loss and cancers.

VITAMIN B5

Vitamin B5 prevents premature ageing and wrinkling of the skin. A deficiency may cause anaemia, baldness and arthritis.

BIOTIN

Biotin is essential for utilisation of protein, carbohydrates and fats. A deficiency can cause dermatitis, baldness and anaemia.

PABA

PABA helps to synthesise folic acid and assists the breakdown of proteins. Effective for the treatment of vitiligo and other skin pigmentation disorders. A deficiency may be involved in causing eczema.

SULPHUR

Sulphur cleanses the blood and tissue of toxic build up, especially of acids which can cause dandruff and acne. Sulphur-rich foods provide keratin, a protein substance which improves the condition of skin, nails and hair.

CALCIUM

Calcium plays an important role in creating the elasticity and firmness of the skin. Calcium-rich foods help prevent acne and the spread of cancerous cells. A calcium deficiency can cause varicose veins, freckles, skin disorders and weak muscles.

SODIUM

Sodium-rich foods nourish the skin, the hair and the eyes. Sodium is essential for functioning of the lymphatic system.

FLUORINE

Fluorine helps preserve a youthful complexion. It is also needed for the teeth and eyes.

IRON

Iron is essential for he distribution of oxygen to all cells of the body.

Herbal treatment

ALTERATIVE HERBS

Alterative herbs have obvious benefits for the skin. Generally speaking, these herbs alter the body's processes of metabolism so that tissues can best deal with the range of functions from nutrition to elimination. Many of these herbs improve the body's ability to eliminate wastes from the body through the kidneys, liver, lungs or skin. The alterative herbs which can benefit the skin are:

- Burdock Root: one of the best remedies for the treatment of dry and scaly skin conditions (psoriasis and eczema). This bitter herb stimulates digestive juices and therefore, improves systemic imbalances which may cause skin problems and dandruff. It also makes a good poultice or compress for external applications;
- Cleavers: a lymphatic tonic which is especially good for dry skin conditions where it can be combined with Yellow Dock and Burdock;
- Nettles: specific in cases of childhood eczema and all other varieties of this condition, especially nervous eczema;
- Figwort: may be used for eczema, psoriasis and any skin condition where there is itching and irritation;
- Red Clover: useful for childhood skin problems including eczema; also useful in more chronic conditions such as psoriasis;
- Other alternatives used for the treatment of skin conditions include Golden Seal, Sarsaparilla, Sassafras, Thuja, Poke Root and Yellow Dock.

VULNERARY HERBS

Vulnerary herbs promote the healing of fresh cuts and wounds. Some of these herbs are astringents and a large part of their healing contribution is due to their ability to arrest bleeding and to condense the tissue.

The most commonly used vulnerary herbs are:

- Aloe;
- Chickweed;
- Comfrey;
- Elder Flower;

- Golden Seal (only use for one to two weeks and don't use if pregnant);
- Horsetail;
- Irish Moss;
- Marigold;
- Marshmallow Root;
- Self-Heal;
- Slippery Elm;
- Witch Hazel.

ANTI-MICROBIAL HERBS

For many skin conditions anti-microbial herbs have to be employed to counter attack microbes that are attacking the skin. Anti-microbials include:

- Chickweed;
- Echinacea;
- Eucalyptus;
- Garlic;
- Marigold;
- Thuja;
- Thyme.

ANTIBACTERIAL AND ANTIVIRAL HERBS

In Chinese and Ayurvedic medicine there is a category of herbs which 'clear heat and attack toxins'. These herbs have antibacterial and antiviral properties, and they assist the processes of detoxification. This category includes such herbs as:

- Blue Flag;
- Burdock Root;
- Dandelion Root;
- Echinacea;
- Pulsatilla;
- Red Clover;

- St John's Wort;
- Sarsaparilla;
- Yellow Dock.

Aromatherapy treatment

The essential oils that benefit the skin include:

- Bergamot;
- Cedarwood;
- Cinnamon;
- Clary Sage;
- Lavender;
- Lemon;
- Neroli;
- Sandalwood;
- Thyme.

Use these oils as bath or body oils. For further information see page xvi.

Traditional Oriental approach

The metal element (which governs the lungs and the large intestine) is responsible for the conditions of the skin which are affected by the health of the lungs and the large intestine. This element nourishes the skin and the hair, the skin acting as a 'third lung', being the outermost layer of the body which is in contact with the air. The pores of the skin open and close to release sweat and oil and they absorb a small amount of oxygen. In both Chinese and Western medicine, lung condition and skin problems are often closely related. Asthma, eczema and skin rashes are commonly associated with colds and lung infections. Dry or oily skin may be indicative of a lung chi imbalance. It is not uncommon for children who have been given suppressive skin treatment for eczema to go on to develop asthma.

Like the large intestine, the skin is very important in the process of elimination. The skin plays a role in eliminating wastes and toxins. The large intestine is also one of the main organs of elimination; if this organ is not functioning optimally then the whole system becomes more toxic. A diet which is high in preserved or processed foods, artificial additives, or mucus-forming foods will greatly challenge the elimination and detoxification processes of the body and can cause or aggravate skin problems.

The skin is also affected by the functioning of the kidneys; when the kidneys are clearing toxins poorly or are expected to handle too much, the skin may have to work harder to clear these waste products. This can lead to skin rashes. In Chinese medicine there is a intimate relationship between the kidneys, the lungs and the skin, especially in regard to fluid distribution.

Proper lung function and a complete breathing pattern coupled with appropriate bowel movements make for healthy skin and hair (particularly if the kidney chi is also strong). Herbs which assist lung function are: Licorice root, Wild Cherry Bark, Slippery Elm, Mullein, Horehound and Irish Moss. Ginger root and Cayenne Pepper also boost lung chi and these herbs, therefore, promote healthy skin and hair.

Dietary and lifestyle recommendations

FOODS FOR THE SKIN
Foods that benefit the skin include: goat's milk, rye, avocados, sea vegetables, whey, apple, cucumber, millet, rice bran and sprouts, banana, berries, dates, figs, oranges, asparagus, beans, cabbage, carrots, lettuce, garlic, apricots, grapes, parsley, capsicum and peaches.

JUICES FOR THE SKIN
Juices that benefit the skin include: carrot, celery and lemon juice; cucumber, lettuce and pineapple juice; or half a glass of cucumber juice mixed with half a glass of water.

ACNE

Description

Acne is a chronic inflammatory disorder of the skin, usually due to hormonal changes and overactive sebaceous glands during adolescence. Acne is more common in males because androgens (the male sex hormones) stimulate the production of keratin and sebum (an oily substance produced by the oil glands). During puberty androgens increase in both sexes, therefore girls in this age group are also susceptible to acne.

Symptoms

Acne appears in a variety of different types, ranging from contagious pimples to deep-seated skin conditions. Acne is accompanied by blackheads, pustules and pimples that are red, swollen and contain pus. The pus is seen as a yellowish or white-tipped centre in some blemishes. In more advanced cases, cysts appear, which are red, swollen lumps beneath the surface of the skin.

Causes

The exact cause of acne is not known, but factors which contribute to or aggravate the condition include: heredity, oily skin, androgens, allergies, stress, over–consumption of junk food, saturated fats, hydrogenated fats, nutritional deficiencies, the use of cosmetics and menstrual cycles. Excessive sweating can encourage acne and some drugs, e.g. oral contraceptives and corticosteroids, can aggravate the condition. A body pH that is too high, or too alkaline, also fosters the nesting and breeding of acne-causing bacteria.

Nutritional supplements for acne

SUPPLEMENT	DOSAGE	COMMENT
Vitamin A	25,000 iu daily. Use emulsion form (if pregnant do not exceed 10,000 iu daily)	Strengthens the protective skin tissue
Vitamin B complex plus	100 mg three times daily	All forms of vitamin B are important for healthy skin tone. Vitamin B combats stress factors and deficiencies that have been associated with acne
Vitamin B3	100 mg three times daily (do not take vitamin B3 if you have a liver problem, gout, high blood pressure)	
Vitamin B6	50 mg three times daily	
Vitamin B5	50 mg three times daily	
Vitamin C with bioflavonoids	3000–5000 mg through the day	Reduces inflammation and boosts immune function
Vitamin E	400 iu daily. Also used as an ointment to prevent scarring	An anti-oxidant that speeds up healing. Helps absorption of vitamin A

Nutritional treatment

Nutritional supplements that may be beneficial in the treatment of acne are included in the table below. See pages xii–xii for information on how to use these supplements.

Herbal treatment

The herbal treatment of acne aims at supporting the body's ability to metabolise fats and carbohydrates, assisting lymphatic drainage and facilitating elimination. Some external applications of poultices, infusions and tinctures can also help. For information on how to use these herbs see pages xiii–xv.

INTERNAL APPLICATIONS

- Alternative herbs that are helpful in treating acne include: Burdock Root, Cleavers, Red Clover and Figwort.
- Lymphatic herbs such as Poke Root and Echinacea and liver cleansing herbs such as Blue Flag and

Nutritional supplements for acne

SUPPLEMENT	DOSAGE	COMMENT
Evening Primrose oil	As directed on label	Keeps the skin soft, repairs damaged skin cells and helps unblock the pores
Zinc	30–80 mg daily	Heals damaged tissue and prevents scarring. Fights bacteria. Activates normal hormone functioning
Chromium yeast	400 mcg daily	Reduces skin infections and improves skin glucose tolerance
Calcium	As directed on label	Helps maintain the acid/alkali balance
Potassium	As directed on label	Deficiency may cause acne
Garlic	Two 500 mg capsules three times daily	Fights bacteria and enhances immune system
Selenium	200 mcg daily	Improves skin elasticity
Acidophilus fibre	As directed on label	Replenishes essential bacteria and assists bowel elimination of toxins

Dandelion can also be useful in the treatment of acne.

- Blue Flag, Echinacea, Burdock and Yellow Dock is an excellent combination of herbs for acne. Mix the herbs equally, infuse with hot water to make a tea, and drink a cup of this tea three times daily. Or you can take 2–4 ml of the tincture daily.
- Burdock, Dandelion and Sarsaparilla are also effective in treating acne. Use these as herbal teas, or tinctures; either separately or mixed in equal parts. See page xiv for further information.

EXTERNAL APPLICATIONS

- Dab the blemishes with undiluted Tea Tree oil, fresh lemon juice or fresh cabbage juice three times daily.
- Cold Sage tea has astringent and antiseptic qualities as well as a drying effect when patted onto the blemishes.
- Golden Seal tincture can also be useful when applied to the acne.
- A lotion of equal parts of infused Marigold, Chickweed and distilled Witch Hazel can soothe the inflammation and repair damaged tissue.
- An anti-flammatory skin wash made from Calendula and Camomile, or a mixture of Yarrow, Elder and Lavender will soothe the skin and reduce the outbreak.

Homeopathic treatment

Treatment that may be prescribed by a homeopath for acne includes:

- Calcarea fluorica;
- Kali bichromicum (for itchy pimples on the face and chest that are brought on by hormonal changes);
- Sulphur (for heat, inflammation and burning pain);
- Hepar sulphuris (for large painful spots filled with pus brought on by puberty);
- Pulsatilla (for acne which is worse at puberty and when menstruation is about to begin).

For information on how to use homeopathics see page xv.

Aromatherapy treatment

The following essential oils can be used as poultices, facials, packs, in baths, steamers, saunas or as massage oils.

- Bergamot;
- Cedarwood;
- Chamomile;
- Eucalyptus;
- Geranium;
- Juniper;
- Lavender;
- Peppermint;
- Tea Tree;
- Rosemary;
- Sandalwood.

For information on how to use these essential oils see page xvi.

Dietary and lifestyle recommendations

- Eat a diet that is high in fibre and low in fat. A high-fibre diet will assist in elimination of toxins through the bowel. Avoid all refined sugars, saturated fats and processed foods. Increase your daily intake of zinc-rich foods including shellfish, soybeans, whole grains, sunflower seeds and a small amount of raw nuts (e.g. almonds, cashews).
- Avoid alcohol, butter, caffeine, cheese, chocolate, cocoa, cream, eggs, fat, fish, fried foods, hot and spicy foods, hydrogenated oils, shortenings, margarine, meat, poultry, soft drinks and wheat. Too much salt intake can also cause acne.
- Improve digestion by taking digestive enzymes or apple cider vinegar with meals.
- Avoid stress as much as possible, as stress can trigger hormonal changes and trigger new outbreaks of acne.
- Avoid wearing make-up, cosmetics and tight clothes as friction can aggravate the inflammation.
- Do not squeeze the spots as this can spread the bacteria to other parts of your body.
- Keep skin clean by washing twice daily with natural, unperfumed soap.
- Maintain a balance between adequate rest, exercise, fresh air and sunlight. Ultraviolet rays from the sun actually sterilise the skin but don't overdo it. A sunlamp may be used three times a week when sunlight is not available; use for ten to 20 minutes at moderate heat.
- An often effective external treatment of moderate cases of acne is the topical application of tretinoin, a derivative of vitamin A which contains the ingredient retin A.

BOILS

Description and symptoms

A boil is a bacterial infection involving a plugged hair follicle and the inflamed tissue around it. A boil begins as a painful red lump that swells and fills with pus, which hardens and forms a yellow head. The pus is made up of white blood cells coming to clear the infection away. The redness is caused by blood bringing nutrients and antibodies to the area and the pain which occurs is due to pressure on nerve endings because of the swelling. Scratching the boil can carry the infection to other parts of the body. Boils most commonly appear on the neck, armpits, breasts, face, buttocks, genital areas and the scalp.

Causes

Poor nutrition, a weakened immune system, immune-suppressive drugs, and chemical deodorants and antiperspirants are some of the common causes of boils. If left untreated a boil usually comes to a head, opens, drains and eventually heals in two to three weeks. The healing can be sped up and the symptoms can be alleviated through the following treatments. Boils are common among children and adolescents.

Nutritional treatment

Nutritional supplements that may be beneficial in the treatment of boils are included in the following table. See pages xii–xiii for information on how to use these supplements.

Herbal treatment

Herbal treatment for boils is directed towards boosting the body's immune system and healing abilities both internally and externally, as well as fighting the invading bacteria.

See pages xiii–xv for information on how to use these herbs.

Internally alterative and anti-microbial herbs are recommended, such as:

- Burdock;
- Echinacea;
- Golden Seal (only use internally for one to two weeks and don't use if pregnant);

Nutritional supplements for boils

SUPPLEMENT	DOSAGE	COMMENT
Vitamin A	100,000 iu for five days, decrease to 50,000 iu for five days, then to 25,000 iu	An anti-oxidant that facilitates tissue healing
Vitamin B complex	100 mg three times daily	Important for healthy skin tone. A deficiency of B2 can cause oily skin
Vitamin C	5000–10,000 mg throughout the day	Boosts immune system and reduces inflammation
Vitamin E	600 iu daily	An anti-oxidant that speeds up tissue healing
Garlic	Two 500 mg capsules three times daily	Fights bacteria and enhances immune system
Coenzyme Q10	60 mg daily	Boosts immune system

- Garlic;
- Pasque Flower;
- Wild Indigo;
- Yellow Dock;
- Red Clover.

These herbs can be taken as a tea, tablets, or a tincture.

CHINESE HERBAL TREATMENT

A Chinese herbal formula for boils includes the following herbs:

- Echinacea;
- Golden Seal (only use internally for one to two weeks and don't use if pregnant);
- Chaparral;
- Honeysuckle flowers;
- Sarsaparilla root;
- Yellow Dock root;
- Ginseng root;
- Ginger root;
- Cinnamon twigs.

Consult a Chinese herbalist for this particular blood-purifying formula taken for boils.

EXTERNAL TREATMENT

- A cabbage leaf poultice can be made by taking the inner leaves of a white cabbage. Remove the stalks and lightly bruise the leaves. Apply to the affected area and hold in place with a light bandage, renew the leaves after an hour.
- Warm poultices of Slippery Elm or Poke Root can also be applied. For more information on how to make and use a poultice see page xv.
- Boil some Fenugreek seed in water and apply the hot pulp to the boil to soften the area and draw the pus to the surface.
- A mixture of honey plus 20–30 drops of Echinacea tincture can be applied to the boil.

Homeopathic treatment

Treatment that may be prescribed by a homeopath for boils include:

- Belladonna for the early stages when the boil is forming;
- Hepar sulphuris for the later stages when the pus is formed;
- Hypericum lotion can be applied externally as a compress (renew it every four to six hours);
- Silica opens boils to expel the pus;
- Sulphur is used for itching boils.

See page xv for information on how to use homeopathics.

Aromatherapy treatment

The essential oil most effective in treating boils is Tea Tree oil. It can be used in a bath or applied directly to the affected area. A combination of Tea Tree and Thyme oil can also be very effective when applied to the boil. See page xvi for information on how to use essential oils.

Dietary and lifestyle recommendations

- Keep the boil wet and warm with a herbal compress (see herbal treatment on pages xiii–xv) or a warm water compress applied for 15 minutes, four or five times daily.

- If you are susceptible to boils wash your skin frequently with an antiseptic soap. When the boil is draining reduce the chances of the infection spreading by showering frequently.
- Vitamin A oil, vitamin B oil or pure honey can be applied directly to the boil. Applying pieces of warm milk-soaked bread to the affected area is an old folk remedy.
- Consult your naturopath or see Chapter Eleven for a cleansing fast to detoxify your system and strengthen your immune system.

IT'S IMPORTANT TO SEE YOUR DOCTOR IF:
- The boil is large (more than 1.5 cm) or recurrent;
- There are red lines radiating from the boil;
- You develop chills and fever.

HERPES Simplex I and Simplex II

Description

Herpes simplex I (cold sores) are caused by a virus. The sores appear three to ten days after exposure and may last up to three weeks. Approximately 60 percent of the population are infected with herpes simplex I and these people remain carriers for the rest of their lives. Although the virus remains within the body for life, the body does become more effective at suppressing it.

Herpes simplex II (genital herpes) is sexually transmitted, the first attack usually coming four to eight days after exposure to the virus. See pages 235–39 for more information on sexually transmitted diseases.

Symptoms

The main symptom of herpes simplex I are small blisters on and around the lips and mouth. They may look like round sores with little holes punched out, which then become scabbed over. You may find them singly or in clumps. They can crust over and weep

Nutritional supplements for herpes

SUPPLEMENT	DOSAGE	COMMENT
L-lysine	1–6 g daily between meals until healed, then 500 mg daily to prevent recurrence (monitor your cholesterol levels while taking L-lysine)	Slows or alters the growth of the virus
Vitamin A	50,000 iu daily in emulsion form (if pregnant do not exceed 10,000 iu daily)	Prevents spreading of infection and facilitates tissue healing
Vitamin C with Bioflavonoids	200 mg three times daily at start of discomfort	Inhibits the growth of the virus and may decrease length of disease
Vitamin B complex	50 mg three times daily	Works with L-lysine as a preventative and keeps virus from spreading
Vitamin E	500 iu daily	Applied topically or taken internally to heal and contain the virus
Zinc chelate	50–100 mg spread throughout the day	Use zinc chelate for genital herpes. Zinc gluconate lozenges for oral herpes
Lactobacillus acidophilus	Three times daily on an empty stomach, take as directed on label	Improves bowel flora

(become runny) toward the end of the herpes infection. The lymph nodes in the area may also become swollen.

The main symptom of herpes simplex II are blisters on the genital area. In men the initial blisters break out on the penis, groin and scrotum area. The early signs are itching or numbing of the penis, fatigue, headaches, fever and sickly feelings may accompany the sores. In women the blisters develop around the rectum, clitoris, cervix and in the vagina. There is often a watery discharge and pain when urinating.

Within 48 hours the blisters erupt and painful ulcers form. These sores crust over and dry out while they are healing.

Recognising the early symptoms that indicate that the virus has been activated is important in taking measures to ensure that other people aren't infected. The early warning signs are local tenderness, a numbing or tingling sensation and a small bump. The virus becomes contagious even at this early stage. The initial outbreaks of the virus may be the most severe, subsequent cases becoming less dramatic in many cases.

Causes

The herpes virus is passed from one person to another by direct contact such as kissing or sharing a utensil.

Acute flare ups of cold sores are triggered by another infection somewhere else in the body which lowers your resistance, windburn, stress and nervous tension.

Genital herpes is sexually transmitted.

Nutritional treatment

Wholistic treatment of cold sores is directed towards strengthening the immune system, supplementing nutritional deficiencies, soothing the nervous system and inhibiting the viral growth. See pages xii–xiii for information on how to use the supplements listed in the table.

Herbal treatment

For information on how to use the following herbs see pages xiii–xv.

- The herbs that are used to treat herpes include: Alfalfa, Cleavers, Echinacea, Golden Seal, Ginseng, Hops (for the nervous system), Licorice, Marjoram, Oats, Poke Root, Peppermint and Red Clover. Aloe Vera and Hyssop are both used to inhibit the growth of the virus. Use these herbs as tablets, teas or tinctures (see page xiv).
- Tea Tree oil is a powerful natural antiseptic and can be applied directly to the affected area. Use either full strength or if too strong, dilute with distilled water.
- External application of Marigold, Marshmallow, Nettle and St John's Wort may be helpful.
- Another treatment is to apply Walnut or Golden Seal extract to the affected area.
- Try a lotion of Echinacea (with or without Myrrh) applied directly to the affected area.
- A herbal mixture made from equal parts of Cleavers, Echinacea, Oats and Poke Root, taken as a tea can have preventative and curative benefits. (See page xiv for information on how to make herbal tea.)

CHINESE HERBS

A Chinese herbal formula for Herpes Simplex I and II removes 'damp or toxic heat' from the Lower Burning space. It includes the following herbs for the liver Meridian:

- Bupleurum;
- Echinacea;
- Yellow Dock;
- Gentian Root;
- Golden Seal;
- Wild Yam;
- Marshmallow Root;
- Myrrh.

This herbal formula cools and de-toxifies the blood and the liver meridian. Consult a Chinese herbalist for this formula.

Homeopathic treatment

For information on how to use the following treatments see page xv.

- For cold sores use Rhus toxicodendron, Lycopodium and Natrum muriaticum.
- For sores on the lips use Natrum muriaticum, Rhus toxicodendron and Sepia.
- For sores caused by exposure to sun, stress, grief or emotional factors use Natrum muriaticum.
- For genital herpes with dry skin and hot, puffy lesions use Natrum muriaticum.
- For genital herpes when the genitals burn and sting with a red itchy rash use Capsicum.
- For genital herpes with bad ulcers and the entire genital area tender and painful use Sempervivum.
- A mixture of Calendula officinalis and Hypericum perforatum can be

applied (one part tincture to three parts distilled water) frequently to the sores as soon as they appear.

Aromatherapy treatment

The following essential oils are helpful in the treatment of herpes:

- Clary Sage;
- Bergamot;
- Lavender;
- Sandalwood;
- Cedarwood;
- Neroli;
- Tea Tree;
- Cinnamon;
- Lemon;
- Thyme.

Tea Tree oil can be applied directly onto the affected area. Dab on with a cotton wool ball, either full strength or diluted. All other oils can be used as bath or body oils.

See page xvi for further information on how to use these oils.

Dietary and lifestyle recommendations

It is important to take a diet high in lysine and low in arginine. Lysine is an amino acid that slows or alters the growth of the herpes virus. Therefore:

- Avoid all chocolate, peanuts, almonds, walnuts, cashews, cereals or grains like rye, corn, oats and barley, soybeans, chicken and beer, as these contain arginine. Eat more fish, shellfish, bean sprouts, brewer's yeast, beans, fruit and vegetables, as these foods are high in lysine. Do not consume citrus fruit or juices while the virus is active.

- Reduce stress.
- Cold sore sufferers should use plenty of 15+ sunscreen around their lips and other susceptible areas.
- To dry out the cold sores either apply ice packs or an over-the-counter product containing zinc oxide, or a cream containing lithium from your health food store. Even calamine lotion can dry out the lesions and speed up the healing process. Vitamin E oil is helpful, so too is lysine cream (available from your health food store).
- If you suffer from genital herpes, wear cotton underpants, don't touch the sores and abstain from sex while the sores are present.

CORNS and CALLUSES

Description and symptoms

Corns and calluses are lumps of thickened and hardened dead skin cells from the outer layers of the skin (the epidermis). They form to protect any part of the body which is exposed to constant irritation, pressure or friction. Corns tend to appear over a toe joint or on the sole of the foot. Soft corns may appear between the toes; they are caused by friction between the bony points of the toes. The moisture of the area between the toes keeps them soft, whereas corns that form on top of the toes are harder.

Calluses are also hardening and thickening of the skin, usually on the feet, knees, elbows or hands. Both corns and calluses can cause inflammation and pain and be very sensitive to touch.

Causes

Corns and calluses are the result of ongoing pressure or friction on an area of skin. Corns are very often caused by friction with shoes but this can be aggravated by poor biomechanics of the foot when walking or running. An acid/alkaline imbalance may be indirectly responsible for corns and calluses. Overeating of fats, sugars and highly processed foods is a common cause of an acid/alkaline imbalance.

Herbal treatment

For information on how to use the following herbs see pages xiii–xv.

- Apply tincture of Sundew directly to corns and calluses to stimulate their removal. Blood Root tincture applied externally is also useful for corns, eczema, ringworm, scabies and warts.
- Alternatively apply Golden Seal tincture and Tea Tree oil to

minimise infection and speed up the healing process.

- A compress of crushed garlic applied to the corn each day can help.

Homeopathic treatment

Treatment that may be prescribed by a homeopath for corns and calluses includes:

- A mixture of Calendula and Hypericum makes a soothing and healing lotion. Apply directly to affected area four times each day.
- Apply Arnica ointment or oil two or three times a day for relief of pain.
- Apply Ruta graveolens ointment twice daily to ease pain.

See page xv for information on how to use these treatments.

Dietary and lifestyle recommendations

- To treat corns and calluses, first soften them by thoroughly soaking in a solution of two tablespoons of sodium carbonate (washing soda) dissolved in a basin of water. Dry the area with a soft towel, rub in a couple of drops of Vitamin E oil then gently remove any rough skin by rubbing with a pumice stone.
- Vitamin E oil mixed with a crushed garlic clove is very effective for softening corns or calluses.
- To relieve pain and soften corns and calluses soak your feet in half a cup of Epsom salts and warm water. Soak feet twice a day for ten minutes each time.
- Eat raw vegetables and juices for three days to cleanse toxins and to assist your acid/alkaline balance. Avoid fried foods, meats, caffeine, sugar and highly processed foods as these are likely to aggravate your condition.
- Wear round-toed shoes and an insole for extra padding, as well as non-medicated corn pads. The salicylic acid in medicated corn pads often causes burning and ulcers.

DANDRUFF

Description

Dandruff is dry, flaky skin that lifts off the scalp when the hair is brushed or combed. The condition can be uncomfortable, and even a little embarrassing, but is usually not serious. There is, however, a disease known as Seborrheic dermatitis where the skin becomes inflamed and itchy and can spread to the eyebrows, ears and other parts of the body.

Symptoms

Dandruff is characterised by scaly dry skin on the scalp, which can be inflamed and itchy.

Nutritional supplements for dandruff

SUPPLEMENT	DOSAGE	COMMENT
Vitamin A	20,000 iu daily	Aids in healing skin tissue
Vitamin B complex	100 mg twice daily	For healthy skin and hair
Vitamin C with bioflavonoids	3000–6000 mg daily	An anti-oxidant that prevents tissue damage and aids in healing
Selenium	As directed on label	An anti-oxidant that helps control dry scalp
Vitamin E	400 iu daily	Promotes circulation
Zinc lozenges	Five daily for one week	Important for the breakdown and absorption of proteins
Kelp	1000–1500 mg daily	Provides essential minerals

Causes

Dandruff is a very common condition which often results from emotional stress, hormonal imbalance or an inadequate diet. Seborrheic dermatitis is caused by overactive sebaceous glands. It is usually triggered by trauma, illness or hormonal imbalance.

Nutritional treatment

Nutritional supplements that may be beneficial in the treatment of dandruff are included in the following table. See pages xii–xiii for more information on how to use these supplements.

Herbal treatment

Herbs that are helpful in treating dandruff include:

- Burdock (for the treatment of skin conditions which result in dry scaly skin);
- Red Clover (used to treat chronic skin conditions);
- Yellow Dock (combines well with Dandelion, Burdock and Cleavers to treat skin complaints);
- Nettles (strengthens and supports the body, Excellent in treating skin conditions);
- Thyme (has mild antiseptic properties).

HERBAL TEAS

- A combination of Rosemary and Sage infused with boiling water can be used as a gentle hair rinse.
- Nettle tea can also be used as a hair rinse.

For information on how to use these herbs see pages xiii–xv.

Homeopathic treatment

Treatment that may be prescribed by a homeopath for dandruff includes:

- Calendula (used externally to treat skin ailments);
- Sulphur (for the treatment of skin conditions);
- Arsenicum album (to treat a dry, scaly scalp).

See page xv for information on how to use these treatments.

Aromatherapy treatment

Recommended oils for the treatment of dandruff are:

- Rosemary;
- Thyme;
- Chamomile;
- Lavender;
- Cedarwood;
- Juniper;
- Rosemary oil massaged into the scalp stimulates circulation and helps eliminate dandruff;
- A combination of Rosemary and Chamomile oil mixed with a base of Almond oil and gently warmed makes an excellent massage oil for the scalp.

See page xvi for information on how to use essential oils.

Dietary and lifestyle recommendations

- Avoid refined sugars and processed foods.
- Personal hygiene is of considerable importance. Keep the hair clean by washing and brushing regularly.

- Try massaging the scalp with warm olive oil combined with a squeeze of lemon juice. Apply to damp hair and leave in for ten to 15 minutes before shampooing.
- Rinse hair with a little vinegar and water instead of plain water.
- Avoid chemical-based shampoos and soap products as these can dry and irritate the skin and scalp.
- Jojoba oil soothes an inflamed scalp and can help in the elimination of dry, scaly skin.

DERMATITIS
Description and symptoms

Dermatitis appears as a rash or inflammation of the skin. The affected area is very often red and swollen with either tiny pimple-like blisters that weep, or dry, scaly skin which is extremely itchy.

Causes

The causes of dermatitis are many and varied. Allergic or contact dermatitis can be caused by a number of substances that irritate the skin. Stress and anxiety can play a large role in either causing or exacerbating the problem.

Household chemicals and cleaners, detergents, shampoos, make-up, moisturisers and even some plants such as poison ivy and nettles can be the triggers for dermatitis.

Metals such as gold, silver and nickel have also been found to cause skin irritation. Sensitivity to sunlight

Nutritional supplements for dermatitis

SUPPLEMENT	DOSAGE	COMMENT
Vitamin A	100,000 iu for one month, decrease to 50,000 iu for two weeks and then to 25,000 iu daily	Aids in healing skin conditions
Vitamin B complex	50–100 mg three times daily with meals	Needed for healing and promoting new cell growth
Vitamin B3	100 mg three times daily	Promotes good blood circulation
Vitamin B6	50 mg three times daily	Promotes red blood cell formulation
Biotin	100 mg three times daily	Promotes healing of the skin
Vitamin C with bioflavonoids	3000 mg daily	Relieves inflammation
Vitamin E	400 iu daily	Relieves dryness and itching
Zinc	100 mg daily (do not exceed this dosage)	Enhances immune function and aids healing
Para Amino Benzoic Acid (PABA)	200 mg four times daily	An anti-oxidant. Helps protect skin against the effects of dryness and sunburn
Sulphate lotion	Use as directed on label	Inhibits dermatitis. Protects the skin against toxic substances

can cause a rash in some people. Prescription drugs and antibiotics can also be associated with triggering dermatitis. Whatever the irritant, prolonged exposure will only make the condition worse.

Nutritional treatment

Nutritional supplements that may be beneficial in the treatment of dermatitis are included in the above table. See pages xii–xiii for information on how to use those supplements

Herbal treatment

There are a number of herbal lotions and ointments that have been proven to be very helpful for treating dermatitis externally, however herbs taken internally are more effective.

INTERNAL USAGE

- The following herbs may be useful in treating the irritation, anxiety and stress associated with dermatitis: Burdock Root, Cleavers, Figwort, Red Clover, Yellow Dock, Chickweed, Comfrey and Nettle.
- Red Clover, Yellow Dock and Nettle are a very effective combination. To make an infusion of any of the herbs, pour a cup of boiling water onto one–three teaspoonfuls of the dried herbs and leave to infuse for ten to 15 minutes. Drink three times a day.
- Another highly effective internal formula is made by combining one part Golden Seal, one part Clivers and one part Burdock. For every 30 g of the herbal mix, dilute with 500 ml water. Take 50–100 ml three times daily. This formula can be taken with juice.

EXTERNAL OINTMENT

- Chickweed combined with Marshmallow makes a very good ointment for the relief of itching associated with dermatitis and eczema. This ointment is available at health food stores.

For more information on how to use herbs see pages xiii–xv.

Homeopathic treatment

Treatment that may be prescribed by a homeopath for dermatitis includes:

- Sulphur;
- Calendula officinalis;
- Petroleum;
- Urtica urens;
- Graphite;
- Rescue Remedy.

For more information on how to use homeopathics see page xv.

Aromatherapy treatment

The following essential oils will provide relief from the symptoms of dermatitis:

- Lavender (promotes healing of the skin and has antibacterial qualities);
- Neroli (calming, healing for the skin, antibacterial);
- Sandalwood (calming, soothing, softens and heals the skin);
- Roman Chamomile (speeds healing, helps where there is inflammation and allergies).

See page xvi for information on how to use essential oils.

Dietary and lifestyle recommendations

Natural therapies can be of great benefit to those suffering from dermatitis. It is important to remember, however, that the skin is one of the four main organs of elimination so a detoxification or cleansing program should be undertaken to gain maximum results.

* Avoid dairy products, gluten, fried foods and processed foods.
* Try a gluten-free diet for six weeks. This can be beneficial in controlling dermatitis.
* Avoid potential allergens such as chemicals, household cleaners, shampoos and certain foods (see above). Some lanolin based ointments can also aggravate skin conditions.
* Sorbelene, vitamin E oil, Avocado oil or Wheat Germ oil are recommended as moisturisers.
* Cotton-lined rubber gloves should be worn when doing dishes or washing.
* Ice packs can help relieve itching.
* Oatmeal and herbal baths can provide temporary relief from irritation.

HIVES

Description and symptoms

Hives, also known as urticaria, is characterised by itchy and inflamed red weals that appear on the body. The condition is usually caused by an allergic reaction, physical irritation or stress.

The body begins to release histamines into the skin and the skin reacts by swelling and becoming red and itchy. The red weals can disappear within minutes or hours but the irritation and itchiness can last for a couple of days or even weeks.

Causes

Allergic responses to certain stimuli can cause the histamine release in the body. These allergens are numerous and varied. A sensitivity to certain foods such as eggs, dairy products, shellfish, or tomatoes can sometimes cause the body to react. Other triggers include pesticides, soaps, detergents and certain chemicals. Viral and bacterial infections or antibiotics such as penicillin can also induce hives.

Nutritional treatment

Nutritional supplements that may be beneficial in the treatment of hives are included in the following table. See pages xii–xiii for more information on how to use these supplements.

Herbal treatment

The following herbs may bring relief from hives:

* Alfalfa (excellent blood tonic as it cleanses the blood and helps free the body of toxins);

Nutritional supplements for hives

SUPPLEMENT	DOSAGE	COMMENT
Lactobacillus acidophilus	As directed on label	Reduces allergic reactions
Kyolic garlic	As directed on label	Helps destroy bacteria
Vitamin C	1000 mg three times daily	Enhances immune response
Vitamin B complex	100 mg daily	Promotes healthy skin
Vitamin D	400 iu daily	Helps to reduce outbreaks of rashes
Vitamin E	600 iu daily	An anti-oxidant that aids circulation
Zinc	50 mg daily	Promotes immune system

- Chamomile (reduces swelling caused by inflammation);
- Chickweed (use externally to relieve itching and irritation);
- Burdock root (used to treat skin conditions);
- Dandelion (diuretic, liver tonic);
- Echinacea (an anti-microbial, speeds healing of wounds when used externally);
- Nettle (strengthens and supports the body. Excellent in treating skin conditions);
- Yellow Dock (used in the treatment of chronic skin conditions. Is a blood cleanser).

For more information on how to use these herbs see pages xiii–xv.

To make a blood cleansing herbal tea, combine Dandelion Root, Burdock and Cleavers. Place one–two teaspoons of the mixture in a cup of water, bring to the boil and simmer for ten to 15 minutes. Drink three times daily.

POULTICE

For external use only, try a poultice made with Black Nightshade leaves. Wash and boil leaves, put them in a cloth and apply to affected area (avoiding the eye area).

Homeopathic treatment

The following homeopathic treatments can be of great benefit to those suffering from hives. Use:

- Apis mellifica for skin rash, red, burning and swelling;
- Dulcamara for lumpy skin rash and hives that are worse when hot or after scratching;
- Rhus toxicodendron for burning, itching, stinging and joint pain;
- Urtica urens for prickly heat.

For more information on how to use homeopathics see page xv.

Aromatherapy treatment

Place a few drops of any of these oils in an oil burner to provide a soothing, relaxing fragrance which benefits the skin.

- Bergamot;
- Lavender;
- Sandalwood;
- Lemon;
- Thyme;
- Clary Sage.

For more information on how to use essential oils see page xvi.

Dietary and lifestyle recommendations

- Try to identify the cause of the condition to minimise further exposure to it.
- Avoid alcohol and all processed foods. It may be beneficial to go on an elimination diet.
- Drink plenty of water.
- Try applying cold compresses or ice to the affected area, as this can help reduce swelling and relieve itching.
- Add baking soda to a cool bath and soak. This can help relieve the symptoms.

IT'S IMPORTANT TO SEE YOUR DOCTOR IF:
- The hives develop in your mouth or throat as this could interfere with your breathing or swallowing and develop into a potentially dangerous situation.

PSORIASIS
Description and symptoms

Psoriasis is an inflammatory disease which appears as patches of silvery scales or red, dry skin on the legs, knees, arms, elbows, scalp, ears and back. Fingernails and toenails can also be affected, becoming pale and pitted or developing ridges. Psoriasis usually follows a pattern of periodic flare ups alternating with periods of remission. People between the ages of 15 and 25 appear to be the most vulnerable and the infection is not contagious.

Psoriasis does not usually itch but it can hurt when cracks appear in the dry patches on the hands or soles of the feet. Psoriasis is a common condition and it affects one in 50 people at some time in their life.

Causes

The underlying cause of the condition is not known, although it appears that psoriasis may be caused by faulty utilisation of fats. A weakened immune system will also allow for flare ups of the condition, so too can a toxic build up in an unhealthy colon. Conditions which can trigger an attack of psoriasis are: stress, anxiety, nervous tension, illness, surgery, viral or bacterial infections, sunburn, cuts, lithium, overuse of drugs and alcohol, chloroquine and beta-blockers.

Nutritional treatment

Nutrients that are of benefit in this condition are included in the following table. See page xii for information on how to use these supplements.

Nutritional supplements for psoriasis

SUPPLEMENT	DOSAGE	COMMENT
Vitamin A	10,000 iu three times daily	Regulates the keratinisation of the skin
Vitamin B12	2000 mcg daily	Use a lozenge or sublingual form
Folic acid	400 mcg daily	Improves the condition of the skin and hair
Vitamin C	2000–10,000 mg daily	Used for formation of collagen and skin tissue
Vitamin E	Up to 1600 iu daily	Fights free radicals which damage the skin
Essential fatty acids • Fish oil or • Flaxseed oil or • Primrose oil	One–two tablespoons daily	Controls the production and storage of arachidonic acid which causes inflammation
Zinc	50–100 mg daily	Important for the breakdown and absorption of proteins
Selenium	200 mg daily	An anti-oxidant
Lecithin	One tablespoon three times daily	Protects skin cells and breaks down fats
Kelp	Five tablets daily or 1000–5000 mg daily	A rich source of minerals and iodine

Herbal treatment

Herbal treatment for psoriasis focuses primarily on alternative herbs to 'cleanse the blood' and detoxify the system. Such herbs include:

- Burdock root;
- Barberry Bark;
- Cleavers;
- Red Clover;
- Dandelion;
- Yellow Dock;
- Sarsaparilla;
- Figwort;
- Thuja.

OINTMENTS

Ointments can help to ease some of the skin dryness, cracking and discomfort. Use a simple ointment base and to reduce the inflammation add Burdock, Golden Seal and Marigold. Use these tinctures either singularly or mixed in equal parts. Ointments made from Comfrey, Chickweed, Paw Paw or Marshmallow are also very useful.

DIURETICS AND NERVE TONICS

Diuretics like Cleavers or Figwort, and nerve tonics like Motherwort, Lime Blossom, Mistletoe, Skullcap or Valerian can all be used in the treatment of psoriasis. Use as teas, tablets or tinctures. See pages xiii–xv for more information on how to use herbs. It is necessary to search for the root cause or causes of the condition in order to prescribe the appropriate use of alterative, diuretic, hepatic and tonic herbs.

POULTICES

A poultice made from Chaparral, Dandelion and Yellow Dock can benefit psoriasis sufferers. See page xv for information on how to make a poultice.

HERBAL BATH

A warm to hot bath with two teaspoons of grated ginger can help ease the condition.

For more information on using herbs see pages xiii–xv.

Homeopathic treatment

Treatment that may be prescribed by a homeopath for psoriasis includes:

- Sulphur for dry, red and itchy patches;
- Graphites for a sticky, yellowish discharge;
- Petroleum jelly for sensitive, cracked and bleeding skin.

For more information on how to use homeopathics see page xv.

Aromatherapy treatment

The following essential oils can provide relief from the symptoms of psoriasis.

- Lavender oil fights inflammation and soothes sore skin.
- Roman Chamomile is a very calming, relaxing oil which reduces redness and soreness.
- Sandalwood oil has a potent calming effect as well as reducing any allergic reactions.

- Use these oils in an oil burner or vaporiser. Ideally they can be used in a sauna or steam room, but if this is not possible try adding a few drops of the essential oil to a hot bath.

See page xvi for more information on how to use essential oils.

Dietary and lifestyle recommendations

- Digestion should be improved by supplementing with digestive enzymes at each meal.
- Increase your intake of high-fibre foods (such as whole-grain cereals, cooked dried beans and peas, fruits and vegetables). Also increase your intake of fish oils (especially salmon, cod, sardines, tuna or mackerel) and onions and garlic.
- Eat more food high in zinc, such as oysters, pumpkin seeds, brazil nuts, almonds, cashews, hazelnuts, walnuts, rice, barley, sunflower seeds, rye, sesame seeds, wheat and olives.
- Reduce your consumption of red meats, eggs, fat, sugar, alcohol and dairy products.
- Apply seawater to the affected area several times a day and expose to sunlight (moderately).
- Keep the skin well moisturised, especially after bathing. Add some vegetable or olive oil to the bath to moisturise the skin.
- To soothe itching dissolve one cup of baking soda in four litres of water. Soak a washcloth in the solution, wring it out then apply to affected area.
- Adding one tablespoon of apple cider vinegar to a cup of water and applying to the skin will also soothe the itching.
- Another remedy to soothe the itching is to take internally two–four teaspoons daily of linseed, safflower, sunflower or wheat germ oil.
- Avoid stressful situations, fatigue, extreme changes in temperature, and injuries to the skin as these can initiate new skin lesions.

SCABIES

Description

Scabies is an infestation of the skin due to a tiny parasite known as sarcoptes scabiei. The parasite burrows into the skin in order to lay her eggs and the condition that follows is one of intense itching. Care must be taken as the rash that develops may become infected from scratching.

Symptoms

Scabies is characterised by small red lumps on the skin which become increasingly itchy, especially at night in bed. The main areas affected are the fingers, palms, wrists, armpits, buttocks and genitals, however it can spread over the entire body.

Nutritional supplements for scabies		
SUPPLEMENT	DOSAGE	COMMENT
Vitamin A	10,000 iu–15,000 iu daily (if pregnant do not exceed 10,000 iu daily)	Construction of skin tissue
Vitamin C	3000 mg daily	Promotes healing of skin
Vitamin E	600 iu daily	Promotes healing
Garlic	Two 500 mg capsules three times daily with meals	A natural antibiotic
Kelp	1000–1500 mg daily	Balances minerals
Zinc	50 mg daily	Aids in tissue repair

Causes

Scabies is caused by a parasite and transmitted from person to person by close personal contact. Scabies is highly contagious so good personal hygiene is of the utmost importance.

Nutritional treatment

Nutritional supplements that may be beneficial in the treatment of scabies are included in the above table.

See pages xii–xiii for information on how to use these supplements.

Herbal treatment

Use these herbs externally for relief from the symptoms of scabies:

- Tansy (apply as lotion or use in the bath);
- Aniseed (apply as a lotion);
- Poke Root (use as lotion);
- Camphor (helps stop itching);
- Blood Root (use as a lotion but do not apply to any broken skin or open wounds).

To make these lotions heat 50 ml of almond oil and add 20–30 drops of the herbal tincture. Simmer for a few minutes, cool and then apply. See pages xiii–xv for information on how to use these herbs.

Homeopathic treatment

Sulphur is a specific homoeopathic for scabies. See your homeopath for an individual treatment.

Aromatherapy treatment

The essential oils that are effective in treating scabies are:

- Lavender (a strong antiseptic and insect repellent);
- Peppermint;
- Rosemary;

- Tea Tree (renowned for its antifungal and antiseptic properties);
- Thyme.

An aromatic bath can be relaxing and detoxifying. Try adding a few drops of any one of the above oils to your bath water and soak for ten minutes. Lavender, Peppermint, Rosemary and Thyme can also be used as body oils. See page xvi for more information on how to use these oils.

Dietary and lifestyle recommendations

- Scabies is a highly contagious condition so therefore it is of the utmost importance to be hygienic.
- Change all bed linen after beginning treatment and wash thoroughly in boiling water.
- Those close to the person who has scabies must be treated as well.
- Soak 150 g of Alder leaves in half a litre of diluted apple cider vinegar and use as a spray to treat scabies.

IMPORTANT

It is important the condition be properly diagnosed by a medical doctor. This is done by taking a scraping of skin from the affected area and examining it under a microscope.

Orthodox treatment often prescribes an insecticide lotion which is applied to the whole body. The treatment is then repeated two weeks later to kill off any remaining eggs in the skin.

TINEA and FUNGAL INFECTIONS

Description, symptoms and causes

Tinea is a term which includes almost every fungal infection of the skin. Fungal infection of the skin is most common in areas of the body where there is a moist, warm environment.

ATHLETE'S FOOT

Tinea pedis (athlete's foot) is a term for fungal infections of the foot. Tinea is also called ringworm, although it is not a worm. The fungi live off the dead skin cells and calluses of the feet, especially on the skin between the toes. Symptoms of athlete's foot include:

- itching, burning and/or stinging between the fingers or toes;
- red areas on skin;
- scaling areas;
- tiny blisters on skin areas and cracks in skin.

The infection is caught from infected skin fragments that may be found on damp floors such as communal showers. Although you can catch athlete's foot, some people seem to have a resistance to it. The fungus that causes athlete's foot spreads rapidly when the skin's beneficial bacteria are destroyed by antibiotics, drugs or radiation. The strength of the immune system is another important factor influencing susceptibility to tinea infections.

JOCK ROT

Fungal infection or tinea in the groin area is commonly called jock rot or jock itch. Jock rot is sometimes caused by the friction of clothing coupled with perspiration, which creates the right environment of heat and moisture for the fungus to thrive. This is why the rash tends to recur in summer and with exercise.

The person may complain of 'itching' and discomfort and there will be spreading, sharply demarcated red, raised areas and weeping areas on the skin in the genital area.

TINEA VERSICOLOR AND TINEA CAPITIS

Tinea versicolor is a fungal skin infection of the tropics which is very common in Queensland and the Northern Territory. The fungus produces small patches of white, depigmented skin caused by sunlight being unable to tan the skin under the fungus.

Tinea capitis is tinea of the scalp.

ORAL THRUSH

Fungal infection of the mouth is referred to as oral thrush, a condition

Nutritional supplements for tinea and fungal infections		
SUPPLEMENT	DOSAGE	COMMENT
Vitamin A	25,000 iu daily (if pregnant do not exceed 10,000 iu daily)	Important for skin healing and immune system
Vitamin B complex	50 mg three times daily	Nourishes the helpful bacteria to regulate the harmful bacteria
Vitamin C with bioflavonoids	5000–20,000 mg daily	Important for immune system
Vitamin E	400–800 iu daily	Important for immune system
Garlic	Two 500 mg capsules three times daily	Neutralises fungal growth and boosts immune system
Acidophilus	As directed on label	Supplies body with helpful bacteria to regulate the harmful bacteria
Zinc	50 mg daily	For skin repair and immune system

in which creamy-looking white patches form on the tongue and the insides of the mouth. If the patches are scraped off bleeding may occur. Oral thrush is most common in infants whose immune system is weak. Oral thrush is a infection caused by Candida albicans.

VAGINAL THRUSH

Fungal infection of the vagina is called a 'yeast infection' and is commonly known as monilia or vaginal thrush. Antibiotics are the main cause of vaginal thrush, disturbing the normal bacterial flora of the vagina, thereby allowing the yeast to multiply more quickly. Thrush may also result from hormonal changes during pregnancy, or during your introduction to the birth control pill, from friction between the thighs, friction with underwear or friction during sex. Thrush is caused by Candida albicans from the gut which comes out onto the skin around the anus.

The symptoms of thrush are:

- a white vaginal discharge;
- intense itching of the vulva and surrounding skin;
- inflammation of the urine opening so that passing urine causes discomfort.

For more information on thrush see Candida albicans, pages 210–213.

Nutritional treatment

Nutritional supplements that may be beneficial in the treatment of fungal infections are included in the table on page 71. See pages xii–xiii for information on how to use these supplements.

Herbal treatment

For information on how to use the following herbs see pages xiii–xv.

HERBAL TEA

Take Echinacea or Red Clover as a herbal tea.

POULTICES, BATHS OR LOTIONS

Apply the following herbs as poultices, baths or lotions for tinea:

- Aloe;
- Blood Root;
- Calendula;
- Echinacea;
- Eucalyptus;
- Garlic;
- Golden Seal;
- Marigold;
- Myrrh;
- Thuja (for ringworm or thrush).

See page xiv for information on how to make a herbal lotion.

FINGER AND FOOT BATHS

- Soak feet in a cooled infusion of Thyme or Sage tea.
- Soak feet in diluted apple cider vinegar when there is itching and redness.
- Use Comfrey root as a warm foot bath or soak feet in a cooled infusion of Thyme or Sage.
- For toenail or fingernail fungus soak nails in a mixture of Pau d'Arco and Golden Seal.

Homeopathic treatment

The homeopathic treatment for fungal infections varies according to the symptoms. Treatments that may be prescribed by a homeopath are listed below, but see your homeopath for a specific remedy.

VAGINAL THRUSH

For vaginal thrush with:

- burning discharge use Borax veneta, Mercurius solubilis, Nitric acidum or Sepia;
- copious discharge use Sepia;
- smelly discharge use Mercurius solubilis or Sepia;
- yellow discharge use Sepia;
- white discharge use Borax;
- greenish discharge use Mercurius solubilis;
- dryness use Sepia;
- itching use Sepia or Nitric acidum;
- soreness and itching use a douche made with five–ten drops of Calendula tincture in cooled Chamomile tea.

ORAL THRUSH

- In babies and children use Borax veneta, Kali muriaticum, Mercurius solubilis, Natrum muriaticum, Sulphuric acid.
- For oral thrush with tongue and gums coated white use Kali muriaticum, or Natrum muriaticum.
- For oral thrush with hot, dry, bleeding gums use Borax veneta.

TINEA CAPITIS

Use Sulphur or Sepia for tinea capitis.

See page xv for information on how to use homeopathics.

Aromatherapy treatment

The following essential oils can provide relief from fungal infections:

- Lavender;
- Myrrh;
- Patchouli;
- Sandalwood;
- Tea Tree.

Sandalwood, Lavender and Patchouli can be used as bath or body oils. Myrrh can be used as a body oil or in an oil burner. Sandalwood and Tea Tree can be applied directly to the skin lesions.

See page xvi for information on how to use these essential oils.

Dietary and lifestyle recommendations

FOR ATHLETE'S FOOT

- Sprinkle baking soda onto your feet as a powder or make a paste with lukewarm water and rub the mixture on your feet. Rinse off after 15 minutes and dry thoroughly.
- Use a hair dryer to dry your shoes and feet.
- Place a small piece of lambswool between the tips of your toes to enable your toes to breathe.

- Swap or rotate your shoes regularly to allow them to dry out. Your can disinfect your shoes with a cloth and a dab of disinfectant.

DIETARY TIPS
- Increase your intake of brussels sprouts and cabbage.
- Avoid all yeast and mould foods for a trial period of five weeks: bread, mushrooms, Vegemite, cheese, soy products, wine, beer, preserved meats, peanuts, peanut butter, dried fruits, vinegar, canned fruit, melons, grapes, tinned foods, olives and salad dressings. Also eliminate sugar and refined carbohydrates.
- Take one dessertspoon of olive oil and one clove of garlic daily.
- Eat a diet consisting of 70 percent raw foods. Eat plenty of fresh vegetables, some broiled fish and some broiled skinless chicken.
- Improve digestion and bowel movements by supplementing with Acidophilus fibre (one–two dessertspoons per day) and digestive enzymes. The herb Gentian is also a good stimulant of gastric acid secretion.

RINGWORM
- Apply crushed or powdered garlic to the affected area and alternate with pure honey.
- Keep the skin as clear as possible and expose the affected area to the air whenever possible.

IT'S IMPORTANT TO SEE YOUR DOCTOR IF:
- The symptoms worsen and you develop further inflammation, swelling and fever.

WARTS

Description and symptoms

Warts are solitary or clustered hard nodes of flesh, most often seen on the hands, fingers or genitals. Warts are divided into three main types:

- genital warts;
- skin warts;
- plantar warts.

Causes

Warts are spread by various strains of the common papovaviruses, spread by humans not by frogs. Warts are mildly infectious but many people never catch them even though they are exposed. Warts often appear on body areas of lowered resistance, along with other infections.

GENITAL WARTS
These are transmitted by sexual or intimate personal contact. In men, the warts may be present on the penis but no warty nodes are observable. Both men and women can be carriers of the virus without even being aware that they are affected. Women may develop warts not only externally on the genitals, but internally where they are

very difficult to detect. The virus can then attack the cervix and infections of this type are associated with cervical cancer. Pap smear tests can detect genital warts, cancer and other gynaecological problems at an early stage.

SKIN WARTS

Once a skin wart has developed it can disappear as spontaneously as it appeared, but it is difficult to predict when it will disappear. Skin warts can remain for a week, a month or even years. The most common areas for skin warts are the knees, elbows, hands and feet.

PLANTAR WARTS

When warts develop on the soles of the feet they are termed plantar warts, which tend to grow inwards rather than outwards. Plantar warts do not tend to spread to other parts of the body. They are bumpy white growths that may resemble calluses or corns except that they often bleed if the surface is trimmed. When treating a patient, a homoeopath or naturopath would take into account the strength of the patient's immune system and also any inherited tendency which could create a susceptibility to warts.

Nutritional treatment

Nutritional supplements that may be beneficial in the treatment of warts are included in the following table. See pages xii–xiii for information on how to use these supplements.

Nutritional supplements for warts

SUPPLEMENT	DOSAGE	COMMENT
Vitamin A	25,000 iu daily for three months, then to 15,000 iu daily (if pregnant do not exceed 10,000 iu daily)	Plays an important role in keratinisation. Can be used externally
Vitamin B complex	50 mg three times daily	Anti-oxidant and important in normal cell multiplication
Vitamin C	4000–10,000 mg daily	To combat viral proliferation
Vitamin D	400–800 iu daily applied externally to warts	Facilitates tissue growth and repair and is an anti-oxidant
Zinc	50–80 mg daily	Strengthens resistance to viruses

Herbal treatment

See pages xiii–xv for more information on how to use herbs.

INTERNAL APPLICATIONS

For internal applications use herbs from the group of lymphatic cleansers. These include the following herbs:

- Cleaver;
- Echinacea;
- Garlic;
- Poke Root;
- Prickly Ash;
- Thuja;
- Wormwood.

EXTERNAL APPLICATIONS

The following herbs can be applied externally as they are or made into a lotion. See page xiv for information on how to make a lotion.

- Aloe Vera gel
- Blood Root tincture
- Clove oil
- Chickweed tincture
- Dandelion (white sap from the flower stem)
- Golden Seal tincture
- Mandrake Root tincture
- Pau d'Arco tincture
- Sundew
- Tea Tree oil
- Thuja tincture
- Wintergreen oil

The juice of Nettle rubbed on a wart of ten to 14 days is an effective treatment. The juice of Buttercup leaves is also used to remove warts.

Rubbing garlic on the warts and eating garlic will also help remove warts.

Homeopathic treatment

Homeopathic remedies for warts include:

- Thuja;
- Calcarea carbonica;
- Natrum carbonicum;
- Antimonium (for plantar warts);
- Causticum and graphites (for warts under and around the fingernails);
- Nitric acidum (for yellow, painful and bleeding warts).

See your homeopath for a specific remedy. For more information on how to use homeopathics see page xv.

Aromatherapy treatment

The following oils benefit the skin:

- Chamomile;
- Frankincense;
- Geranium;
- Lavender;
- Neroli;
- Rose otto.

All these oils can be used as bath or body oils. See page xvi for more information.

Dietary and lifestyle recommendations

- Apply a paste made from castor oil and baking soda to the warts, cover it with a bandage and leave in place overnight. Repeat each night for three to four weeks.
- Apply vitamin A oil (from a capsule) to the warts each day for three to four weeks.
- Apply a paste made from crushed vitamin C tablets mixed with water to the warts and cover with a Bandaid or pad.

IT'S IMPORTANT TO SEE YOUR DOCTOR IF:
- You are a woman and you suspect you have genital warts, as they have been linked to cervical cancer.

CHAPTER THREE

THE NERVOUS SYSTEM
Maintenance of the brain, spinal cord and peripheral nerves

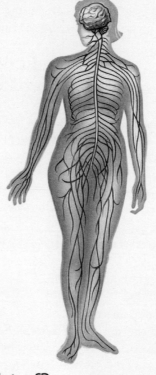

What does it consist of?

The nervous system is made up of the central nervous system (the brain and the spinal cord) and the peripheral nervous system (the cranial nerves and the spinal nerves). Peripheral nerves are either sensory nerves or motor nerves. Sensory nerves from the peripheral nervous system bring sensations *to* the central nervous system where they are integrated and interpreted and responses are sent *from* the central nervous system to peripheral motor nerves to carry out the response. The body and the brain are constantly buzzing with billions of electrical and chemical signals. Most nerve signals are unconscious and they keep the human body safe and functioning properly.

The brain controls both conscious and unconscious bodily functions. The brain and the spinal cord are surrounded by cerebro-spinal fluid which nourishes and protects the central nervous system. The brain is also protected by the cranial bones and the cranial meninges, which are a three-layered membrane covering the brain.

What does it do?

The mind–body connection is more apparent in the nervous system than any other body system. The nervous system is responsible for the physical sensations of pain, touch, temperature, taste, smell, sight and hearing. It is also responsible for the psychological processes of memory, interpretation and association, which colour our experience of physical sensations and our responses to them.

In Chinese medicine the mind, the emotions and the spirit are seen as importantly integrated with the body; in fact they are part of a continuum of energies which are interrelated. The condition of the physical body affects the emotions, the mind and the spirit, and vice versa. A holistic approach to health and healing acknowledges this interconnectedness between mind and body. Any disease which manifests in the body also has mental, emotional and spiritual aspects.

What goes wrong with it?

Disorders of the nervous system are understood by Western medicine as:

- damage to the nerve pathways;
- damage to the brain;
- damage to the blood supply to the brain;
- problems with the chemical and electrical signals within the brain.

Psychological problems such as depression and anxiety are often caused by chemical imbalances within the brain. These chemical imbalances can be manipulated by taking certain drugs or nutrients.

Traditional Oriental approach

From the perspective of Chinese medicine the brain's functions are related to and affected by all the organs and meridians of the body, but chiefly associated with the heart, spleen and kidneys.

Nutritional treatment

See pages xii–xiii for information on how to use vitamins and minerals.

VITAMIN B COMPLEX

- Vitamin B1 is often referred to as the morale vitamin due to its relation to a healthy nervous system. It also has a beneficial effect on mental attitude. The body rapidly uses up vitamin B1 during times of depression, worry, anxiety and emotional stress. Vitamin B1 deficiency is related to depression, emotional instability, irritability, poor memory, low energy, lack of concentration and nightmares.
- Vitamin B2 is essential for nerve tissue repair. Deficiency can lead to

Parkinson's disease, depression, trembling and various nervous disorders.

- Vitamin B3 promotes a good sleeping pattern and is vital for the proper functioning of the nervous system. Vitamin B3 deficiency leads to: insomnia, irritability, depression, personality changes, dementia and tremors.
- The brain contains one the highest concentrations of vitamin B5. Vitamin B5 improves a poor memory and protects the body in times of stress. Deficiency of vitamin B5 can lead to insomnia, nerve disorders (which may produce pins and needles in the hands and feet), fatigue, apathy and depression.
- Vitamin B6 helps to maintain a balance of the minerals potassium and sodium, which is essential for the entire nervous system. Vitamin B6 deficiency leads to nervousness of the hands, numbness and cramps in the arms and legs, slow learning, inability to concentrate, irritability, depression, Parkinson's disease and headaches.
- Vitamin B12 is known as the energiser. Deficiency of vitamin B12 leads to fatigue, diminished reflexes, stammering, poor memory and concentration, nervous irritability, a pins and needles sensation and schizophrenia.

MINERALS

- Magnesium nourishes the white nerve matter of the brain and spinal cord, and is involved in muscle impulse transmission and neurotransmission. It helps to build a good memory. Deficiency leads to neuritis, muscle twitch, tremors, personality changes, confusion, depression and irritability.
- Phosphorus strengthens the spinal cord and the brain and is needed for healthy nerves and efficient mental activity. Phosphorus compounds called lecithin are found in the white matter of the nerves. The B vitamins are activated by phosphorus. It is essential for the maintenance and repair of the entire nervous system. Deficiency leads to mental and physical fatigue, nervous disorders and seizures.

AMINO ACIDS

- Tryptophan is a precursor to the brain neurotransmitters serotonin and melatorim. Tryptophan regulates sleep and mood patterns.
- Tyrosine increases the neurotransmitters dopamine and noradrenalin.
- Valine is essential for the nervous system.

Herbal treatment

There are many herbs which benefit the nervous system. See pages xiii–xv for information on how to use herbs.

RELAXANTS

Relaxants are used in cases of stress and tension for nervousness and inability to relax.

The main relaxants are:

- Black Cohosh;
- Catnip;
- Chamomile;
- Hops;
- Hyssop;
- Lavender;
- Lime Blossom;
- Linden;
- Mistletoe;
- Motherwort;
- Passion Flower;
- Rosemary;
- St John's Wort;
- Skullcap;
- Valerian;
- Wild Yam.

NERVE TONICS

These are used to strengthen, repair and nourish the nervous system in cases of shock, stress or nervous debility, and after illness.

The main nerve tonics are:

- Damiana;
- Ginseng;
- Lemon Balm;
- Oats;
- Skullcap;
- Vervain.

STIMULANTS

Stimulants are generally useful for treating depression, fatigue and poor circulation.

The main stimulants are:

- Chilli;
- Coffee mate;

- Gotu Kola;
- Peppermint;
- Tea;
- Tea (black);
- Vervain.

SEDATIVES

Sedatives are useful for treating insomnia, excitability, anxiety and hyperactivity.

They include:

- Hops;
- Passion Flower;
- Valerian;
- Wild Lettuce.

Aromatherapy treatment

The following oils are all useful in treating disorders of the nervous system.

- Basil is a nerve tonic which stimulates the brain and is useful for depression.
- Benzoin relaxes the nerves and is useful for emotional exhaustion.
- Bergamot has an uplifting effect on the nervous system and is used for depression and anxiety.
- Cedarwood is used for calming anxiety and nervous tension.
- Chamomile is a calming herb for insomnia, hysteria and relaxing the muscles.
- Clary Sage eases nervous and muscular tension and pain, and is also useful for anxiety, depression and nervousness.

- Frankincense is a calming nerve tonic used for relaxation and meditation.
- Jasmine treats problems of the nervous system and as an antidepressant it disperses depression, tension and fear.
- Lavender soothes frayed nerves, and its calming effect will induce a restful sleep. It is useful as an antidepressant and for clearing the head, headaches and migraines.
- Marjoram is useful for anxiety, grief and insomnia. It is a strong sedative herb which can calm the emotions and provide sleep for insomniacs.
- Neroli has a very calming influence on the nervous system. It is used for stress, anxiety, depression, nervous tension, hysteria, palpitations and insomnia.
- Patchouli is a stimulant to the nervous system that lifts anxiety and depression.
- Peppermint cools the emotions, clears the mind and is useful for depression and headaches.
- Rose is an antidepressant which soothes the nerves, calms anger and is used for depression and insomnia.
- Sandalwood has a strong calming effect on the nervous system. It eases anxiety and nervous tension, as well as promoting confidence and meditation.
- Sage relaxes the nervous system, promotes the memory and eases muscular and nervous tension. (Avoid using during pregnancy.)

See page xvi for information on how to use essential oils.

Dietary and lifestyle recommendations

FOODS

To nourish and strengthen your nervous system, incorporate a range of the following foods into your diet.

- apples
- apricots
- asparagus
- avocados
- bananas
- broccoli
- brussels sprouts
- cabbage
- capsicum
- carrots
- cauliflower
- celery
- cherries
- cucumber
- dates
- egg yolk
- figs
- fish
- goat's milk
- grapes
- lemons
- lettuce
- melons
- olives
- onions
- oranges
- papaya
- parsley
- peaches
- pears
- peas
- pineapples
- plums
- spinach
- tomatoes
- yeast

JUICES

To help repair your nervous system try:

- Celery, carrot and prune juice;
- Prune juice;
- Sesame, sunflower or almond with avocado butter (blended into a thick juice);
- Radish and prune juice;
- Lettuce and celery juice (especially for insomnia).

ALZHEIMER'S DISEASE

Description

Alzheimer's disease is characterised by the destruction of nerve cells in certain areas of the brain associated with mental function. Pathological changes occur in the cerebral cortex, including the formation of plaque and tangles of nerve fibres. The first signs of dementia are memory loss and disorientation.

Alzheimer's disease is an extremely distressing disorder for all involved, especially the family and friends of the patient. As the disease progresses the patient becomes more and more confused, unsure of where they are and often they don't recognise people close to them, such as family members. In the later stages the patient can suffer from loss of speech, difficulty with swallowing and incontinence, finally becoming in need of full-time care.

Senile dementia can occur in the later stages of a number of disorders, such as Huntington's chorea, Parkinson's disease, cerebrovascular disease, chronic meningitis, chronic alcoholism and vitamin B deficiency.

Symptoms

The main symptom of Alzheimer's disease is memory loss. Other symptoms include reduced physical activity, lack of concentration, apathy, insomnia, lack of energy and disorientation.

Causes

Exposure to heavy metals such as aluminium may be a predisposing factor in developing Alzheimer's disease. Nutritional factors must also be taken into consideration; deficiencies in vitamin B, folic acid and zinc can cause dementia. There can also be some hereditary links.

In order to diagnose Alzheimer's disease a number of tests must be undertaken, such as blood tests, X-rays and electroencephalograms. Neurological and physiological tests can also be done to diagnose the progress of the disease. It is important to rule out other conditions when diagnosing Alzheimer's disease.

Nutritional treatment

Nutritional supplements that may be beneficial in the treatment of Alzheimer's disease are included in the following table. See page xii for more information on nutritional treatment.

Herbal treatment

See pages xii–xiii for information on how to use herbs.

RELAXANTS
These are used for stress, tension and inability to relax:

- Black Cohosh;
- Catnip;

Nutritional supplements for Alzheimer's disease

SUPPLEMENT	DOSAGE	COMMENT
Vitamin A	25,000 iu daily	Nourishes brain and nervous system
Vitamin B complex Vitamin B Vitamin B3 Vitamin B12	See your doctor about injections of B vitamins. Injections work quickly and give good results	Deficiency can cause depression and mental dysfunction. Important for brain function
Folic acid	800 mcg daily	Essential for the production of energy and the formation of red blood cells
Vitamin C with bioflavanoids	6000–10,000 mg through the day	Enhances immune function
Vitamin E	400 iu daily	Anti-oxidant
Magnesium chelated with calcium	750 mg daily	Has a definite calming effect
Potassium phosphate	As directed on label	Needed for electrolyte balance
Zinc	50–100 mg daily	Helps stop plaque formation

- Chamomile;
- Lavender;
- Lime Blossom;
- Mistletoe;
- Motherwort;
- Passion Flower;
- Rosemary;
- St John's Wort;
- Skullcap;
- Valerian;
- Wild Yam.

- Damiana;
- Ginseng;
- Lemon Balm;
- Oats;
- Skullcap;
- Vervain.

NERVE TONICS

Nerve tonics are used to strengthen, repair and nourish the nervous system. These include:

SEDATIVES

These are used for treating insomnia and anxiety:

- Hops;
- Passion Flower;
- Valerian;
- Wild Lettuce.

For a more comprehensive treatment it is recommended you consult a qualified herbalist as Alzheimer's disease can be greatly helped by strengthening the nerves and toning the whole nervous system.

Aromatherapy treatment

There are number of aromatherapy oils used for nervous system disorders, including:

- Basil;
- Bergamot;
- Chamomile;
- Clary Sage;
- Jasmine;
- Lavender;
- Marjoram;
- Peppermint;
- Rose;
- Sage.

These oils should not be used internally. Place a few drops in a warm bath, in a massage oil or in a vaporiser. See page xvi for information on how to use essential oils.

Dietary and lifestyle recommendations

- Avoid antacids that contain aluminium.
- Avoid cooking with aluminium utensils or eating or drinking from aluminium.
- Check for heavy metal toxicity through hair analysis.
- Check for food sensitivities.

- It is important to eat a well balanced diet, with plenty of green leafy vegetables, fruits, legumes and lean meat.
- Avoid free radicals such as cigarette smoke, radiation, pollution etc.
- Keep occupied with activities that stimulate brain cells.
- Physical activity is also recommended.
- Bach Flower remedies can be useful in treating some of the symptoms of Alzheimer's disease. Consult your herbalist.
- Contact your nearest Alzheimer's Association for information and support.

ANOREXIA NERVOSA

Description

Anorexia nervosa is an eating disorder, the chief feature of which is a profound loss of weight. The majority of sufferers are between the ages of 12 and 18 years. Some anorexia nervosa sufferers refuse to eat anything, some take laxatives after eating and some make themselves vomit after eating. Some do all three of the above. The sufferers (95 per cent of whom are female) have an aversion to food based on an inappropriate body image which leads them to feel overweight, or have a fear of becoming overweight, or have a fear of becoming overweight even though they're actually starving themselves. The fixation on being obese often causes them to exercise excessively. Many sufferers are also bulimic, which means binge eating followed by self-induced vomiting.

Symptoms

The anorexia nervosa sufferer can become seriously emaciated and undernourished. There is often an accompanying loss of menstrual periods as well as personality changes, extreme weakness, dizziness, swelling of the neck, ulcers of the oesophagus, erosion of the tooth enamel (from constant vomiting), broken blood vessels of the face, heart damage from potassium deficiencies, a low pulse rate and low blood pressure, as well as weak resistance to infection from lowered immunity.

Causes

Originally anorexia nervosa was thought to be strictly a psychological disease. Research has isolated the family background as one of the major causes. Some associated factors include a family history of physical, emotional, mental or sexual abuse, alcoholism, depression, divorce or parental domination. Teasing by parents, siblings or peers about their body shape or developing sexuality can play a role in making the sufferer obsessed with being fat.

In recent years research has revealed some physical causative factors as well. Chemical imbalances and severe zinc deficiency have been found in many cases as well as an inability to absorb vitamin A.

Treatment of anorexia nervosa is a sensitive issue. Often parental pressure to seek help will only serve to worsen the condition as the patient may be storing resentment and anger towards their parents from previous family trauma.

Herbal Treatment

For information on how to use the following herbs see pages xiii–xv.

APPETITE STIMULANTS

Herbs that may be helpful to stimulate the appetite include:

- Angelica (use as a tincture – 2 ml three times daily – or a tea);
- Burdock (use as a tincture – 2–5 ml three times daily, or as a decoction – 150 ml three times daily);
- Ginseng (use in tablet form three times daily);
- Centaury (use as a tea);
- Golden Seal (use as a decoction or in tablet form. Not recommended during pregnancy or if you suffer from hypertension);
- Gentian (use as a tincture – 2 ml three times daily);
- Peppermint (use as a tea);
- Ginger (use as a tea);
- Lovage;
- Gotu Kola.

HERBAL TEA

A mixture a digestive herbs and nerve tonics – Chamomile, Gentian and Skullcap – taken as a tea three times daily is recommended for anorexia nervosa.

ANTI-SPASMODIC HERBS

Anti-spasmodic herbs and relaxing herbs are also useful:

- Valerian (use as a tea or in tablet form);
- Vervain (use as a tea);
- Passion Flower (acts as a gentle sedative – use as a tea or in tablet form);
- Hops (the flowers and leaves can be placed inside your pillow case to aid sleep);
- Motherwort (use as a tea or tincture).

LIVER STIMULANTS

Herbs to stimulate the liver and tonify the blood are recommended. These include:

- Dandelion (the roasted root can be used as a coffee substitute);
- Milk Thistle (use as a tea or tincture);
- Red Clover (use as a tea);
- Wild Yam (to be taken as a decoction – 50 ml three times daily).

NUTRITIVE HERBS

Take nutritive herbs such as:

- Alfalfa (seeds available from health food stores. They should be sprouted and eaten raw);
- Fenugreek (available in seed form. Can be sprouted and used in salads);
- Rosehips (use as a tea);
- Slippery Elm powder (the powder is available from health food stores. Mix with water as recommended on packet).

BACH FLOWER REMEDIES

The Bach Flower remedies include:

- Mimulus;
- Hornbeam;
- White Chestnut;
- Star of Bethlehem.

Homeopathic treatment

Treatment that may be prescribed by a homeopath for anorexia nervosa is listed below. Consult your homeopath for a specific remedy.

- Use China officialis if the patient has loss of appetite with anaemia and sunken eyes, is craving cold drinks and spicy foods, and has a bitter taste in their mouth.
- Use Ferrum metallicum if the patient has loss of appetite alternating with hunger, and a pale face which flushes easily.
- Use Natrum muriaticum if the patient is anaemic, catches colds easily, if their lips and mouth are dry and cracked, and they have an extreme thirst and bitter taste in their mouth.
- Thuja may also be prescribed for some sufferers of anorexia nervosa. Consult your homeopath for a specific dosage.

For information on how to use homeopathics see page xv.

Aromatherapy treatment

Choose any of the essential oils listed on pages 82–3 and see page xvi for information on how to use them.

Dietary and lifestyle recommendations

- Begin to eat small, frequent meals and fruit or vegetable juices. Brewer's yeast can be added to these juices as it is an excellent source of B vitamins.
- Make sure you eat a well balanced, high-fibre diet which contains no sugar or white flour products.
- Eat lots of rice as it will stimulate your appetite.
- Avoid processed foods, additives and preservatives, junk food and fast foods.
- Seek help from a counsellor, hypnotherapist, kinesiologist or find a support group to help deal with any self-esteem, anger, resentment or depression problems.

ANXIETY

Description

It is normal to be anxious about many situations which arise in everyday life, particularly situations which threaten our security and well-being. Anxiety becomes a problem when it is persistent or when it is brought on by routine situations which the majority of people would take for granted, such as going shopping, catching a bus, meeting new people or using electrical appliances. These persistent, irrational or exaggerated fears should be treated because they can lead to serious physical and psychological disorders. Unfortunately, many sufferers are also anxious about seeking help so it may be necessary for friends and relatives to give support.

Anxiety disorders can be either acute or chronic. Acute anxiety manifests as 'panic attacks'. During a panic attack the sufferer may experience shortness of breath, a smothering sensation, heart palpitations, sweating, nausea, trembling, numbness or tingling sensations in the arms and legs, hot flushes and/or chills. The sufferer may believe that they are experiencing a heart attack or a stroke. Panic attacks are often triggered by stress (including the fear of having an attack) and certain emotions, or they occur in response to certain foods, drugs or illness.

Chronic anxiety is a more generalised form of this disorder; the symptoms are less severe but still very distressing. Some people with chronic anxiety also suffer from panic attacks.

Depression is often linked with anxiety and usually requires treatment aimed specifically at alleviating it, in addition to the treatment designed to relieve anxiety. See Depression, pages 92–7.

Symptoms

Generally, the physical symptoms of anxiety may include: digestive problems, headaches, high blood pressure, insomnia, muscular tension, skin problems, a rapid pulse, palpitations, breathlessness or hyperventilation, tightness in the chest, a feeling of faintness, sweating, fatigue, weakness, nausea, diarrhoea, abdominal pain, loss of appetite and compulsive behaviour such as overeating.

Causes

Causes of anxiety may include: inability to cope with stress and conflict, illness, a genetic predisposition, environmental and life stresses, hormonal imbalances (e.g. hyperthyroidism), lack of interests, poor diet, lack of exercise, fluctuating blood sugar levels, excess coffee intake, alcohol, drugs, relationship and financial problems, or excess of heavy metals.

Nutritional treatments

Nutritional supplements that may be beneficial in the treatment of anxiety are included in the following table. See pages xii–xiii for information on how to use these supplements.

Herbal treatment

For information on how to use the following herbs see pages xiii–xv.

RELAXANTS

The most effective relaxant herbs for anxiety are:

- Chamomile;
- Lady's Slipper;
- Lime Blossom;
- Mistletoe;
- Passion Flower;
- Skullcap;
- St John's Wort;
- Valerian.

HERBAL TEAS

- Skullcap and Valerian can be taken together in equal parts and drunk as a tea three times daily. This tea can be taken at bedtime to promote sleep and prevent panic attacks at night. The only disadvantage to this relaxing tea is its taste. Sweeten with honey or a touch of maple syrup. (These herbs are available from health food stores in tea form.)
- Another calming combination is a teaspoon of hawthorn flowers, infused together with a fig and prune in a cup of boiling water.
- Drink ginger tea two or three times daily and use ginger as a spice in cooking.
- St John's Wort is a mood elevator which improves feelings of anxiety.

Homeopathic treatment

Treatments that may be prescribed by a homeopath for anxiety vary according to the symptoms. Try:

- Aconite for sudden panic attacks;

Nutritional supplements for anxiety

SUPPLEMENT	DOSAGE	COMMENT
Vitamin B complex plus	*As directed on label*	*Essential for health of entire nervous system*
Vitamin B1 plus	*50 mg three times daily*	*Has a beneficial effect on mental attitude*
Vitamin B6 plus	*50 mg three times daily*	*Balances the minerals potassium and sodium*
Vitamin B3	*500 mg two times daily*	*Vital for proper functioning of the nervous system*
Calcium	*2000 mg daily*	*Facilitates nerve transmission and acts as a natural tranquilliser*
Magnesium	*300–1000 mg daily*	*Deficiency may cause anxiety, depression, insomnia and irritability*
Zinc	*50–100 mg daily*	*Deficiency can cause depression, moodiness and sleep problems. Has a calming effect on the nervous system*
L-tryptophan	*300–4000 mg daily (tryptophan can aggravate aggressive behaviour)*	*A percursor of vitamin B3, melatonin and serotonin. Deficiency associated with anxiety, depression and insomnia*
L-tyrosine	*500 mg three times daily, on an empty stomach. Do not take if you suffer from melanoma or are taking a MAO inhibitor drug.*	*Increases the neurotransmitters dopamine and noradrenalin. Important for anxiety and depression*

- Arsenicum album for more prolonged experiences of anxiety, restlessness, tiredness and insecurity;
- Calcarea, Pulsatilla and Ignatia for fear of the opposite sex;
- Lycopodium and Gelsemium for fear of public places;
- Natrum muriaticum if the person is dwelling on negative or morbid thoughts;

- Tarentula for difficulty with relaxing and sleeping;
- Other homeopathic treatments commonly used for anxiety are Sweet Marjoram, Silica, Argentum, Causticum and Nitricum.

See your homeopath for a specific remedy. For information on how to use homeopthics see page xv.

Aromatherapy treatment

For information on how to use the following oils see page xvi.

- Clary Sage, Frankinsense, Sandalwood, Lavender, Geranium and Bergamot oil mixed with Sweet Almond oil and added to the bath create a soothing and calming effect for anxiety.
- Orange Blossom (Neroli) oil burnt in an oil burner has wonderful sedative properties. Jasmine, Lavender and Sage oils are also very calming when used in an oil burner. (Avoid using Sage oil during pregnancy.)

Dietary and lifestyle recommendations

- Avoid alcohol, caffeine (tea, coffee, cola, chocolate) and sugar as these have been found to aggravate anxiety and panic attacks.
- Include the following foods in your diet: apricots, asparagus, avocados, bananas, broccoli, brewer's yeast, brown rice, dried fruits, figs, egg yolk, fish (especially salmon),

garlic, green leafy vegetables, soy products, onions and whole grains.
- To avoid large fluctuations of your blood sugar level eat small frequent meals rather than fewer, bigger meals. Avoid eating when emotionally upset.
- Drink soda water as it increases the carbon dioxide levels in your body.
- Get regular exercise. Try brisk walking, jogging, bicycle riding or swimming; any type of moderate, not too strenuous, exercise will do.
- Find a friend or family member who is a good listener. Talking abut your concerns and fears often helps to release them.
- Check with you naturopath or health care provider for mercury or heavy metal toxicity, chemical sensitivity or candida albicans.

See Chapter Eleven on relaxation and breathing techniques.

DEPRESSION

Description

Short-term depression is a natural reaction to a death in the family, loss of a job, a marriage or relationship break-up, or some other traumatic situation. Depression in this sense is a form of grieving. Depressive disorders are long-term or prolonged forms of depression.

Depression can develop into bi-polar disorders which involve alternating episodes of depression and mania. During a manic episode the sufferer has symptoms of hyperactivity, rapid speech, changing topics frequently, an overactive mind and sleeplessness. The treatments offered in this chapter are more effective for depression than mania.

Symptoms

Sufferers of depression will display some of the following symptoms:

- long lasting feelings of sadness despair and hopelessness;
- insomnia or hypersomnia (sleeping too much);
- lack of energy and feelings of fatigue, accompanied by sluggish speech and movements;
- changes in appetite; either lack of appetite with weight loss, or excess appetite with weight loss, or excess appetite with weight gain;
- feelings of worthlessness, inadequacy, or self-reproach and guilt;
- irritability or anxiety, restlessness;
- headaches and backaches;
- loss of sexual desire and lack of interest in pleasure activities;
- digestive disorders and constipation;
- recurring thoughts of death and suicide.

Causes

There are a wide range of causative factors and triggers for depressive episodes. These include:

- chemical imbalances in the brain which may have genetic or psychological origins;
- thyroid disorders;
- food allergies, nutritional deficiencies;
- stress and anger which is turned inward towards the self instead of being released;
- lack of exercise;
- hypoglycaemia;
- underdeveloped social skills leading to feelings of loneliness and inadequacy.

Nutritional treatment

Nutritional supplements that may be beneficial in the treatment of depression are included in the following table. See pages xii–xiii for information on using these supplements.

Herbal treatment

A herbal repertory for the treatment of depression would include the following herbs:

- Balm;
- Borage;
- Celery (one to two glasses of juice per day);
- Chamomile (use as a tea);
- Ginger (use as a tea);
- Kola;
- Kava Kava;
- Licorice (use as a tea);
- Oats (broth – 20 g oat flakes in one litre water, boil gently for half an hour. Strain, serve);

Nutritional supplements for depression

SUPPLEMENT	DOSAGE	COMMENT
Vitamin B complex plus	100 mg three times daily	Essential for the functioning of the entire nervous system
Vitamin B3 (Niacin)	50 mg three times daily	Promotes a good sleeping pattern and it is important in energy production
Vitamin B5	100 mg three times daily	Protects the body and nervous system in times of stress
Vitamin B6	100–500 mg daily	Necessary for the conversion of L-tryptophan into serotonin
Vitamin B12	1000 mcg daily	Known as the energiser vitamin, B12 deficiency can lead to fatigue, depression and schizophrenia
Vitamin C	1000 mg twice daily	Deficiency of vitamin C can lead to chronic depression, tiredness and irritability
L-tryptophan	4–6 g daily (avoid protein for 90 minutes before and after taking it and take with fruit juice)	Influences brain serotonin levels
L-tyrosine	2 g three times daily	Influences brain dopamine and noradrenalin levels
L-phenylalanine	150–200 mg daily	A precursor to tyrosine
Calcium	1500 mg daily	Has a calming effect on the nervous system
Magnesium	1000 mg daily	Nourishes white nerve matter of the brain and spinal cord and works with calcium
Zinc	50 mg daily (use the chelated form)	Deficiency can lead to depression
Folic aid	400 mg daily	Important in the synthesis of noradrenaline and serotonin

Nutritional supplements for depression		
SUPPLEMENT	DOSAGE	COMMENT
Biotin	5000 mcg daily	Aids in utilisation of B-complex vitamins. A deficiency can cause loss of appetite, hair loss, depression, muscle pain and nausea
Selenium	600 mcg daily	An essential trace mineral and anti-oxidant related to vitamin E
Chromium	300 mcg daily	A fat mobiliser which provides energy
Lecithin	As directed on label	Prevents mental fatigue, nervous breakdown, and other forms of mental stress
GABA	750 mg daily	Has a calming, tranquillising effect on the mind

- Peppermint (use as a tea);
- Rosemary (internally as a weak tea. 50 ml three times daily);
- Skullcap (use as a tea);
- Siberian Ginseng;
- St John's Wort (use as a herbal tincture or tea);
- Valerian (use as a tea or in tablet form);
- Vervain (tea is available from health food shops);
- Wormwood.

These herbs can be used as teas, tablets or tinctures. See page xiv for details.

St John's Wort is a mood elevator which improves feelings of anxiety, depression and inadequacy. Take this herb as a tincture (2–4 ml) or a tea. St John's Wort also helps sleep problems.

HERBAL TEAS

- If the depression is accompanied by general fatigue use the following herbal combination: Kola, Damiana, Lavender, Oats and Rosemary. Valerian can be added to make the combination more powerful.
- Borage makes a refreshing and invigorating tea which is very useful in relieving mild depression.
- Lemongrass tea is helpful for headaches, insomnia and depression.

These herbal teas are all available from health food stores. Use as recommended on packet. For information on how to use these herbs see page xiv.

Aromatherapy treatment

The following essential oils may be beneficial in the treatment of depression.

- Bergamot is an anti-depressant and a gentle relaxant. Use as a body or bath oil.
- Basil is a nerve tonic which clarifies the mind. Use as a body or bath oil, or in an oil burner.
- Clary Sage is a relaxant which helps insomnia, anxiety and nervousness. Use as a body or bath oil.
- Geranium is a very calming oil for tension, stress and depression. Use as a bath or body oil, or in an oil burner.
- Frankincense eases anxiety and nervousness. Use as a bath or body oil, or in an oil burner.
- Lavender soothes frayed nerves, helps insomnia and relaxes aches and pains. Use as a bath or body oil.
- Lemon has a mild sedative action and also stimulates the immune system. Use as a bath or body oil.
- Rose is an anti-depressant which is very soothing for the nerves. Use as a bath or body oil, or in an oil burner.
- Sandalwood eases anxiety and nervous tension with its potent calming effect on the nerves and the stomach. Use as a bath or body oil, or in an oil burner.

See page xvi for information on how to use these oils.

Homeopathic treatment

Treatment that may be prescribed by a homeopath for depression includes:

- Arsenicum if the person is feeling restless, insecure, tired and anxious and may be exhibiting a compulsive behaviour such as extreme tidiness;
- Calcarea for someone who is mentally disoriented, forgets things and fears they may be going insane;
- Ignatia amara for depression caused by suppressed grief;
- Lycopodium for a depressed person who is worried about the future but shows little emotion;
- Natrum muriaticum if a person is dwelling on morbid or negative thoughts and hates to be consoled or sympathised with. Is also used for depression caused by suppressed grief;
- Pulsatilla for a person who is sensitive, shy, lonely, introspective, moody, jealous, gentle, irritable and from whom depression is worse in the evening, in a stuffy room, or from suppressed grief;
- Sepia for a person who is angry, anxious, confused, depressed, forgetful and dislikes company;
- Tarentula if the person finds it difficult to rest even in bed, with a hyperactive nervous system from stress;
- Zinc for a person who has difficulty thinking because of nervous exhaustion. Their thoughts wander and they may be slow to respond.

See page xv for information on how to use homeopathics.

Dietary and lifestyle recommendations

- Your diet should include lots of raw fruit and vegetables, and complex carbohydrates, soybeans and soy products (e.g. soymilk), brown rice, millet, green leafy vegetables (for their folic acid), whole grains (except wheat products), low-fat dairy products, cereals and fish (especially salmon). Seafood is high in the trace mineral selenium.
- Eat foods which contain tryptophan: chicken, turkey, fish, dried beans and peas, soybeans, nuts, peanut butter, brewer's yeast, avocado, dates, bananas, figs, grapefruit, oranges, papaya, peach, pears, pineapple, strawberry and tomato.
- Eat garlic, onions, hot chilli peppers, honey and licorice.
- Avoid sugar, meat, fried foods, alcohol, caffeine and processed foods.
- Moderate forms of exercise in the sun and fresh air, such as brisk walking, jogging, cycling and swimming, can be of great benefit to sufferers of depression. Keep your mind occupied with creative thoughts and get plenty of rest.
- Find a good counsellor and a support group so that you can express your feelings without indulging nor denying them. Expose your negative thinking and behavioural patterns and let them go.
- Consult your naturopath or kinesiologist to check for food allergies.

EPILEPSY

Description

Epilepsy is a disease characterised by recurring seizures in which the electrical activity of the brain cells gets temporarily out of control. A sudden surge of activity occurs in the brain causing a seizure or fit. Some people are born with epilepsy, while others acquire the disease later in life after a brain infection, tumour or injury. In 75 percent of cases the seizures begin in childhood and are characterised by staring spells and a few seconds of mental absence. In the remaining 25 percent of cases, the seizures start later in life. Seizures may be partial (limited to one area of the brain) or generalised (spread over a wide area of the brain). Partial seizures are divided into simple or complex, while generalised seizures are described as grand mal or petit mal.

Symptoms

SIMPLE PARTIAL SEIZURE

In simple partial seizure jerking begins in the fingers and toes and progresses up through the body. The fit only involves one side of the body and the patient remains conscious during the seizure. The jerking can vary greatly in severity to the extent that one arm and/or leg contracts and relaxes, thrashing about outside the conscious control of the patient.

COMPLEX PARTIAL SEIZURE

In a complex partial seizure consciousness is lost to the extent that the person has little or no memory of the seizure. The patient may experience a distinctive warning sign or aura before this type of seizure. The aura may include flashes of light, strange smells, buzzing noises, sweats, flushes and hallucinations, as well as 'butterflies' in the stomach. The seizure usually takes the form of a blank stare, difficulty in talking or swallowing, and a chewing motion, like lip-smacking.

GRAND MAL SEIZURE

The person will lose consciousness, fall to the ground, and the whole body will become stiff, then begin to twitch and jerk. The person may urinate, pass faeces and become blue. The seizure usually lasts two or three minutes and is followed by disorientation, confusion, fatigue and memory loss.

PETIT MAL SEIZURE

Again the person loses consciousness, but this only lasts from a few seconds to a minute or more. There may be some twitching movements but nothing as violent as a grand mal attack. The person may stumble momentarily or drop to the ground and rapidly recover. The attack may happen while the person is mid-sentence and appear as an unusual break in speaking of a few seconds. The person is often unaware that they have had an attack.

Causes

Epileptic attacks may be triggered by a variety of factors: flickering lights, certain foods, emotional upsets, stress, infections, fever, hunger, hypoglycaemia, lack of sleep, nutritional imbalances and head injuries. A number of people have a single fit only; in children this is often a fit associated with a very high fever.

Nutritional treatment

Nutritional supplements that may be beneficial in the treatment of epilepsy are included in the table below. Please note dosages recommended are for adults.

- For a child 12–17 years old give three-quarters the dosage.
- For a child six to 12 years old give half the dosage.
- For a child up to six years old give one-quarter the dosage.

See page xii for information on how to use these supplements.

Herbal treatment

A herbal repertory for epilepsy would include:

- Alfalfa (taken in capsule form 2000 mg daily);
- Black Cohosh (tincture – 2–4 ml three times daily or decoction);

- Hyssop (tincture – 3 ml three times daily or tea);
- Lobelia;
- Passion Flower (extract, tincture or tablet form);
- Skullcap;
- Valerian.

ANTI-SPASMODIC HERBS

The anti-spasmodic herbs Valerian, Vervain, Passion Flower and Mistletoe are useful in treating epilepsy. These herbs can be taken as a tincture (ten–30 drops) or as herbal teas (three cups daily). For best results the herbs should be used alternately. To make the tea, pour a cup of boiling water onto one–three teaspoonfuls of the dried herb and leave to infuse for ten to 15 minutes.

For more information on how to use these herbs see pages xiii–xv.

Homeopathic treatment

Treatment that may be prescribed by a homeopath for epilepsy includes:

- Aconite if the fit is brought on by fright, anxiety or fever;
- Belladonna if the person is angry, anxious, confused and/or excitable, and while fitting becomes wide-eyed, staring, red-faced and feverish;
- Chamomile if the fit is brought on by anger, or by teething in children (especially if one cheek is hot and red, the other cheek is pale and white);
- Cuprum metallicum if the convulsions are violent, the face and lips turn blue and the fingers and toes may be twitching;
- Glonoin if the face is red, the mind confused or forgetful, the head is hot and congested and the fingers and toes are widespread;

Nutritional supplements for epilepsy

SUPPLEMENT	DOSAGE	COMMENT
Folic acid	50 mg daily	Important for the synthesis of noradrenalin, serotonin, choline and tyrosine
Vitamin B6	50 mg three times daily	Important for synthesis of serotonin, dopamine, noradrenalin and GABA. Needed for normal brain function
Magnesium	700–1000 mg daily in divided doses (use magnesium chloride form)	Vital role in neuromuscular transmission; deficiency may cause muscle spasms and convulsive seizures

Nutritional supplements for epilepsy

SUPPLEMENT	DOSAGE	COMMENT
Manganese	50 mg daily	Common deficiency associated with epilepsy
Zinc	50–80 mg daily	Common deficiency associated with epilepsy. Protects the brain cells
Choline	1–20 g daily	Essential for the transmission of nerve impulses from the brain through the central nervous system
Vitamin E	300 iu daily, slowly increase to 1500 iu daily (emulsion form recommended)	Known to help seizures in children and may also control seizures in adults
Vitamin B complex	As directed on label	Essential vitamins for functioning of entire nervous system
L-taurine	500 mg three times daily	Helps control seizures
L-tyrosine	500 mg three times daily (take with 50 mg vitamin B6 and 100 mg vitamin C for better absorption)	Important for proper brain function
Vitamin C with bioflavonoids	2000–7000 mg daily in divided doses	Vital for the adrenal glands functioning and therefore helps in dealing with stress

- Ignatia amara if the fit is brought on by emotional upset, the face is pale and twitching starts in the face.

For more information on how to use homeopathics see page xv.

Aromatherapy treatment

The following essential oils will provide relief from the symptoms of epilepsy.

- Chamomile
- Hyssop
- Rose
- Sandalwood

Use in a warm bath (five–10 drops of oil), or as a body oil for massage (60 drops to 100 ml of almond oil).

Hyssop and Sandalwood can also be used in an aromatherapy burner.

See page xvi for more information on how to use these oils. See a qualified herbalist or aromatherapist before using essential oils if you suffer from epileptic seizures.

Dietary and lifestyle recommendations

- Avoid alcohol, caffeine, nicotine, peanuts and black tea as these have been shown to trigger seizures. Avoid artificial sweeteners such as aspartame.
- Include in your diet green leafy vegetables, yoghurt, eggs, raw nuts and seeds, soybeans, red grapes, seaweed (nori), peas, cheese and raw milk.
- Many small meals throughout the day are preferable to a few larger meals.
- Drink fresh vegetable juices made from carrots, green beans, peas and green leafy vegetables.
- Eat calcium-rich foods such as chick peas, almonds, sesame seeds, pistachio nuts, dried figs, sunflower seeds, mung beans, olives, broccoli, broadbeans, spinach and prunes. Kelp (seaweed) is also highly recommended.
- Take an Epsom salts bath twice a week.
- Get moderate exercise such as walking or swimming to improve circulation to the brain.

- Check for food and for chemical sensitivity or heavy metal poisoning; ask your naturopath about a hair analysis.
- Reduce stress through breathing exercises, relaxation programs and meditation. See Chapter Eleven on breathing and relaxation.

HEADACHES and MIGRAINES

Description

Headaches are often brought on by stress and tension resulting in muscular contraction in the neck area causing insufficient blood supply to the brain. There are, however, numerous different types of headaches which vary in severity and result from any number of causes. The three most common headaches are:

TENSION HEADACHES

These are often brought about by stress causing muscle tightness in the shoulders and neck.

SINUS HEADACHES

These result from changes in the weather, allergies or a head cold causing pain behind the eyes.

MIGRAINE HEADACHES

These can produce severe throbbing pain on one side of the head which is often accompanied by nausea, vomiting, blurred vision and light sensitivity. Migraine headaches may last for hours or even days.

Symptoms

The following symptoms can vary depending on the severity and type of headache.

- A feeling of pressure or tightness around the head
- Tension in the neck and shoulders
- A dull ache behind the eyes and around the forehead
- Sensitivity to light
- Throbbing in the temples and all over the head

Causes

It is of fundamental importance to try to locate the cause of the headache. The causes can vary from digestive disorders, menstruation, a slipped disc, high or low blood pressure, food additives, vitamin and mineral deficiencies, eyestrain, allergies, chemicals or stress. Headaches can also be the result of more serious diseases.

Nutritional treatment

Nutritional supplements that may be beneficial in the treatment of headaches are included in the following table. See pages xii–xiii for information on how to use these supplements.

Herbal treatment

Herbs that may be beneficial in the treatment of headaches are listed below. See pages xiii–xv for information on how to use the following herbs.

- Balm helps with digestive troubles, and is an anti-depressant used for treating stress and tension.
- Cayenne strengthens the heart, arteries and nerves. It is a general tonic for the digestive system.
- Chamomile helps with anxiety, insomnia and digestive problems.
- Elder Flower used to treat sinus headache.
- Lady's Slipper helps ease nervous pain and anxiety. Relieves emotional tension.
- Lavender is a calming antidepressant.
- Marjoram is a treatment for tension headaches.
- Skullcap is a nervine tonic and sedative. Relaxes and revives the central nervous system.
- Feverfew is a primary remedy for treating migraine headaches. Feverfew should not be used during pregnancy.
- Valerian is helpful in treating migraine.
- To avert a headache or a migraine try a five minute foot bath, as hot as possible, using either Chamomile, Feverfew or Lemon Balm.

Nutritional supplements for headaches and migraines

SUPPLEMENT	DOSAGE	COMMENT
Vitamin A	*10,000–50,000 iu*	*Liver detoxification*
Vitamin B complex	*50 mg three times daily*	*Aids nerve function*
Vitamin B3 (Niacin)	*100–3000 mg daily*	*Used to treat headaches*
Vitamin B6	*50 mg three times daily*	*Essential for normal brain function*
Vitamin C with bioflavonoids	*2000 mg daily*	*Anti-stress function*
Vitamin E	*400 iu daily*	*Improves circulation*
Magnesium	*300–1000 mg daily*	*Vasodilation of blood vessels*
Potassium	*3–8 mg daily*	*Aids nerve function*

HERBAL TEAS

- For the relief of tension headaches combine one teaspoon Valerian and one teaspoon Skullcap. Infuse in a cup of boiling water for ten to 15 minutes. Drink when needed.
- For the relief of headaches combine Lavender, Lady's Slipper and Valerian. Infuse one–two teaspoons of the herbs with boiling water for ten to 15 minutes. Drink when needed.

Homeopathic treatment

Treatment that may be prescribed by a homeopath for headaches includes:

- Natrum muriaticum for pre-menstrual headache, eye strain, mental exhaustion, sinus headache and frontal headache with pressure over eyes;
- Silica for pain that starts in nape of neck over head and settles in one eye. Also used if the head feels cold and every draught of air is felt and if the head sweats profusely;
- Ignatia for nervous headache that comes on at the end of the day after stress and for head congestion. Ignatia works better if it is applied hot;
- Aconitum napellus for sudden, violent headaches that feel as if a tight band were around the head. Also used for throbbing in temples that moves from one side to the other, restlessness, anxiety and thirst;
- Argentum nitricum if the head feels enlarged and there is pressure pain on one side. It is good for headaches that feel worse for mental effort and violent movement.

For more information on how to use these homeopathic treatments see page xv.

Aromatherapy treatment

Any of the following essential oils can be mixed with a base oil (such as almond, hazelnut, wheat germ, grapeseed, olive or safflower) and used as a massage oil to relieve neck, shoulder and head tension.

- Basil
- Chamomile
- Eucalyptus
- Ginger
- Lavender
- Lemongrass
- Melissa
- Peppermint
- Rose
- Rosemary

These oils can also be used as a bath. Place a few drops in a hot bath to provide relief from tension and stress-related headaches.

You can also use one or a combination of the above oils as a foot bath to provide relief from migraines and headaches.

Dietary and lifestyle recommendations

- Try to avoid migraine and headache triggers including chemicals, pollutants, food additives or colourings, caffeine and chocolate.
- Try to avoid situations that cause stress and anxiety.
- Make a note of foods eaten prior to an attack to see if you can trace any allergies.

- Place an ice pack on your head while the headache is still a dull throb. This can be an effective way to end the headache before it takes hold.
- A long hot shower or hot pack can be of benefit for tension headaches. Heat helps soothe the muscles and increase the blood supply.
- Exercise is an excellent way of reducing stress, and therefore avoiding stress-induced headaches.
- Yoga and meditation are also great stress busters. They provide the sufferer with the breathing and relaxation techniques necessary to avoid or reduce the severity of headaches.
- Orthodox treatment often involves pain-killers of some description. It is important to avoid these if possible as they provide only temporary relief. Treating and locating the cause provides long-term benefits.

INSOMNIA

Description and symptoms

Each person has an individual sleep pattern and the amount of sleep needed each night varies from one person to another. Some people require only three or four hours, most require seven or eight hours, while others may need ten hours. As we age we are inclined to need less sleep.

Insomnia is an extremely common complaint that can be divided into two categories:

- Sleep onset insomnia – difficulty falling asleep.
- Sleep maintenance insomnia – waking during the night with difficulty returning to sleep.

Causes

Insomnia can result from a wide variety of causes: psychological factors such as anxiety, tension, grief, fear and stress; alcohol; coffee; hypoglycaemia; muscle aches; indigestion; breathing problems; drugs such as some appetite suppressants, antidepressants, beta-blockers and thyroid hormone replacement drugs; sinus problems; digestive problems and constipation.

Nutritional treatment

Nutritional supplements that may be beneficial in the treatment of insomnia are included in the following table. See pages xii–xiii for information on how to use these supplements.

Herbal treatment

The following herbs can be taken in tea, tincture, tablet or capsule form. It is best to rotate your usage of these herbs, not relying solely on any one herb. See pages xiii–xv for information on how to use these herbs.

- Chamomile
- Cowslip
- Hops
- Jamaican Dogwood
- Kava Kava
- Lime
- Passion Flower
- Skullcap
- Valerian
- Vervain
- Wild Lettuce

HERBAL TEAS
- Lemon Balm and Hops tea has a extremely relaxing effect.
- Another useful mixture for insomniacs is Passion Flower and

Nutritional supplements for insomnia		
SUPPLEMENT	DOSAGE	COMMENT
Vitamin B complex plus	As directed on label	Helps promote relaxation
Vitamin B3 plus	500 mg three times daily	Particularly for sleep-maintenance insomnia
Vitamin B6	50 mg three times daily	Involved in synthesis of serotonin
Inositol	500 mg daily	Has a calming effect
Calcium	1500–2000 mg daily (in divided doses after meals and before bedtime)	Has a calming effect on the nervous system

Nutritional supplements for insomnia		
SUPPLEMENT	DOSAGE	COMMENT
Magnesium	*1000 mg daily*	*Facilitates muscular relaxation and balances function of calcium*
L-tryptophan	*2 mg daily*	*Precursor of serotonin*
Vitamin E	*400 iu daily*	*Assists the functioning of the entire nervous system*
Vitamin C	*1 g daily*	*Important for the nervous system and adrenal glands*

Valerian (equal portions of each) tea, drunk before going to bed.

- Kava Kava is an excellent herb for insomnia. Take as tincture, tablet or tea.
- The nervous system relaxants Catnip, Chamomile, Lime Blossom and Red Clover are calming teas which can be taken before going to bed.
- Catnip and Chamomile tea is a good combination to drink throughout the day.

HERBAL BATH

- A Chamomile or Valerian root bath is very relaxing in the evening and promotes a restful sleep. Make a strong pot of the tea and then strain it into the bathwater.
- Try a relaxing bath with the essential oils of Chamomile and Geranium.

Homeopathic treatment

Treatment that may be prescribed by a homeopath for insomnia depends upon the symptoms. For insomnia:

- before midnight use Conium maculatum, Kali carbonicum;
- after midnight use Arsenicum album, Rhus toxicodendron, Silica, Phosphoric acid;
- after 2 am use Nitric acidum;
- after 3 am use Bellis perennis, Magnesia carbonica, Nux vomica;
- that takes the form of restless sleep, use Aconite nopellus, Arsenicum album, Belladonna, Pulsatilla, Silica, Sulphur;
- caused by anxiety, use Arsenicum album, Kali phosphoricum;
- caused by grief, use Natrum muriaticum;
- caused by mental strain, use Kali phosphoricum, Nux vomica;
- caused by repeating thoughts, use Pulsatilla;
- caused by worry, use Calcarea carbonica.

See page xv for information on how to use homeopathics.

Aromatherapy treatment

Add the following essential oils to an oil burner for relief from the symptoms of insomnia.

- Clary Sage
- Cypress
- Frankincense
- Juniper
- Lavender
- Orange Blossom
- Rose Otto
- Vetiver
- Ylang Ylang

HERBAL PILLOW

Hops and Lavender are very useful herbs to make into a herbal pillow to promote sleep.

See pages xiv and xvi for information on how to use these oils.

Dietary and lifestyle recommendations

- Avoid black tea, coffee, salt, alcohol and chocolate.
- Don't eat a heavy meal within three hours of going to bed.
- Avoid foods that are high in fat and heavily spiced.
- Avoid foods which contain tyramine (particularly in the evening) including: smoked foods, bacon, cheese, chocolate, eggplant, ham, potatoes, sugar, sausage, spinach, tomatoes and wine.

- Begin a regular exercise program that elevates your heart rate for at least 20 minutes.
- Eat natural food sources of the amino acid tryptophan. Foods that contain tryptophan include: avocado, banana, dates, figs, grapefruit, oranges, papaya, peach, pear, persimmon, pineapple, strawberries, yoghurt, tuna, turkey and milk. Eat these foods especially in the evening.
- Keep the bedroom comfortable, at the right temperature, airy and quiet. Use linen sheets.
- Take a warm bath an hour or two before bedtime, but not right before bedtime as this can be too stimulating.
- Reduce your stress, anxiety and worrying by counselling or learning a relaxation technique such as meditation (see Chapter Eleven).
- If you have legitimate worries allocate a specific time of day for worrying, scheduling, planning etc.

MENINGITIS

Description

Meningitis occurs when an infection – either viral, bacterial or fungal – travels via the bloodstream and infects the three membranes that cover the brain, the meninges. The meninges are situated between the skull and the brain and act to contain the fluid in which the brain is supported. Meningitis is an extremely serious condition which can progress very quickly and become life threatening within hours. It is of the utmost importance to seek orthodox medical treatment immediately. A diagnosis is made by taking a sample of the cerebro-spinal fluid from the lower back to see if certain cells are present.

Symptoms

Symptoms include: fever, headache, nausea, vomiting, tiredness and irritability, muscle weakness and neck stiffness. Sometimes a red blotchy skin rash can occur.

Infants with meningitis will have fever, vomiting and a high-pitched cry. They will have difficulty feeding and the fontanelle on top of the head will be swollen or bulging.

Causes

Causes are many and varied. Complications from mumps, glandular fever, herpes or rubella viruses can all cause viral meningitis. The infection spreads via the nose and throat, the bloodstream or from other places in the body. It is also highly contagious.

Bacteria such as meningococcus, pneumococcus and streptococcus can cause bacterial meningitis. Bacterial meningitis is a more serious condition than viral meningitis with comparatively milder symptoms.

Complications that can occur through meningitis are: deafness, brain damage, heart and kidney damage, arthritis, paralysis, coma and even death. Orthodox medical treatment recommends aggressive antibiotic treatment.

The following natural therapies recommended are to support orthodox medical treatment, not to replace it.

Nutritional treatment

Nutritional supplements that may be beneficial in the treatment of meningitis are included in the following table. See pages xii–xiii for information on how to use these supplements.

Herbal treatment

For patients recovering from meningitis it is recommended a herbalist be consulted to provide treatment according to individual needs. See pages xiii–xv for information on how to use the following herbs.

CLEANSING HERBS

Herbs used to cleanse the system following drug therapy include:

- Cleavers;
- Echinacea;
- Gentian;
- Golden Seal (only use internally for one to two weeks and don't use of pregnant);
- Nettle;
- Oats;
- Wormwood.

ANTI-MICROBIAL HERBS

Anti-microbial herbs are used to combat infections and revitalise the body. These include:

- Echinacea;
- Eucalyptus;
- Garlic;
- Myrrh;
- Nasturtium;
- Thyme;
- Wild Indigo;
- Wormwood.

Homeopathic treatment

The following homeopathics are recommended as an emergency treatment if meningitis is suspected. See page xv for information on how to use these homeopathics. However for a more comprehensive treatment consult your doctor.

- Arnica if the symptoms begin after head injury.
- Belladonna for fever, high temperature, sudden onset of symptoms and a throbbing headache.

- Bryonia for severe headache that is made worse by eye movement.
- Pulsatilla for lingering fever, restlessness and irritability.

Aromatherapy treatment

See page xvi for information on how to use the following essential oils.

- A few drops of Basil oil in a warm bath is great for the nerves. It also stimulates the brain and relaxes the body.
- Eucalyptus oil, used as an inhalant, clears the head and nasal passages if you are congested.
- Myrrh oil, used either as an inhalant or massage oil, is beneficial in treating flu symptoms and mucus conditions.

Nutritional supplements for meningitis

SUPPLEMENT	DOSAGE	COMMENT
Vitamin A	50,000 iu for five days 25,000 iu for seven days 10,000 iu daily after that	Anti-oxidant needed for healing membranes
Vitamin C with bioflavonoids	3000–10,000 mg daily	Anti-bacterial action
Calcium	2000 mg daily	To relieve irritability and protect against bone loss
Zinc	One tablet three times daily	An immune booster
Kyolic garlic	Two capsules three times daily with meals	Natural antibiotic

Dietary and lifestyle recommendations

If the characteristic symptoms of meningitis develop, seek orthodox medical advice immediately.

When the patient is on the road to recovery it is important to eat a well-balanced diet and get plenty of rest. A course of nutritional supplements, homeopathy and herbs can also help enhance the immune system.

MULTIPLE SCLEROSIS

Description

Multiple Sclerosis (MS) is the progressive destruction of the myelin sheath that surrounds, insulates and protects nerves. As the sheath breaks down it forms scleroses which are hardened scars or plaques. The destruction of the nerve covering causes nerve conduction to be slowed down and short circuited. This scrambles and confuses the signals from the brain to the body.

Among the early symptoms of MS are:

- muscular weakness;
- heaviness or stiffness which causes leg-dragging, clumsiness and a tendency to drop things;
- sensations of pins and needles, tingling and/or numbness;
- visual impairment which includes blurred vision, double vision, haziness, eyeball pain and problems with light and colour perception;
- loss of balance and co-ordination, light-headedness and a feeling of spinning;
- nausea and vomiting;
- incontinence and loss of bladder sensation;
- loss of sexual function.

Symptoms

Symptoms vary according to which portions of the nervous system are affected. Usually the first symptoms occur in early adult life, the average age of onset being 33 years. The frequency of episodes is greatest during the first three to four years of the disease (although a first attack may not be followed by another attack for ten to 20 years). More women are affected than men; 60 percent of sufferers are female.

Causes

The causes of multiple sclerosis are not clearly understood. The predominant theories involve two main factors:

- The body's reaction to a virus (possibly the measles virus).
- An auto-immune response in which the body becomes allergic to itself and starts attacking its own cells.

The more holistic theories see MS as being associated with such causative factors as:

- diets which are high in gluten and dairy products, saturated fats, alcohol and cholesterol (food allergies and malabsorption problems may also play a role);
- Chemical poisoning of the nervous system by pesticides, pollution, industrial chemicals, food preservatives and heavy metals (e.g. mercury poisoning from mercury amalgam dental fillings).

Nutritional treatment

Nutritional supplements that may be beneficial in the treatment of multiple sclerosis are included in the following table. See page xii for information on how to use these supplements.

Herbal treatment

A herbal repertory for the treatment of multiple sclerosis would include the following herbs. See pages xiii–xv for information on how to use these herbs.

- Evening Primrose oil (500 mg capsule three times daily) taken over an extended period of time enables the myelin sheath to rebuild, therefore, protecting the nerves.

MUSCULAR STIFFNESS
- Use a Horseradish compress for muscular stiffness.

Nutritional supplements for multiple sclerosis

SUPPLEMENT	DOSAGE	COMMENT
Vitamin B complex plus	100 mg three times daily	Necessary for both immune system and nervous system
Vitamin B1	100 mg three times daily	Has a beneficial effect on mental attitude. Deficiency may lead to poor memory, emotional instability, low energy and depression
Vitamin B6	50 mg three times daily	Assists the nervous and immune functions
Vitamin B12	250 mcg per wek	Assists with normal nerve function
Vitamin C	3000 mg daily	Necessary for the production of the anti viral protein called interferon. Strengthens immune system and detoxifies.

Nutritional supplements for multiple sclerosis

SUPPLEMENT	DOSAGE	COMMENT
Vitamin E	600 iu daily	Destroys free radicals and protects the nerves
Vitamin D	1000 iu daily	Assists in regulating the immune system.
Selenium	200 mcg daily	Inhibits lipid peroxidation and protects the myelin sheath covering the nerves
Calcium	2000 mg daily	Facilitates nerve transmission (use chelated form)
Magnesium	1000 mg daily	Required for efficient calcium absorption
Flaxseed oil	One tablespoon daily	Supplements linoleic acid
Cod liver oil	One tablespoon daily	Supplements linoleic acid
Garlic	Two capsules three times daily or as directed	Protects the nervous system and strengthens the immune system

- A bath of Sage, Mugwort, or Strawberry leaves will help with stiff muscles and aching joints.

NERVE RELAXANTS
- Lobelia
- Skullcap
- Valerian root

LIVER DETOXIFIERS
- Burdock
- Dandelion
- Echinacea
- Golden Seal
- Pau d'Arco
- Red Clover
- Sarsparilla
- St John's Wort

- Yarrow
- Violet Leaves

Aromatherapy treatment

For information on how to use these essential oils see page xvi.

- Mix one part Juniper oil with nine parts olive oil and massage into areas affected by muscular paralysis, stiffness and soreness.
- Choose aromatherapy oils from the introduction to the Nervous System (see page 82).

Use these essential oils as bath oils, body oils or in an oil burner.

Dietary and lifestyle recommendations

- Maintain a low fat diet and totally exclude saturated fats.
  Saturated fats include meats, dairy products, margarine, coconut and palm oil, shortening, chocolate, dried foods and egg yolks.
- Take a normal allowance of protein, although meat is not advised. Use the following protein sources: fish, legumes, grains, vegetables, nuts and soy products.
- Take cold water fish (mackerel, sardines, salmon and herring) for the Omega 3 fatty acids. Omega 3 oils are important for maintaining normal nervous system functioning and production of the myelin sheath.
- Supplement Omega 3 Oils by taking one tablespoon of Flaxseed oil and one tablespoon of cod liver oil daily. Use coldpressed, virgin olive oil for cooking (not the omega 3 oil).
- Avoid chocolate, salty foods, spicy foods, coffee, alcohol and cigarettes, dairy products, fried foods, meat, oats, barley, sugar, wheat, processed, canned or frozen foods.
- Eat plenty of dark, leafy greens, raw sprouts and alfalfa.
- Drink at least eight glasses of quality water daily.
- Get tested for food allergies, especially milk and gluten.
- Take a fibre supplement to keep your colon clean and your bowels moving.
- Have a regular massage.
- Get regular, moderate exercise (walking and swimming) and keep yourself mentally stimulated, but not stressed.
- Get 15 minutes of all-over sun three to five times per week.
- *Taking Control of Multiple Schlerosis*, by Prof. George Jelinek, is essential reading.

NEURALGIA and NEURITIS

Description and symptoms

Neuralgia is pain in a peripheral nerve while neuritis is the inflammation and/or deterioration of a peripheral nerve or a group of nerves.

Neuralgia and neuritis are closely related, often occurring together. Neuritis can result in muscle weakness and atrophy, loss of sensations, pins and needles and diminished reflexes. The incidence of neuritis is highest in men between the ages of 30 and 50. The radial, medial (carpal tunnel syndrome) and ulna nerves of the arms are the three nerves most commonly affected by neuritis.

Nutritional supplements for neuralgia and neuritis

SUPPLEMENT	DOSAGE	COMMENT
Vitamin B1	100 mg twice daily	Deficiency is associated with neuritis and trigeminal neuralgia
Vitamin B3	50 mg twice daily	Maintains healthy nerves (do not take if you have a liver disorder, gout or high blood pressure)
Vitamin B6	50 mg twice daily	Deficiency may cause neuritis
Folic acid	1000 mcg daily	Deficiency may cause neuritis
Vitamin B12	2000 mcg twice daily	Deficiency may cause neuritis. Facilitates mylenation of nerve fibres
Calcium chelated with Magnesium	2000 mg daily 400–1000 mg daily	Calcium is important in nerve impulse conduction. Magnesium also plays an important part in neuro-transmission
Essential fatty acids (e.g. Flaxseed oil)	As directed on label	Facilitates nerve damage repair
Potassium	5 g daily	Important for nerve and heart function

Causes

Neuralgia may be caused by pinching of the nerve between other tissues; by reduced blood supply to the nerve; by an infection of the nerve (such as shingles); by a traumatic injury to the nerve or by arthritis. It may also be caused by emotional problems, stress, alcohol and drugs. Some examples of neuralgia are: migraines, shingles and trigeminal neuralgia.

Neuritis may be caused by a vitamin deficiency (especially B vitamins); by metabolic imbalances; by traumatic injury; by an infection of the nerve; by diseases such as gout, diabetes and leukaemia; and by toxic levels of metals such as lead and mercury.

Nutritional treatment

Nutritional supplements that may be beneficial in the treatment of neuralgia and neuritis are included in the above table. See pages xii–xiii for information on how to use these supplements.

Herbal treatment

The following herbs can be used as teas, tablets, or tinctures. See pages xiii–xv for information on how to use these herbs.

ANTI-SPASMODIC HERBS

Anti-spasmodic herbs can be used to relax the muscles. These include:

- Black Haw;
- Cramp Bark;
- Hops;
- Rosemary;
- Wild Lettuce;
- Wood Betony.

NERVINES

Nervines or nerve tonics include:

- Feverfew (don't use if pregnant);
- Kava Kava;
- Lobelia;
- Passion Flower;
- Skullcap;
- Valerian;
- White Willow bark;
- Oats (taken as a tincture or as a porridge is a nerve tonic which feeds nervous tissue. It can even be taken as an infusion in the bath);
- Gotu Kola (is an Ayurvedic herb, considered to be the prime nervine tonic, used to treat insomnia, stress, nervousness and other nervous system disorders. Take Gotu Kola as a tea, tablet or tincture).

ANTI-INFLAMMATORY HERBS

Anti-inflammatory herbs include:

- Bilberry;
- Calendula;
- Chamomile;
- Marshmallow Root;
- St John's Wort;
- Yarrow;
- Yucca.

HERBAL TEAS

- Herbal teas for neuralgia and neuritis include: Ginseng, Hops, Jamaican Dogwood, Passion Flower, St John's Wort and Valerian.
- For shingles take Echinacea and Marigold as a tea or tincture daily for at least three months.

For information on how to use herbal teas see page xiv.

HERBAL LINAMENTS AND OILS

- Herbal liniments and oils for neuralgia and neuritis include: Rosemary, Lavender and St John's Wort.

Homeopathic treatment

Treatment that may be prescribed by a homeopath for neuralgia and neuritis varies according to the symptoms. See page xv for information on how to use these homeopathics.

- Use Aconite if the nerve pain flares up in cold wind, or is worse at night, or if the affected part of the body feels congested as well as numb.

- Use Arsenicum if the nerve pain flares up in dry cold, or if the person feels chilly, or if they look pale and anxious.
- Use Colocynthis if the attack is brought on by cold or damp, if the condition is aggravated by anger or excitement, or if the pain is violent and better for the application of heat.
- Use Hypericum for shooting pains that are worse for cold and pressure, and if the condition is due to accident or injury.
- Use Lachesis if the pain is worse for heat, worse during the morning, worse for pressure, worse after sleep and worse on waking.
- Use Magnesia for cramping pain, that is better for heat or firm pressure, and worse for cold, touch, being uncovered and walking in fresh air.
- Use Ranunculus if the pain affects the rib cage or above the right eye.
- Use Spigelia for pain above the left eye which worsens on movement.

Aromatherapy treatment

Try any of the essential oils on pages 82–3 and see page xvi for information on how to use these oils as body or bath oils, or in an oil burner.

You can also try four drops of Lavender oil on a little brown sugar an hour before each meal.

Dietary and lifestyle recommendations

It is important to well-balanced diet of fruit, vegetables, nuts, seeds and whole grains. If there is an infection present, such as herpes, then your protein, calorie and fluid intake should be increased.

- Avoid coffee, caffeine, carbonated drinks, cigarettes and alcohol.
- Try some mild exercise, such as walking, to increase circulation and oxygenate the tissues.
- Try some deep-tissue massage and/or acupuncture.

PARKINSON'S DISEASE

Description

Parkinson's disease is a slow progressing neurological disorder caused by a degeneration of the nerve cells in the brain.

Symptoms

The main symptoms of Parkinson's disease are muscle tremor causing involuntary movement of hands and head, stiffness and weakness of the limbs and slowness of movements.

As the disease progresses everyday tasks become more difficult. A deterioration in handwriting is noticeable, walking turns into shuffling, speech becomes slower and a general feeling of depression and anxiety can take over.

Other symptoms include involuntary dribbling, constipation and bladder problems. In the early stages of the disease, the patient's motor functions are affected, however their cognitive functions are not impaired.

Causes

Symptoms first appear when there is a lack of the neurotransmitter dopamine in the brain. The underlying cause, however, is unknown.

Nutritional treatment

Nutritional supplements that may be beneficial in the treatment of Parkinson's disease are included in the following table. See pages xii–xiii for information on how to use these supplements.

Herbal treatment

Those suffering from Parkinson's disease often have an accumulation of toxins in the body. Herbs are beneficial in detoxifying and cleansing the body. They can be taken internally as herbal

Nutritional supplements for Parkinson's disease

SUPPLEMENT	DOSAGE	COMMENT
Vitamin C plus	3000–6000 mg daily	Anti-oxidants that may slow progression of the disease
Vitamin E plus	3200 iu daily	
Selenium	200 mcg daily	
Vitamin B complex	50 mg three times daily with meals	Important for brain function
Vitamin B6	50–75 mg three times daily with meals (consult your doctor before taking this vitamin)	Dopamine production in the brain depends on adequate supply of this vitamin
Multivitamin mineral complex	As directed on label	To correct nutritional and deficiencies
Lecithin granules	One tablespoon three times daily	Improves brain function and protects nerve cells
Calcium and Magnesium	800–1400 mg daily 350 mg daily	Important for neuromuscular transmission

teas, cold drinks and tinctures. They can also be taken externally in foot baths, infused in massage oils and rubbed into affected areas, or simply by absorbing the herbal benefits through aromatherapy. See pages xiii–xv for more information on using the following herbs.

The following herbs have detoxifying effects on the liver:

- Burdock root;
- Dandelion root;
- Milk Thistle.

These herbs are particularly good for cleansing the blood:

- Hawthorn;
- Licorice;
- Red Clover;
- Sarsaparilla;
- Yellow Dock.

TENSION-REDUCING HERBS
Herbs used for treating stress and anxiety include:

- Chamomile;
- Ginseng;
- Lime Blossom;
- Mistletoe;
- Oats;
- Skullcap;
- Valerian.

A herbal tea for anxiety and muscle tension can be made from one part Skullcap and one part Valerian. This tea can be drunk three times daily or when needed.

ANTI-DEPRESSIVE HERBS
The following herbs are excellent anti-depressives:

- Damiana;
- Ginseng;
- Lady's Slipper;
- Lavender;
- Skullcap;
- St John's Wort;
- Vervain.

NERVINES
For nervous tension try a combination of:

- Hawthorn;
- Hops;
- Lime Blossom.

These herbs can be made into a herbal tea and taken three times daily.

Homeopathic treatment

Treatment that may be prescribed by a homeopath for Parkinson's disease includes:

- Mercurius for increased saliva, trembling of limbs, nervousness and depression;
- Agaricus for trembling and twitchiness, and stumbling when walking;
- Rhus toxicodendrom for stiffness, aches and pains, a cramp that is made worse by immobility but improves when moving and a metallic taste in the mouth.

See page xv for information on how to use homeopathics.

Aromatherapy treatment

The following essential oils may provide relief from Parkinson's disease.

- Basil is a nervine and anti-depressant. Use as a bath oil or an inhalant.
- Black Pepper is used for stiff joints, anxiety, depression, bad circulation and constipation. Use as a massage oil (combined with a base oil of Apricot or Avocado) or as an inhalant.
- Cedarwood is used for nervous tension and anxiety. Place a few drops in a warm bath and soak or combine with a base oil and use as a relaxing massage oil.
- Clary Sage is used for tension, stress, nervousness and depression. Use it as a bath oil or a massage oil.
- Geranium assists circulation, calms tension and depression, and helps with urinary problems. Use as a bath oil, a massage oil or compress.
- Juniper is used for kidney and urinary tract problems. Use as a bath oil, massage oil or compress.
- Rosemary will help circulation, muscles, joints and memory. Use as a bath oil, or massage oil or in an oil burner
- Ylang Ylang assists circulation, anxiety and depression. Use as a bath oil or massage oil.

It is important never to use the essential oils neat on the skin. They should be mixed with a base oil such as Apricot, Avocado or Grapeseed and stored in a dark glass bottle. The usual ratio is one drop of essential oil to 2 ml of base oil.

See page xvi for more information on using essential oils.

Dietary and lifestyle recommendations

- Avoid saturated fats.
- Reduce exposure to toxic metals, pesticides and tobacco smoke.
- Avoid deadly nightshade vegetables such as tomatoes.
- Include exercise and movement therapy into your daily routine as this will help you maintain physical strength and muscle tone.
- Take time out to relax with meditation.

IMPORTANT

It is important the patient undergoes a thorough physical examination to properly diagnose the condition. Although there is no cure as yet for Parkinson's disease, the treatment is focused on relieving the symptoms and maintaining independence for as long as possible. Drug therapy is most often used to treat people with this condition.

SCIATICA

Description and symptoms

Sciatica is a type of neuritis characterised by severe pain along the path of the sciatic nerve. Inflammation or injury of the nerve causes pain, that passes from the back or thigh down its length in to the leg and sometimes to the foot and toes.

Causes

Among the possible causes of sciatica are a herniated (slipped) disc, inflammation of the nerve or sprained joints. Damage through injury to the lower back, arthritis, bursitis and irritable bowel syndrome are other possible causes. See pages 295–98 for more advice and information on sciatica.

Nutritional treatment

Nutritional supplements that may be beneficial in the treatment of sciatica are included in the following table. See pages xii–xiii for information on how to use these supplements.

Herbal treatment

The following herbs can be used in tablet, tea or tincture form. For information on how to use these herbs see pages xiii–xv.

- St John's Wort can be used internally or in the treatment of neuralgic and sciatic pain as an external massage oil.
- Valerian aids in anxiety reactions that can accompany pain.
- Yellow Jasmine is a strong pain reliever that should only be used on the advice of a recognised herbalist.
- Wild Lettuce is a pain reliever.

POULTICES
Herbal compresses and poultices are recommended for sciatica.

Nutritional supplements for sciatica		
SUPPLEMENT	DOSAGE	COMMENT
Calcium and	1500–2000 mg daily	Needed for strengthening bones
Magnesium	700–1000 mg daily	Aids absorption of calcium and magnesium
and Vitamin D	400 iu daily	Important in the utilisation of calcium
Multivitamin mineral complex	As directed on label	Supplies a range of nutrients and important for the healing of connective tissue
Vitamin B complex	As directed on label	Nourishes the entire nervous system
Vitamin E	200–400 iu daily	Anti-oxidant

- An old remedy for sciatica is a poultice made of shredded cabbage leaves.

HERBAL BATH

A handful of dried herbs such as Lavender Flower, Lemon Balm and Rosemary leaves can be placed in a muslin bag and suspended from the hot water tap so the water flows through it. This provides you with a fresh infusion for a relaxing therapeutic bath.

Homeopathic treatment

For homeopathic treatment of sciatica, use the same treatments that are recommended for neuralgia (see page 115).

Aromatherapy treatment

Aromatherapy oils that can be used for the relief of sciatic pain include:

- Rosemary for the relief of nerves, circulation, rheumatic pain, muscular and joint pain.
- Eucalyptus for the relief of rheumatic pain.
- Patchouli is a nervine, anti-inflammatory, sedative and relaxing essential oil.
- Lavender is a healing and nervine muscle relaxant that is a sedative and calming.
- Sage is a nervine and relaxant that helps relieve nervous and muscular tension pain.

These oils can be used in a warm bath, or mixed with a base oil such as Almond, Grapeseed or Wheat Germ and massaged into the affected area. See page xvi for information on how to use these oils.

Dietary and lifestyle recommendations

- Rest and apply hot or cold compresses to the affected area.
- Massage, acupuncture, hydrotherapy and chiropractic work may help alleviate pain.
- Stretching exercises such as yoga are highly recommended, especially as an ongoing preventative measure.
- Relax in a warm herbal bath.

STRESS

Description

Stress can be the underlying causative factor in many disease states from asthma and allergies through to heart disease. Stress that is suffered on a long-term basis can be debilitating both to the body and mind. The term 'stress' refers to any reaction to a physical, mental or emotional stimulus that upsets the body's natural balance. A certain amount of stress or challenge is useful as a motivating factor to stimulate us, but when the stress is excessive, ongoing or of an unhealthy kind it can stretch our body and mind beyond the capacity to cope.

Symptoms

The stress response causes the body to produce the hormones adrenalin, noradrenalin and corticosteroids; these hormones produce muscular tension, an increased heart and breathing rate and a hyperactive mind.

Some longer-term symptoms of stress may be: high blood pressure, high cholesterol level, neck and backaches, dizziness, diarrhoea or constipation, irritability or tearfulness, fatigue, insomnia, lack of concentration, chronic headaches, memory loss, low self-esteem, social withdrawal, cold hands, lowered sexual drive, loss of appetite or overeating, gastrointestinal disorders and a weakened immune system.

The increased production of adrenalin is responsible for most of these symptoms of stress. The stress response causes the body to release adrenalin as a reaction to a perceived threat, whether the threat is real or imaginary.

Causes

Many of the stress-related disorders result from Vitamin B-complex deficiencies; B vitamins are essential for the proper functioning of the nervous system and are depleted by the stress response. Stress also promotes the body to produce free radicals that damage body tissue when oxidised.

The stress response may be triggered by work issues, emotional issues, lack of sleep, financial problems, grief, noise, traffic, crowds, changes in routine or lifestyle, pollution, excessive alcohol consumption and smoking.

Nutritional treatment

Nutritional supplements that may be beneficial in the treatment of stress are included in the following table. See pages xii–xiii for information on how to use these supplements.

Herbal treatment

A herbal repertory for stress would include the following herbs from the categories of nervine relaxants and tonics. The following herbs can be used as teas, tablets or tinctures.

* Balm
* Borage
* Catnip
* Chamomile
* Damiana
* Ginseng
* Golden Seal (only use internally for one to two weeks and don't use if pregnant)
* Hops
* Kava Kava
* Lady's Slipper
* Lavender
* Lime
* Mistletoe
* Passion Flower
* Pau d'Arco
* Skullcap
* St John's Wort
* Valerian

See pages xiii–xv for information on how to use these herbs.

HIGH BLOOD PRESSURE

For high blood pressure use Hawthorn berries and Lime blossom. These herbs may also be used with Hops and Mistletoe in the form of tinctures or infusions (see pages xiii–xv for more information).

TRAUMA

For immediate relief in traumatic situations take Valerian, Passion Flower, Jamaican Dogwood, Wild Lettuce or Lady's Slipper. The Bach Flower remedy 'Rescue Remedy' is also good for trauma.

LONG-TERM STRESS

For medium to long-term stress it is necessary to feed the adrenal glands as this enables the system to recover from stress faster. Use the following herbs:

- Borage;
- Ginseng;
- Licorice (also useful for peptic ulcers and gastritis);
- Siberian Ginseng.

SPASM-REDUCING

Chamomile is a gentle anti-spasmodic and anti-inflammatory which soothes the digestive tract and assists in sleeping.

Nutritional supplements for stress

SUPPLEMENT	DOSAGE	COMMENT
Vitamin A	25,000 iu daily	An anti-oxidant
Vitamin B complex plus	100 mg daily	B, A, C, and E vitamins are anti-oxidants which disarm free radicals caused by stress
Vitamin B6 plus	Injection form of 1 cc weekly or as prescribed by your doctor	B vitamins (especially B12) are depleted by stress and are necessary for the functioning of the nervous system
Vitamin B12 plus		
Vitamin B5	500 mg daily	
Vitamin C with bioflavonoids	3000–10,000 mg taken throughout the day	Used up by the adrenal glands during stress response and needed to produce anti-stress hormones
Vitamin E	400 iu daily	An anti-oxidant and necessary for immune function

Nutritional supplements for stress

SUPPLEMENT	DOSAGE	COMMENT
Zinc	50 mg daily	Necessary for immune function. It also protects the cells from free radicals
Calcium and Magnesium	2000 mg daily 1000 mg daily	Depleted by stress response. Deficiency can cause anxiety, depression and fear
L-tyrosine	1000 mg twice daily in morning and evening	Precursor of adrenalin, dopamine and noradrenaline. Also regulates blood pressure
GABA	750 mg twice daily (take with 50 mg inositol)	Tranquillises and nourishes the brain
Lecithin granules or capsules	Two capsules with meals or as directed on label	Protects nervous system and brain function
Fibre (oat bran or psyllium husks)	As directed on label	Cleanses the bowel
Brewer's yeast	As directed on label	A rich source of B vitamins

SEDATIVE

Hops is a sedative and hypnotic herb used to ease nervousness, restlessness, tension, anxiety and insomnia. For insomnia it can be combined with Valerian and Passion Flower. As a tincture take 1–4 ml three times daily, or as an infusion take a cup at night to induce sleep.

NERVINE

Valerian keeps the nervous system strong and prevents it from being overwhelmed. It is also useful for stress-related headaches and insomnia. Valerian can be combined with Skullcap for tension. Take 2–4 ml of Valerian three times a day or two–three cups of the herbal tea daily.

Skullcap and Oats are excellent nervine tonics which nourish and condition the nervous system.

Homeopathic treatment

Treatment that may be prescribed by a homeopath for stress varies according to the symptoms.

- Use Aconitum napellus if you have restless sleep, anxious dreams, a red face, palpitations or hot sweat.
- Use Argentum nitricum if you have mental strain, are fearful, restless, panic stricken or if you have a red tongue tip.

- Use Arsenicum album if you look pale and anxious, are weak and exhausted, and suffering from palpitations and restlessness.
- Use Calcarea carbonica if you are tending towards self-pity, weeping easily about your problems and if you feel a failure. Your worry and overactive mind may cause insomnia.
- Use Gelsemium for mild anxiety with social withdrawal, if you're depressed but can't cry; and fearful of public speaking, crowds and death.
- Use Ignatia for stress following an emotional upset such as a broken relationship.
- Use Nux vomica for stress produced by overwork and over indulgence, including smoking, eating and drinking too much.
- Use Phosphoric acid for stress due to grief or bad news.
- Use Picric acid for stress due to overwork.

See page xv for information on how to use these homeopathics.

Aromatherapy treatment

Make the following bath or body oils by mixing one drop of the essential oil with 2 ml of either sweet almond oil or peach kernel oil.

- Basil can be used as a body oil, a bath oil or in an oil burner. Basil is a nerve tonic which clarifies the mind and acts as an anti-depressant.
- Bergamot can be used as a body or bath oil. It is an anti-depressant and gentle relaxant.
- Chamomile can be used as a body or bath oil. It is soothing and calming for anxiety and insomnia, and it relaxes the muscles.
- Clary Sage can be used as a body or bath oil. It is a relaxing oil used for anxiety, stress, nervousness and ulcers.
- Frankincense can be used as a bath oil, a body oil or as incense. Frankincense eases anxiety and soothes nervous tension.
- Jasmine can be used as a bath or body oil, as a perfume or in the oil burner. It is an anti-depressant which calms the nerves and relieves anxiety.
- Lavender can be used as bath or body oil. Lavender soothes frayed nerves, relaxes and eases aches and pains and is useful for headaches and migraines.
- Marjoram can be used as a bath oil, body oil or in the oil burner. It is used for anxiety, grief, headaches and insomnia.
- Patchouli can be used as a bath oil, a body oil or in the oil burner. It is a nerve stimulant which relieves stress and lifts anxiety and depression.
- Rose can be used as a bath or body oil. Rose soothes the nerves, calms anger and is used for depression and insomnia.

See page xvi for information on how to use these oils.

Dietary and lifestyle recommendations

- Change your diet so that it consists of 50–75 percent raw foods. These can include: melons, papaya, lettuce, blackcurrants, spinach, cherries, oats, whole grain breads and cereals. Honey, onions and all carbohydrates (pasta, potatoes, beans, bread, cereal) have a calming effect on the brain.
- Avoid caffeine, alcohol, tobacco, and refined and processed foods. Test for dairy allergies by eliminating dairy products for three weeks then slowly reintroduce as you check for reoccurring stress symptoms.
- Avoid artificial sweeteners, fizzy drinks, chocolate, eggs, fried foods, port, red meat, sugar, white flour products and foods containing preservatives.

- See Chapter Eleven on fasting, relaxation, and breathing.
- Get regular (not too strenuous) exercise such as bushwalking, swimming and cycling. Also practice some stretching exercise like yoga or tai chi which have a deep breathing component.
- Soak yourself in a warm bath (not too hot) with one of the aromatherapy oils (five–ten drops) for at least 15 minutes to relax muscles and increase peripheral circulation.
- Buy a pet, have a good laugh or a great cry, treat yourself to a regular massage and some satisfying sexual pleasure.
- Seek out a compatible counsellor or support group so that you don't withdraw deeper into isolation.

CHAPTER FOUR

THE CIRCULATORY SYSTEM

Maintenance of the heart, blood pressure, blood vessels and circulation

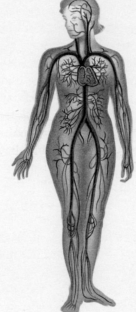

What does it consist of?

The circulatory system consists of the heart, blood vessels and the blood.

What does it do?

Blood is pumped out from the heart through tough, elastic tubes called arteries. Another network of tubes called veins return blood to the heart. Linking the smallest arteries and veins are tiny blood vessels called capillaries. Oxygenated blood from the lungs circulates through the arteries to the capillaries. Oxygen is released in the capillaries and passes into the fluid that bathes surrounding tissues. Deoxygenated cells take up this oxygen and use it to produce energy. The deoxygenated blood returns from the capillaries to the heart where it is pumped to the lungs to receive more oxygen.

Blood transports oxygen, nutrients from digestion and waste products excreted from cells. It helps to regulate the body's water content, temperature and the acid/alkali balance. The blood also carries specialised cells and proteins which repair tissues damaged by injury and fight against infections.

The heart is a four-chambered organ which receives deoxygenated blood from the veins and pumps it to the lungs. It then receives oxygenated blood from the lungs and pumps it to the arteries which take the blood to every cell in the body. The heart and the blood vessels have the job of transporting blood (carrying oxygen and nutrients) to the cells and removing waste products from the cells. If these functions are impaired in some way then tissue damage and/or organ dysfunction will quickly result.

What goes wrong with it?

In our society the circulatory system is a common site for illness, often fatal ones, as our lifestyle, diet, use of tobacco and alcohol, stress, and lack of exercise all affect the condition of the heart, blood vessels and blood. Prevention is far better than having to deal with a circulatory disorder that has developed. The foods, supplements and herbs recommended in this chapter specifically nourish, repair and strengthen the circulatory system.

Traditional Oriental approach

In Chinese medicine the heart is associated with the fire element, and is called the 'ruler of the body'. The heart is seen as the organ responsible for our spirit in the sense of our enthusiasm, motivation, joy and will. The Oriental sense of spirit involves both aspects of mind and emotions. If the heart is strong the circulation will be good; the mind will be clear, happy and peaceful; the emotions will be balanced and the sleeping pattern will be regular.

Symptoms of a disturbance of heart chi may include:

* insomnia;
* poor memory;
* restless sleep with excessive dreaming;
* poor long-term memory;
* unclear speech;
* anxiety;
* circulatory problems;
* blood pressure problems;
* hot flushes;
* hyperactivity.

The heart energy can become excessive and too hot or it can become deficient and depleted.

To cool a hyperactive, manic, excessively excited or anxious heart chi use:

* Chamomile tea or tincture;
* Hibiscus or Mint herbal teas or tinctures;
* orange or lemon juice;
* brown rice;
* whole grain oats and wheat.

Foods rich in calcium and magnesium will also help to cool an overheated heart, such as:

- almonds;
- beans;
- broccoli;
- cabbage;
- calcium in low-fat dairy products;
- carrots;
- cashews;
- celery;
- chick peas;
- figs;
- green vegetables;
- hazelnuts;
- leeks;
- lentils;
- lettuce;
- magnesium in kelp;
- millet;
- olives;
- oranges;
- parsley;
- peanuts;
- sesame seeds;
- soy beans;
- spinach;
- walnuts;
- wheat bran;
- wheat germ.

To strengthen the heart chi use the herbs:

- Borage;
- Ginseng;
- Golden Seal;
- Motherwort;
- Tansy;
- Valerian.

Other recommended foods include:

- apricots;
- beetroot;
- cabbage;
- cauliflower;
- corn;
- garlic;
- mustard;
- peaches;
- plums;
- raspberries;
- red lentils;
- strawberries;
- sunflower seeds.

Nutritional treatment

The following vitamins and minerals are of great benefit to the circulatory system. See pages xii–xiii for more information on how to use these supplements.

VITAMIN B1

Thiamine (vitamin B1) deficiency may result in a lack of oxygen absorption by the blood. A deficiency also makes it difficult for a person to digest carbohydrates and leaves too much pyruvic acid in the blood. This can cause lack of concentration, laboured breathing, irregular heartbeat and cardiac damage. The heart muscles are weakened and cardiac failure may occur.

VITAMIN B3

Niacin (vitamin B3) helps to control the release of fats from the body and regulates the fat levels of the blood, which can prevent high cholesterol and arteriosclerosis. Niacin is essential for good circulation as it widens blood vessels and removes fats from arterial walls.

VITAMIN B6

Vitamin B6 assists in the formation of red blood cells and the cells of the immune system. Deficiency of vitamin B6 causes disturbances of the bone marrow, which then causes anaemia. Deficiency can also allow cholesterol to accumulate in the walls of the arteries.

VITAMIN B12

Vitamin B12 is essential for the production of red blood cells. Deficiency will impair the development of the blood cells in bone marrow which may lead to anaemia of the large red blood cells. Injections of vitamin B12 can be used to treat pernicious anaemia.

VITAMIN C

Vitamin C converts cholesterol into bile acids, strengthens the blood capillaries and promotes a constant flow of enzyme reactions which are essential for the heart function. Vitamin C enables the body to store folic acid which prevents anaemia. Lack of vitamin C may lead to hardening of the arteries and easy bruising.

VITAMIN E

Vitamin E assists in supplying the red blood cells with pure oxygen. It plays an essential role in cellular respiration of all muscles, especially the heart. Vitamin E prevents coagulation of the blood by preventing blood clots from forming. It strengthens the capillary walls, protects the red blood cells and improves blood circulation.

A deficiency of vitamin E may lead to anaemia, arteriosclerosis, hypertension, easy bruising and varicose veins. Vitamin E improves blood circulation by enlarging blood vessels which provides oxygen and nourishment to all body cells.

POTASSIUM

Potassium combines with iron to utilise oxygen in the body and is essential to keep the heart in a healthy condition. It strengthens the heart muscle and assists in purifying the blood via the kidneys. Potassium works with sodium to help normalise the heartbeat. Deficiency may lead to a slow and irregular heartbeat.

IODINE

Iodine makes thyroxine (the thyroid hormone which regulates cholesterol levels) and assists the body to burn up excess fat. A deficiency may lead to irregular heartbeat, hardening of the arteries, or rapid pulse and palpitations.

COBALT

Cobalt is an integral part of vitamin B12 and is necessary for normal functioning and maintenance of red blood cells. Deficiency of cobalt may be responsible for pernicious anaemia.

COPPER

Copper is involved in the production of haemoglobin (the portion of the red blood cells that carries the oxygen). It is also an important anti-oxidant.

CALCIUM

Calcium functions most effectively when combined with magnesium, phosphorus, and vitamins A, C and D. It is essential for healthy blood and it regulates the heartbeat. Calcium is required for the smooth functioning of the heart muscles.

Deficiency may lead to irregular heartbeat, palpitations, increased cholesterol levels, slow pulse rates and varicose veins.

MAGNESIUM

Magnesium deficiency may lead to irregular heart rhythm, coronary heart disease, blood clots in the heart, heart failure and damage to the small arteries.

FOLIC ACID

Folic acid assists in the proper growth and replication of red blood cells in the bone marrow. It is required for the absorption of iron and calcium, and for the prevention of blood disorders, anaemia, arteriosclerosis, and leukaemia.

INOSITOL

Inositol assists the action of the heart by cleansing the blood of excessive fats. It is needed for the growth and survival of cells in the bone marrow. Deficiency may lead to an elevated cholesterol level.

Herbal treatment

Use the following herbs as teas, tablets or tinctures. For more information on how to use these herbs see pages xiii–xv.

TONICS FOR CARDIAC SUPPORT

These are herbs which directly affect the heart function; either by affecting the heart's rhythm or strength of contraction. Heart tonics include the herbs:

- Broom;
- Bugleweed;
- Figwort;
- Ginseng;
- Hawthorn;
- Lily of the Valley;
- Motherwort.

NERVINES OR SEDATIVES

These herbs are useful when stress or anxiety are factors in heart problems.

- Balm
- Chamomile
- Hops
- Lime Blossom
- Motherwort
- Skullcap
- Valerian
- Wood Betony

STIMULANTS

- Black Pepper
- Cayenne pepper
- Chilli
- Cinnamon
- Garlic
- Ginger

- Ginko Biloba
- Horseradish
- Licorice Root
- Nettle
- Rosehips

Aromatherapy treatment

The following essential oils are very beneficial for the circulatory system.

- Black Pepper is a stimulating herb for circulation. Use as a body oil or burn in an oil burner.
- Cinnamon stimulates the heart and helps digestion. Use as a body oil or in an oil burner.
- Cypress is good for circulatory problems, varicose veins, aching legs and swollen ankles. Use as a bath or body oil or in an oil burner. It can also be used locally as a compress. (Aviod cypress if you have high blood pressure.)
- Garlic is used for heart disease, high cholesterol or high blood pressure. Use as a compress.
- Geranium improves the circulation and is used for tired and aching limbs. Use as a body or bath oil, burn in an oil burner or use as a compress.
- Hyssop helps regulate high or low blood pressure. Use as a bath or body oil, burn in the oil burner or use as a compress.
- Lemon aids circulation. Use as a bath or body oil.
- Neroli aids circulation and is used to treat palpitations. Use as a bath or body oil.

- Thyme is a good general tonic which aids circulation and the immune system. Use as a bath or body oil.

Dietary and lifestyle recommendations

FOODS
The following foods are all beneficial to the circulatory system.

- alfalfa sprouts
- apricots
- avocados
- bananas
- beetroot
- berries
- brewer's yeast
- buckwheat
- carrots
- cauliflowers
- celery
- chives
- cucumber
- currants
- dates
- figs
- garlic
- grapes
- leeks
- lemons
- lettuce
- onions
- papaya
- parsley
- peaches
- peas
- pineapples
- plums
- potatoes
- radish
- spinach
- sundried olives
- watercress
- wheatgerm

JUICES
Try to drink at least one of these juices daily.

- lettuce, carrot and parsley
- blackberry and parsley
- grape juice
- hawthorn berry tea
- beetroot juice
- spinach juice
- parsley juice (mix a handful in other juices)

- carrot and celery juice
- tomato and parsley juice
- prune juice
- orange juice
- strawberry, orange and pineapple juice

ANAEMIA

Description

Anaemia is a disorder in which the amount of haemoglobin in the blood is reduced. The red blood cells become fewer and paler. Due to a lack of haemoglobin they contain less oxygen than normal cells.

Symptoms

This lowering of oxygen to all body cells causes a decrease in energy levels resulting in symptoms such as fatigue, general weakness, breathlessness, pale lips, eyelid linings and skin, headaches, brittle nails, sore tongue, chronic diarrhoea or malabsorption and poor immunity.

Causes

The most common cause of anaemia is iron deficiency, or too little iron in the blood. The problem may also lie in the impaired absorption of nutrients necessary for the health and proper function of the blood cells. Blood loss due to haemorrhage or heavy periods often results in iron deficiency. The overuse of anti-inflammatory medica-tions such as aspirin may also cause internal bleeding. This excessive use of aspirin is more common in elderly patients. It is important to confirm the diagnosis of anaemia with a blood test so the underlying cause can be uncovered.

Nutritional treatment

Nutritional supplements that may be beneficial in the treatment of anaemia are included in the following table. See pages xii–xiii for information on how to use these supplements.

Herbal treatment

For information on how to use the following herbs see pages xiii–xv.

DIGESTIVES

Herbs used to aid digestion and stimulate the body's natural processes are:

- Condurango;
- Gentian;
- Wormwood.

DEMULCENTS

Malabsorption is a common condition amongst anaemia suffers. It occurs when the small intestine is unable to absorb food or specific minerals.

Herbs that soothe and heal the lining of the intestine are called demulcents. These include:

- Comfrey Root;
- Marshmellow Root;
- Slippery Elm.

Nutritional supplements for anaemia

SUPPLEMENT	DOSAGE	COMMENT
Vitamin B12	2000 mcg three times daily	Essential in the production of red blood cells
Vitamin B6	100 mg daily	Aids cellular reproduction and helps absorption of vitamin B12
Vitamin C	3000–10,000 mg daily	Important for iron absorption
Vitamin E	600 iu daily	Prolongs the life span of red blood cells
Folic acid plus biotin	800 mcg twice daily	Needed for red blood cell information
Iron	As prescribed by a physician	To restore iron (use ferrous gluconate)
Zinc	30 mg daily (do not exceed this amount)	Zinc and copper work together in the production of red blood cells
Copper	2 mg daily	
Brewer's yeast	As directed on label	Rich in nutrients and is a good source of Vitamin B

ANTI-INFLAMMATORY HERBS

Anti-inflammatory herbs can also be used, such as:

- Meadowsweet;
- Wild Yam.

ASTRINGENTS

Astringents include:

- Agrimony;
- Bayberry.

CALMATIVES

Calmatives can also be used, such as:

- Cardamom;
- Chamomile;
- Hops.

Homeopathic treatment

Treatment that may be prescribed by a homeopath for anaemia varies according to the symptoms. Use:

- China officinalis for anaemia that is accompanied by loss of appetite, pasty face and loss of body fluids;
- Ferrum metallicum for pale face, breathlessness and exhaustion;
- Calcarea carbanica for exhaustion, breathlessness and dizziness;
- Calcarea phosphoric for post childbirth anaemia, headache and heavy periods;
- Kali carbonicum if you are weak, tired, chilly, anxious or fearful.

See page xv for information on how to use these treatments.

Aromatherapy treatment

Use the following essential oils as bath or body oils.

- Benzoin is a warming, energising oil that aids circulation.
- Chamomile is soothing, calming and relaxing.
- Lemon is an appetite stimulant, eases indigestion, is uplifting and aids circulation.
- Ginger is a good general tonic.
- Thyme assists circulation and the immune system.

See page xvi for information on how to use these oils.

Dietary and lifestyle recommendations

- Avoid tea and coffee. They contain chemicals that block iron absorption.
- Avoid calcium supplements when taking iron.
- Take an iron supplement, preferably one that contains ferrous gluconate.
- Citrus juice taken with iron supplements helps absorption.
- The acid contained in spinach makes the iron difficult to absorb.
- Get plenty of rest until your iron levels increase and you have more energy.

- Have a complete blood test to determine if you have an iron deficiency before taking iron supplements. Excess iron can cause damage to the liver, heart and immune cell activity. Use iron supplements only under supervision from your doctor.

VEGETARIANS AND VEGANS

It is important to eat a well-balanced diet containing foods high in iron. These include lean meat, poultry, fish, cereals, vegetables and fruit. Vegetarians and vegans are more likely to suffer from iron deficiency anaemia than those who eat a diet consisting of animal products. It is therefore important for these individuals to make sure they are getting enough iron from other foods such as:

- beetroot;
- chick peas;
- dandelion;
- dates;
- fresh fruit and vegetables;
- lentils;
- lima beans;
- parsley;
- sesame seeds;
- soybeans;
- wheatgerm.

ANGINA PECTORIS

Description and symptoms

Angina is characterised by pressure-like pain in the chest area that can be felt after physical exertion. Stress, anxiety and high blood pressure usually go hand in hand with angina. The pain may radiate to the neck and jaw, into the shoulder-blades and down the arms, usually lasting about 20 minutes.

Causes

The most common cause of angina pectoris is an insufficient blood supply to the heart muscle, usually resulting from atherosclerosis. Atherosclerosis is a build-up of fatty deposits in the lining of the arteries. This accumulation of fat and cholesterol in the blood is known as atheroma or plaque. The plaque thickens the arterial walls, impeding the blood flow to the heart and therefore depriving the heart of sufficient oxygen. This results in tight pain in the chest area called angina pectoris. Other causes of angina can be hyperthyroidism and severe anaemia.

Nutritional treatment

Nutritional supplements that may be beneficial in the treatment of angina are included in the following table. See pages xii–xiii for information on how to use these supplements.

Herbal treatment

The following herbs must only be used under qualified supervision from your natural health practitioner. See page xiii–xv for information on how to use them.

- Lily of the Valley aids the body where there is difficulty breathing due to congestive heart conditions.
- Hawthorn berries are a tonic for the circulatory system and primarily used in the treatment of high blood pressure, atherosclerosis and angina pectoris.
- Motherwort can be used in all heart conditions that are associated with anxiety and tension.

Homeopathic treatment

Treatment that may be prescribed by a homeopath for angina varies according to the symptoms. Use:

- Aconitum napellus for rapid heart rate, pain in left shoulder or pressure on heart;
- Apis mellifica for stinging, burning pain anywhere in body including the heart. Swelling of lower limbs and shortness of breath;
- Arnica for irregular heartbeat or a feeling of the heart being squeezed.

See page xv for information in how to use homeopathics.

Nutritional supplements for angina pectoris

SUPPLEMENT	DOSAGE	COMMENT
Coenzyme Q10	50–100 mg three times daily	Improves cardiac function
Vitamin A	25,000 iu daily	Enhances immunity, protects cells and slows down ageing
Vitamin B complex	100 mg three times daily	Lowers cholesterol and improves circulation
Vitamin C powder	Two–three teaspoons daily	Strengthens veins and arteries
Vitamin E (use this supplement only under supervision from your physician)	200 iu increased slowly by 100 iu weekly until daily dosage is 800–1000 iu	Strengthens immune system and destroys free radicals
Lecithin	One tablespoon with meals	Helps break down cholesterol and fats in the blood
Calcium and Magnesium	1500 mg daily 750 mg daily	Important for the proper function of the cardiac muscle
Acidophilus fibre	One dessertspoon daily	Lowers cholesterol
Copper chelate	3 mg daily	Deficiency may be linked to heart problems
Zinc chelate	50 mg daily	Aids healing

Aromatherapy treatment

The following essential oils may provide relief from the symptoms of angina.

- Black Pepper is good for blood circulation. Use as a body oil or burn in an oil burner.
- Garlic will help high cholesterol and heart disease. Use as a compress over the chest area.
- Cinnamon stimulates the heart and may be either used in an oil burner or as a body oil.
- Neroli aids circulation and is used to treat palpitations. Use in the bath or as a massage oil.

See page xvi for information on how to use these essential oils.

Dietary and lifestyle recommendations

- Reduce total dietary fat intake. Increase your consumption of fish oils or polyunsaturated oils such as Linseed, Sunflower or Wheatgerm oil.

- Avoid tea, coffee, sugar, alcohol, tobacco, butter, red meat, processed and refined foods.
- Reduce your salt intake.
- Eat more garlic, ginger, onions and lecithin, as they all help reduce cholesterol.
- Exercise regularly. This may include 40 minutes of aerobic exercise three times per week. Yoga and meditation are also highly recommended to build strength and reduce stress and anxiety.
- Avoid constipation by eating a diet high in fibre.
- Drink plenty of filtered water. Avoid soft drinks.

ARTERIOSCLEROSIS and ATHEROSCLEROSIS

Description, symptoms and causes

Atherosclerosis (hardening of the arteries) is a degenerative condition of the arteries, characterised by an accumulation of fats (mainly cholesterol) within the artery. Cholesterol forms plaques which gradually increase in size and begin to narrow the passageways of the arteries. Although any artery may be affected, the most commonly affected arteries are: the aorta, and the coronary and cerebral vascular systems which supply blood to the heart and brain.

Degeneration of the arteries in the body, making them hard and inelastic, is arteriosclerosis, or hardening of the arteries. Atherosclerosis causes high blood pressure and can ultimately lead to angina, heart attack, stroke and sudden cardiac death. Although arteriosclerosis causes high blood pressure, high blood pressure can also cause arteriosclerosis. Fatty plaques usually form in parts of the arteries that have been weakened or over-stretched by high blood pressure. This narrows the arteries.

The narrowing of the arteries increases the blood pressure even further. If an artery becomes hardened, it is less able to cope with pressure changes within the blood stream and more likely to rupture, causing a leak of blood. If the leak occurs into vital organs such as the brain, it may lead to a stroke. If the tiny arteries which supply blood to the heart muscle are involved, angina occurs. Peripheral atherosclerosis affects the blood flow to the leg and foot, causing numbness, weakness and heavy feeling in the legs.

Arteriosclerosis and atherosclerosis can be caused by hypertension, diabetes, smoking, a family history of the disease or high cholesterol levels.

Most important in the treatment of atherosclerosis and arteriosclerosis is the reduction of blood cholesterol levels. Dietary and lifestyle modifications (especially in relation to stress) are the only really effective preventative (or curative for less severe cases) treatment.

Nutritional treatment

Nutritional supplements that are beneficial in the treatment of arteriosclerosis and atherosclerosis are included in the following table (see pages 140–41). See pages xii–xiii for information on how to use these supplements.

Herbal treatment

Herbs that are of benefit in the treatment of atherosclerosis and arteriosclerosis include:

- Cayenne;
- Chickweed;
- Fenugreek;
- Ginko Biloba;
- Hawthorn Berries;
- Lime Blossom;
- Mistletoe;
- Yarrow.

TINCTURES AND TEAS
- Lime Blossom has a specific action against the aggregation of cholesterol plaques. Take 1–2 ml of the tincture three times a day or three cups of the tea daily.
- Hawthorn Berries are one of the best cardiac tonics which also improve the circulation. They are used to treat high blood pressure, angina and arteriosclerosis. For high blood pressure combine Hawthorn Berries with Lime Blossom, Mistletoe and Yarrow. Take 2–4 ml of the tincture three times daily or three cups of the tea daily.

- Ginko Biloba can be taken as a tea, tincture or tablet to protect the arteries.

See pages xiii–xv for information on how to use these herbs.

Homeopathic treatment

Treatment that may be prescribed by a homeopath for atherosclerosis and arteriosclerosis includes:

- Argentum nitricum for high blood pressure, nervous strain due to overwork and worry about the future;
- Carbo vegetabilis for poor circulation;
- Crataegus as a heart tonic.

See page xv for information on how to use homeopathics.

Aromatherapy treatment

The following essential oils may provide relief from atherosclerosis and arteriosclerosis. See page xvi for information on how to use these oils.

- Ylang Ylang is a sedative and nervine oil. It regulates the heart and has a balancing effect on high blood pressure. Use as a body or bath oil or burn in an oil burner.
- Cypress improves blood circulation, especially to arms and legs. (Avoid use if you have high blood pressure.) Use as a bath or body oil, compress or burn in an oil burner.

- Juniper is an nervine oil which also improves circulation. Use as a bath or body oil or compress.
- Hyssop is a mild sedative and nerve tonic. It helps regulate blood pressure, either high or low. Use as bath or body oil, compress or burn in an oil burner.

Dietary and lifestyle recommendations

- Garlic, onions and ginger counteract plaque formation, and lower total serum cholesterol levels and triglycerides. Ginger has an even stronger effect than garlic and onions.
- Alfalfa sprouts decrease LDL (low density lipoproteins i.e. 'bad' cholesterol).

Nutritional supplements for arteriosclerosis and atherosclerosis

SUPPLEMENT	DOSAGE	COMMENT
Vitamin B3	100 mg three times daily	Lowers blood cholesterol and metabolises fats. Increases the 'good' cholesterol (HDL)
Vitamin B6	50 mg daily	Decreases the blood levels of triglycerides and cholesterol
Vitamin B complex	100 mg three times daily	May improve the ratio of unsaturated to saturated fatty acids in the blood
Vitamin C with bioflavonoids	1 g three times daily	Helps breakdown triglycerides and strengthens the arterial walls. Lowers total cholesterol and lipids, and increases 'good' cholesterol (HDL)
Vitamin E	600 iu three times daily	Reduces plaque formation and increases 'good' cholesterol (HDL)
Folic acid	5 mg daily	Reduces homocysteine and therefore helps prevent atherosclerosis
Calcium	1500 mg daily, at bedtime	Decreases total fats and inhibits plaque formation
Magnesium	750 mg daily, at bedtime	May be deficient in atherosclerosis
Selenium	200 mcg daily	May prevent plaque formation. Assists the function of vitamin E

Nutritional supplements for arteriosclerosis and atherosclerosis

SUPPLEMENT	DOSAGE	COMMENT
Selenium	*200 mcg daily*	*May prevent plaque formation. Assists the function of vitamin E*
Potassium orotate	*600 mg daily equiv. to 120 mg of potassium*	*May prevent plaque formation*
Zinc chelate	*50 mg daily*	*Promotes 'good' cholesterol (HDL). Aids in cleansing the blood and healing arteries*
Coenzyme Q10	*100 mg daily*	*Improves cardiac function, prevents angina and improves tissue oxygenation*
Omega 3 and 6 fatty acids (Max EPA) *Omega 3 (linseed, salmon, cod liver and mackerel oils)* *Omega 6 (safflower, corn, sunflower and peanut oils)*	*5–10 g daily or as directed on the label*	*Lowers cholesterol levels and prevents plaque formation. Also reduces blood pressure*

- Taking 20 mg of brewer's yeast daily lowers LDLs and increases HDLs.
- Lecithin increases the solubility of cholesterol and thereby decreases the possibility of plaque formation. Take one–three teaspoons of lecithin granules daily.
- Take three cups of low-fat yoghurt daily as it reduces total cholesterol levels.
- Reduce your dietary intake of animal fats (such as butter) and hydrogenated vegetable oils (such as margarine). Avoid fried foods, gravies, pies, fast foods, red meat, sweets, cakes, ice-cream, salt, and all foods containing white flour and white sugar.
- Avoid stimulants such as coffee, tobacco and colas.
- Eliminate alcohol and highly spicy foods. Don't use decaffeinated coffee as it raises cholesterol.
- Eat more raw fruits and vegetables and wholegrain cereals to increase dietary fibre.
- Increase intake of fish oils or polyunsaturated oils such as Linseed, Sunflower oil and Wheatgerm oil.
- Eat plenty of dark green, leafy vegetables, legumes, nuts, seeds, soybeans and wheat germ as these are high in vitamin E.
- Reduce or stop smoking as this is a potent risk factor for atherosclerosis.

- Eat more cherries, blueberries and raspberries.
- Take one teaspoon of organic apple cider vinegar in water with meals.
- Reduce your exposure to stressful situations and learn a stress management technique or breathing skill such as: yoga, tai chi, relaxation or meditation.
- Get regular daily exercise of moderate intensity, e.g. walking or swimming.

CHOLESTEROL

To lower cholesterol increase your intake of the following foods:

- apples or grapefruit (as pectin lowers cholesterol);
- carrots (for their pectin and their affect on maintaining healthy arteries);
- grapes or grape juice;
- kidney beans;
- lima beans;
- navy beans;
- soybeans and other legumes.

See also information on high cholesterol on pages 151–54.

HARDENED ARTERIES

Foods which benefit hardened arteries include:

- avocado;
- bananas;
- beetroot;
- carrot;
- celery;
- grapes;
- lemons;

- lettuce;
- oranges;
- olives;
- parsley;
- potatoes;
- radish;
- spinach.

BRUISING

Description

A bruise occurs due to the rupturing of tiny blood vessels (called capillaries) beneath the skin. Blood leaks out of the broken capillaries and collects under the skin. See also information on bruising on pages 279–82.

Symptoms

The symptoms of bruising include: blotchy, superficial discolouration, swelling, pain and black and blue marks. The skin starts out red and inflamed, then becomes dark and bluish in colour, and finally it turns yellowish as the tissues are repaired and the blood is reabsorbed.

Causes

Bruising is caused by injuries, weakened blood vessels and blood cell abnormalities. But there are several other predisposing factors which may cause easy bruising: a diet low in fresh raw foods, anaemia, obesity, menstruation, heavy nicotine intake, vitamin C deficiency, zinc and bioflavonoid deficiencies and haemophilia.

If easy bruising cannot be definitely linked with one of the predisposing factors then it may indicate the presence of cancer.

Nutritional treatment

Nutritional supplements that may be beneficial in the treatment of bruising are included in the following table. See pages xii–xiii for information on how to use these supplements.

Herbal treatment

EXTERNAL TREATMENTS
External treatments include:

- Cold Witch Hazel tincture.
- Comfrey, Calendula, Cypress (avoid if you have high blood pressure).

Nutritional supplements for bruising

SUPPLEMENT	DOSAGE	COMMENT
Vitamin C with bioflavonoids	3000–10,000 mg throughout the day	Strengthens the capillaries to prevent easy bruising
Vitamin B complex	100 mg three times daily	Anti-oxidant which is important for healing and tissue repair
Vitamin E	500 iu twice daily	Anti-oxidant needed for tissue repair and blood circulation
Vitamin A	10,000 iu twice daily	Anti-oxidant which enhances the adhesion between cells
Zinc	75 mg daily in lozenge form	Strengthens capillaries and is also necessary for tissue repair
Calcium and Magnesium (chelated form)	750–1000 mg daily 400–500 mg daily	Important for blood clotting and regulation of blood vessels as well as healing
Coenzyme Q10	As directed on label	Important for tissue repair
Iron	As directed on label	Especially for anaemia
Alfalfa (vitamin K)	As directed on label	Important for tissue repair and blood clotting
Selenium	200–500 mcg daily	Anti-oxidant and assists vitamin E

- Arnica (never use on broken skin) or Yarrow can be used as an ointment, tincture or compress.
- Bruised cabbage leaves also make an effective compress.

INTERNAL TREATMENTS
Internal treatments include:

- Horsechestnut, Yarrow, Horsetail or Rosehip tea can be drunk as a preventative measure if prone to easy bruising;
- Dandelion and Yellow Dock teas can be taken as an additional source of iron.

See pages xiii–xv for information on how to use herbs.

Homeopathic treatment

Treatment that may be prescribed by a homeopath for bruising includes:

- Arnica for black eyes, painful bruising, swelling or traumatic injuries;
- Bellis perennis for black eyes, painful bruising, bumps and lumps remaining, and bruising from over-exertion or traumatic injury;
- Ledum for black eyes, skin discolouration and bruising from traumatic injuries;
- Sulphuric acid for bluish-black discolouration, and slow-healing bruises;
- Use Arnica, Rescue Remedy, Hamamelis and Ruta as external homeopathic treatment on broken skin.

See page xv for information on how to use these homeopathics.

Aromatherapy treatment

The following essential oils can be used as a bath or body oils or as a compress for relief from bruising.

- Cypress (avoid if you have high blood pressure)
- Hyssop
- Lavender
- Sweet Marjoram

See page xvi for information on how to use these essential oils.

Dietary and lifestyle recommendations

VITAMIN C
Eat a diet high in vitamin C and bio-flavonoids. Include such foods as:

- broccoli;
- buckwheat;
- capsicum;
- citrus fruits;
- dark green leafy vegetables.

ZINC
For their zinc content include the following foods in your diet:

- asparagus;
- brewer's yeast;
- garlic;
- lentils;
- lettuce;
- millet;
- nuts;
- olives;

- onions;
- pumpkin seeds;
- rice;
- soy beans;
- wholegrains.

CHILL THERAPY

Apply an ice pack (or pack of frozen vegetables) wrapped in a towel to the affected area for 15 minutes, then leave for ten minutes before reapplying the ice pack. Continue this chill therapy during the first 24 hours after the bruising, then use warm packs to dispense the blood. Wrap a compress to the affected area and elevate it if possible to decrease blood flow to the area.

IT'S IMPORTANT TO CONSULT YOUR DOCTOR IF:

- Bruising is frequent as this could indicate cancer.

CIRCULATORY PROBLEMS

Description and symptoms

Circulatory problems include thrombosis and thrombophlebitis.

A thrombus develops when blood clots within a vein or an artery. The thrombus can partially or completely block the blood vessel causing a deficiency of oxygen and nutrients downstream from the blocked vessel. The thrombus may even begin to break up and travel through the large veins to the heart and the lungs and may block blood supply to these organs. If the thrombus blocks blood flowing to the heart a heart attack can result; if it blocks blood flowing to the brain a stroke occurs. For more details on thrombosis see atherosclerosis (pages 138–42) and high cholesterol (pages 151–54). A deep venous thrombus in one of the veins of the thigh or lower leg muscles is another serious form of thrombosis. Blockage of superficial veins of the legs causes varicose veins (see pages 164–66).

The symptoms of deep venous thrombosis include constant or cramping pain and tightness in the calf even after a short walk.

Phlebitis refers to inflammation of a vein. This problem is usually associated with the formation of a thrombus and mostly occurs in the extremities, especially the legs. When both a thrombus and inflammation of the veins occur together the condition is called thrombophlebitis. The inflammation of the vein causes symptoms such as swelling, redness and a feeling of hardness and soreness to the touch. This can result in chronic venous insufficiency (weakness of the veins) with swelling, discolouration, increased pigmentation, dermatitis and ulceration of the leg.

Causes

The causes of superficial and deeper thrombosis may be poor circulation, physical trauma, prolonged periods of standing, cholesterol deposits (athero-sclerosis), cancer, operations, lack of exercise, infection or intravenous drug use. Diabetes, pregnancy, varicose veins, being overweight and smoking can also increase the likelihood of blood clotting. Clotting may be due to blood platelet adhesion or aggregation as well as red blood cell aggregation.

Nutritional treatment

Nutritional supplements that may be beneficial in the treatment of circulatory problems are included in the following table. See pages xii–xiii for information on how to use these supplements.

Herbal treatment

For information on how to use the following herbs see pages xiii–xv.

LOCAL INFLAMMATION
For local inflammation and pain use the following herbs, applied externally, as a tincture or compress:

- Arnica;
- Comfrey;
- Golden Seal (only use internally for one to two weeks and don't use if pregnant);
- Marigold;
- Hawthorn berries;
- Witch Hazel.

CIRCULATION
To improve circulation use the following herbs taken internally, as a tea or tincture:

- Angelica;
- Bayberry;
- Chamomile;
- Dandelion;
- Ginko Biloba;
- Nettle;
- Prickly Ash;
- Wild Yam.

HERBAL COMBINATIONS
- A combination of Prickly Ash, Ginger and Hawthorn berries is also very useful.
- Also try a combination of the following kitchen herbs and spices: cayenne, ginger, horseradish and mustard.
- Ginger, Skullcap and Valerian aid the circulation by dilating the blood vessels.

Homeopathic treatment

THROMBOSIS
Treatment that may be prescribed by a homeopath for thrombosis includes:

- Vipera for inflammation of the veins causing a bursting sensation. This is also relieved by elevating the affected limb.
- Bothrops lanciolatus for symptoms mainly on the right side. Used also in the treatment of paralysis caused by stroke.

THROMBOPHLEBITIS
- Arnica for use where thrombophlebitis has followed an injury involving the affected vein.

- Pulsatilla used to treat a person who suffers from varicose veins in which thromophlebitis is common.

Aromatherapy treatment

The following essential oils may provide relief from circulatory problems. See page xvi for information on how to use these oils.

- Black Pepper – use as a bath oil or inhalant.
- Clary Sage – use as a bath oil or body oil.
- Cypress – use as an inhalation, bath oil, body oil or compress (avoid if you have high blood pressure).

- Ylang Ylang – use as a bath oil or body oil.

Dietary and lifestyle recommendations

Exercise is very important. The most helpful form of exercise is walking as it improves the blood flow to the legs and the venous return of blood from the legs. An hour of walking each day may bring on some of the symptoms of thrombosis but will ultimately improve your circulation.

- Eat low-fat foods.
- Avoid red meat, full fat dairy products and salty or fried foods.

Nutritional supplements for circulatory problems

SUPPLEMENT	DOSAGE	COMMENT
Vitamin B3	100 mg three times daily	Lowers blood cholesterol and metabolises fats
Vitamin B6	50 mg daily	Improves oxygenation of tissues and metabolises fats
Vitamin C with bioflavonoids	5000–8000 mg daily in divided doses	Improves circulation and prevents the tendency to clot
Vitamin E	100 iu daily for one week, then increase to 400 iu daily	Can dissolve existing clots, improve circulation and prevent clots from spreading
Coenzyme Q10	100 mg daily	Improves venous circulation to prevent clotting
Calcium and Magnesium	1000 mg daily 1,000 mg daily	These minerals work together to prevent and reduce clotting
Zinc	50 mg daily	Important mineral for tissue healing

Nutritional supplements for circulatory problems

SUPPLEMENT	DOSAGE	COMMENT
Garlic	As directed on label	Prevents infection, improves circulation and reduces clotting
Lecithin granules	One tablespoon three times daily before meals	Powerful fat-dissolving agent which breaks down cholesterol
Essential fatty acids • Flaxseed oil or • Evening Primrose oil or • Linseed oil	Three teaspoons daily	Essential fatty acids improve circulation and prevent clotting

- Eat cold water fish like salmon, herring and mackerel, tuna and sardines.
- Quit smoking and reduce your alcohol intake as these habits can constrict your blood vessels.
- Lay down with your feet and legs elevated for 30 minutes each day.
- Avoid wearing tight-fitting clothes or socks that prevent your blood from returning to the heart and then circulating down to the toes and feet.

HAEMORRHOIDS

Description

Haemorrhoids (also known as piles) are ruptured or swollen veins located around the rectum that may also extend out of the anus. They are sometimes described as varicose veins in the rectum. Haemorrhoids may appear as an intermittent, painless swelling around the anus or in more severe cases they may be extremely tender and painful and bleed frequently.

Symptoms

The most common symptoms of haemorrhoids include itching, pain, inflammation, swelling and bleeding. Once a haemorrhoid has been experienced a weakness will be present in the veins involved and even after one attack has been resolved it may flare up from time to time. Bleeding haemorrhoids can produce severe anaemia due to blood loss.

Causes

Haemorrhoids can be caused by:

- a genetic weakness of the veins around the rectum and anus;
- prolonged periods of standing or sitting or lifting heavy objects;
- pregnancy;
- constipation;
- a low fibre diet;
- straining during defaecation;
- obesity, lack of exercise, poor tone of the abdominal muscles.

Nutritional treatment

Nutritional supplements that may be beneficial in the treatment of haemorrhoids are included in the following table. See pages xii–xiii for information on how to use these supplements.

Herbal treatment

EXTERNAL APPLICATIONS
- Insert a peeled clove of garlic into the rectum before going to bed (this may sting a little a first).
- Apply a potato wedge directly to the affected area to reduce the swelling.
- Try Witch Hazel, Calendula, Pilewort, Golden Seal and St John's Wort ointments.

INTERNAL APPLICATIONS
Take the following herbs internally as a tea or tincture.

- Butcher's Broom

- Gotu Kola
- Horsechestnut
- Nettle
- Pilewort
- Self-Heal
- Slippery Elm (use powder or tablets)

CONSTIPATION
For constipation take:

- Barberry;
- Dandelion Root;
- Golden Seal (only use internally for one–two weeks and don't use if pregnant);
- Rhubarb Root;
- Senna Pods;
- Yellow Dock.

See pages xiii–xv for information on how to use these herbs.

Homeopathic treatment

Treatment that may be prescribed by a homeopath for haemorrhoids includes:

- Hamamelis or Nitric acidum for bleeding piles;
- Hamamelis, Nitric acidum or Kali carbonicum for large piles;
- Nitric acidum for piles with a burning pain;
- Hamamelis for piles which feel sore and bruised;
- Nitric acidum for piles which are worse after a bowel movement;
- Hamamelis or Nux vomica for piles caused by pregnancy;
- Hamamelis or Kali carbonicum for piles caused by childbirth.

Nutritional supplements for haemorrhoids

SUPPLEMENT	DOSAGE	COMMENT
Vitamin E	200–600 iu daily or as a suppository or ointment	Prevents and dissolves blood clots. Suppositories can lubricate the area and reduce pain
Vitamin C with bioflavonoids	1000–3000 mg daily	Improves strength of veins and assists normal healing and clotting of blood
Vitamin A	10,000 iu daily	Strengthens and heals the walls of blood vessels
Vitamin B complex	100 mg daily	Assists the digestive process and takes pressure off the rectum
Zinc	15–30 mg daily	Improves the strength of blood vessel walls
Calcium chelate and Magnesium	1000 mg daily 500–750 mg daily	Important minerals for normal blood clotting
Psyllium husks or guar gum	As directed on label	Bulking compounds which reduce straining with bowel movements

See page xv for information on how to use homeopathics.

Aromatherapy treatment

The following essential oils may bring relief from haemorrhoids.

- Cypress oil and Myrrh oil are specifically useful for haemorrhoids. Cypress oil can be used as a bath or body oil, burnt in an oil burner or used as a compress on the affected area (don't use if you have high blood pressure). Myrrh oil can be burnt in an oil burner or used as a body oil.

- Frankincense and Juniper oils can also be helpful for haemorrhoids. Juniper can be used as a compress and Frankincense as a bath or body oil or burnt in an oil burner.

See page xvi for information on how to use essential oils.

Dietary and lifestyle recommendations

- Avoid fats and red meats as these are especially hard to process by the lower digestive tract.
- Tune in to your digestive and eliminative processes, especially

20 to 30 minutes after breakfast and dinner, when there is a reflex between the stomach and the bowel.

- Don't delay going to the toilet when nature calls. On the other hand, don't sit on the toilet for long periods of time as this can also create strain on the bowel. Avoid using perfumed or coloured toilet paper as the chemicals in these products can create irritation.
- Regular, moderate exercise helps to move food through the bowels more quickly and efficiently. Include walking, jogging, cycling or swimming for 20 to 30 minutes three times a week into your routine. Deep breathing also promotes the movement of food through your intestines.
- Keep your fluid intake up to around six to eight glasses a day (mostly water).
- A warm Sitz bath (i.e. partial immersion of the pelvic region including anus and buttocks) can alleviate the discomfort.

HIGH-FIBRE DIET

A diet that is high in fibre is recommended. Your diet should include:

- beans;
- blackberries;
- bran;
- cereals;
- cherries;
- corn;
- fruits (apples, pears);
- nuts;
- oats;
- rice;
- rye;
- vegetables (especially beets, broccoli, cabbage, green beans);
- wheat.

IT'S IMPORTANT TO SEE YOUR DOCTOR IF:

- There is a change in your bowel movements or if the haemorrhoids persist as there may be some other cause for the bleeding, e.g. colon cancer, anal fissures or intestinal polyps.

HIGH CHOLESTEROL

Description

Research has consistently shown that elevated levels of cholesterol are associated with heart disease and strokes. But all cholesterol is not necessarily hazardous to our health. The human body needs cholesterol to protect nerves and to build new cells and hormones. Serum cholesterol is the amount of cholesterol in your bloodstream, and your serum cholesterol is made up of:

- LDL (low density lipoprotein), which is the 'bad' cholesterol that clogs your arteries and carries cholesterol to the body tissues;
- HDL (high density lipoprotein), which is the 'good' cholesterol that cleans the artery walls and

transports the cholesterol to the liver for metabolism and excretion.

The human body can produce all the cholesterol it needs, in fact, all body cells produce cholesterol but the liver and the intestines produce the majority of our healthy cholesterol. Cholesterol is needed to form sex hormones, adrenal hormones and bile salts. Problems start when we consume too much additional cholesterol through our diet in the form of animal fats and eggs. Fruit, vegetables, grains and fish are sources of the 'good' cholesterol which help to keep our arteries clean.

Symptoms

Elevated cholesterol levels (particularly LDL) lead to plaque-filled arteries which hinders the flow of blood to the heart, brain, limbs and kidneys. High cholesterol levels are also associated with high blood pressure, gallstones and impotence.

Causes

The causes of high cholesterol are:

- a high fat diet;
- faulty fat metabolism;
- an hereditary or genetic predisposition to the accumulation of LDL.

Dietary changes alone are thought to be able to lower the cholesterol level by 50–75 percent. Nutritional and herbal supplements have also proven to be beneficial.

Nutritional treatment

Nutritional supplements that may be beneficial in the treatment of high cholesterol are included in the following table. See pages xii–xiii for information on how to use these supplements.

Nutritional supplements for high cholesterol

SUPPLEMENT	DOSAGE	COMMENT
Vitamin C with bioflavonoids	2000–50,000 mg daily throughout the day	Has an important role in metabolism and regulates the arterial walls
Vitamin B complex	As directed on label	Vitamins B12 and B6 are important for fat metabolism. B1 and B3 lower cholesterol
Vitamin E	200–1000 iu daily	Controls the serum cholesterol level and aids circulation. Raises the level of 'good' cholesterol

Nutritional supplements for high cholesterol

SUPPLEMENT	DOSAGE	COMMENT
Essential Fatty Acids Omega 6 oils include: • *Safflower* • *Corn* • *Sunflower* • *Peanut* *Omega 3 oils include:* • *Linseed* • *Salmon* • *Cod Liver* • *Mackerel*	*One–three teaspoons per day*	*These fatty acids reduce LDL levels and increase HDL levels*
Coenzyme Q10	*60 mg daily*	*Reduces damage to the arteries and veins*
Calcium and Magnesium	*500 mg daily*	*Calcium reduces serum cholesterol levels. Magnesium deficiency produces spasm of the coronary arteries*
Chromium	*200 mcg daily*	*Regulates blood sugar and lowers cholesterol*
Selenium	*200 mcg daily*	*Deficiency is associated with increased risk of heart disease*
Zinc	*150 mg daily*	*Lowers serum cholesterol*
Lecithin	*One tablespoon three times daily before meals*	*Increases the solubility of cholesterol*

Herbal treatment

Take the following herbs as a tea or a tincture:

- Hawthorn berries;
- Lime Blossom;
- Golden Seal (only use internally for one–two weeks and don't use of pregnant).

See pages xiii–xv for information on using herbs.

Dietary and lifestyle recommendations

- Having smaller meals more frequently without increasing your overall caloric intake can be helpful in lowering cholesterol.

- Eat breakfast every morning, particularly fruit, juices, cereals or wholegrains, bran and low-fat yoghurt.
- Take moderate exercise and practice a relaxation, meditation, or breathing technique.

FOODS THAT LOWER CHOLESTEROL

Increase your intake of the following herbs, spices and foods:

- alfalfa leaves and sprouts (decrease cholesterol levels and 'shrinks' cholesterol plaques);
- berries;
- bran;
- cayenne (chilli);
- dietary fibre (brown rice, barley, bran, beans, oats, oat bran, and fruit);
- eat fish at least five times per week, especially sardines and salmon;
- eggplant;
- garlic;
- ginger;
- grapefruit;
- grapes;
- kidney beans;
- lima beans;
- olive oil;
- onions;
- soybeans;
- yoghurt.

FOODS TO AVOID

Meat, dairy products and eggs are the primary dietary sources of cholesterol. Avoid or severely minimise these foods. Also avoid alcohol, chocolate, cakes, lollies, coffee, gravies, fizzy drinks, white bread, tea and refined or processed foods.

HYPERTENSION

Description

Hypertension is characterised by an abnormal elevation of blood pressure.

Blood pressure is the excessive force exerted by the blood against the walls of the blood vessels. Our blood pressure rises temporarily during exercise or emotional stress, however after relaxation our blood pressure will return to normal. Hypertension is when blood pressure does not return to normal but remains elevated.

About 90 percent of hypertension arises for no apparent reason and has been labelled 'essential or primary hypertension'. The other ten percent is called secondary hypertension and is associated with arteriosclerosis, high cholesterol and kidney disease.

Symptoms

Symptoms of hypertension include headaches, dizziness, fatigue, palpitations, shortness of breath, vision disturbances, anxiety and fluid retention.

Causes

Secondary hypertension can be associated with disorders such as arteriosclerosis, elevated blood cholesterol levels, diabetes mellitus, kidney disease and cardiovascular disease.

Essential hypertension can be attributed to caffeine consumption, alcohol intake, smoking, exposure to heavy metals such as lead, obesity, stress and anxiety, lack of exercise, poor eating habits and a high intake of fats and salt.

Hypertension can predispose the patient to coronary artery disease and stroke if left untreated.

Nutritional treatment

Nutritional supplements that may be beneficial in the treatment of hypertension are included in the following table. See pages xii–xiii for more information on how to use nutritional supplements.

Herbal treatment

See pages xiii–xv for information on how to use these herbs. The herbs most commonly used in the treatment of hypertension include:

- Hawthorn berries (as a tonic for the circulatory system they are primarily used in the treatment of high blood pressure, atherosclerosis and angina pectoris);
- Mistletoe (a relaxing nervine that acts to reduce heart rate and strengthen capillary walls);

Nutritional supplements for hypertension

SUPPLEMENT	DOSAGE	COMMENT
Calcium and Magnesium	1500 mg daily 500 mg daily	Important for lowering blood pressure
Garlic	Two 500 mg capsules three times daily	Helps lower blood pressure
Coenzyme Q10	100 mg daily	Improves heart function
Essential fatty acids • Flaxseed oil • Olive oil • Primrose oil	Take as directed on label	For circulation and lowering of blood pressure
Vitamin C	3000 mg daily	Reduces blood clotting tendency
Zinc chelate	100 mg daily	Important for the functioning of the glands
Selenium	200 mcg daily	Deficiency has been associated with heart disease
Vitamin B complex	100 mg twice daily	Important for circulation and lowering blood pressure

- Lime Blossom (used to reduce nervous tension and is considered as a specific treatment for high blood pressure).

Other herbs that are used in the treatment of hypertension include:

- Cramp Bark;
- Fennel;
- Motherwort;
- Parsley;
- Rosemary;
- Valerian.

These herbs can be used as a tea or tincture.

It is, however, important to seek advice from your natural health practitioner for a specific treatment to meet your individual needs.

Aromatherapy treatment

See page xvi for information on how to use essential oils. The following essential oils may provide relief from the symptoms of hypertension.

- Rosemary to calm nerves, uplift and stimulate. A few drops of Rosemary oil in a base oil of Almond, Grapeseed or Apricot makes an aromatic massage oil.
- Lavender is a beautiful calming, balancing nervine that has antibacterial and anti-depressant qualities. Excellent for use as a massage oil, bath oil or in an oil burner.
- Ylang Ylang is renowned for its relaxing effect on the nervous system. It also has a balancing effect on blood pressure. Combined with a base oil of avocado it makes a wonderful body oil.

The essential oils recommended for the treatment of angina pectoris (pages 136–38) are also of benefit for sufferers of hypertension. If you have high blood pressure consult a qualified aromatherapist or herbalist before using essential oils.

Dietary and lifestyle recommendations

- Follow a strict salt-free diet. This is vital for lowering blood pressure.
- Do eat plenty of fruit and vegetables. This can include fresh juices such as apple, carrot, celery, citrus, beetroot and watermelon.
- Increase your consumption of fibre; oatbran is an excellent source.
- Vitamin D supplementation can help lower high blood pressure in women.
- Potassium-rich foods or supplementation should be increased to reduce the risk of stroke. See page 353 for a list of foods that are a natural source of potassium.
- Garlic, ginger, celery and onions can all help lower blood pressure.
- Take up meditation and/or yoga to help clear the mind and relax the body.
- Supplement tea and coffee with Dandelion coffee as a natural alternative.

HYPOTENSION

Description

Hypotension is characterised by an abnormal drop in blood pressure. It is often associated with hyperglycaemia, hypothyroidism or anaemia.

Symptoms

The symptoms of low blood pressure are fatigue, dizziness, light headedness, sensitivity to heat and cold and headaches. Some people experience a feeling of dizziness or even blackouts when rising to quickly from bending over or sitting down. This is usually a symptom of low blood pressure.

Causes

Low blood pressure may occur with an injury resulting in blood loss (shock), heart failure, dehydration, malnutrition or pregnancy.

Nutritional treatment

Nutritional supplements that may be beneficial in the treatment of hypotension are included in the following table. See pages xii–xiii for information on how to use nutritional supplements.

Herbal treatments

Use the following herbs as teas, tablets or tinctures. See pages xiii–xv for more information on how to use herbs. Herbs used to treat low blood pressure are:

- Broom;
- Gentian;
- Hawthorn berries;
- Kola;
- Oats;
- Wormwood.

Nutritional supplements for hypotension		
SUPPLEMENT	DOSAGE	COMMENT
Vitamin A	10,000 iu daily	Resists infection and enhances antibody production
Vitamin B complex	50–100 mg daily	Important in carbohydrate and protein metabolism
Vitamin C	2000 mg daily	For adrenal insufficiency
Vitamin E	400 iu daily	Improves circulation
Manganese	As directed on label	Often people with low blood pressure have low levels of this mineral in their blood

Aromatherapy treatment

The following essential oils may provide relief from the symptoms of hypotension:

- Black Pepper (use as a body oil or in an oil burner);
- Clary Sage (use as a bath or body oil);
- Cypress (use as a bath or body oil, or in an oil burner – avoid using if you have high blood pressure);
- Geranium (use as a bath or body oil, or in an oil burner);
- Lemon (use as a bath or body oil);
- Ylang Ylang (use as a bath or body oil).

See page xvi for information on how to use essential oils.

Dietary and lifestyle recommendations

- Eat a well-balanced diet with an emphasis on complex carbohydrates.
- Eat at least six times a day.
- Avoid tea, coffee, alcohol and refined foods.
- Take time to exercise regularly.
- Drink plenty of water.
- The dietary and lifestyle recommendations for hypoglycaemia (page 160) are also useful in the treatment of hypotension.

HYPOGLYCAEMIA

Description

Hypoglycaemia occurs when there is an abnormally low level of sugar in the blood. Also see hypoglycaemia on pages 257–59.

Symptoms

The main symptoms of hypoglycaemia include:

- shakiness;
- weakness;
- rapid pulse;
- headaches;
- irritability.

In diabetic patients a coma can occur when blood sugar levels drop, so immediate hospitalisation is recommended.

Causes

Hypoglycaemia is often caused by an inadequate diet which is too high in refined carbohydrates. Overeating of refined, sugary foods can result in a temporary rise in blood sugar levels followed then by a large drop.

Hypoglycaemia is also associated with diabetes when too high a dose of insulin is received or as a result of overactivity when too much sugar has been used up. It is important when treating hypoglycaemia to look at the lifestyle of the patient. Irregular meals, an unbalanced diet, stress, irregular sleep patterns, alcohol, caffeine, tobacco and other stimulants can also precipitate an attack of hypoglycaemia.

Nutritional treatment

Nutritional supplements that may be beneficial in the treatment of hypoglycaemia are included in the following table. For information on how to use nutritional supplements see pages xii–xiii.

See your natural health practitioner for a more individual treatment program.

Herbal treatment

Use the following herbs as teas, tinctures or tablets. For more information on how to use herbs see pages xiii–xv.

* Bilberry and Wild Yam are useful in regulating insulin levels.

Liver tonics used to regulate sugar metabolism are:

* Dandelion root;
* Milk Thistle;
* Vervain;

Nutritional supplements for hypoglycaemia

SUPPLEMENT	DOSAGE	COMMENT
Chromium or Brewer's yeast	300 mcg daily As directed on label	Normalises blood sugar and metabolism. Helps stabilise blood sugar levels
Vitamin B complex	100 mg daily	Important for proper absorption and digestion of food
Vitamin B1	30 mg daily	Helps digestion
Vitamin B3	30 mg daily	Aids in proper absorption of food
Vitamin C	3000–8000 mg daily to be taken through the day	For adrenal insufficiency
Vitamin E	400 iu daily	Improves circulation
Magnesium and Calcium	750 mg daily 1500 mg daily	Important for proper metabolism of sugars
Manganese	As directed on label	Helps maintain blood glucose levels
Zinc	50 mg daily	Needed for proper insulin release

- Wild Yam;
- Yellow Dock.

Professional advice is recommended before taking any herbal treatments as treatments can vary depending on individual conditions.

Aromatherapy treatment

The following essential oils can be used in the treatment of hypoglycaemia.

- Juniper – use as a bath oil or massage oil. Juniper is recommended for digestion, kidney function and circulation.
- Sandalwood is digestive, calming, relaxing and soothing. A few drops in a hot bath is recommended.
- Clary Sage can be used as a body oil or in a bath. It is a wonderfully relaxing stress relieving essential oil.

All the above essential oils can also be used in an oil burner. See page xvi for information on how to use essential oils.

Dietary and lifestyle recommendations

- Avoid alcohol, caffeine and tobacco as they can cause blood sugar levels to rise and fall dramatically.
- Try to eat six to eight small meals a day to avoid a low blood sugar reaction.

- To diagnose hypoglycaemia a glucose tolerance test is recommended. See your physician for more information.

DIET
Eat a diet high in fibre and complex carbohydrates such as fruits, vegetables and wholegrains, including:

- artichokes;
- bananas;
- barley;
- cabbages;
- carrots;
- lettuce;
- oats;
- olives;
- onions;
- paw paw;
- peas;
- spinach;
- sunflower seeds;
- sweet potatoes;
- turnips.

PALPITATIONS
Description and symptoms

Palpitations is a term that usually refers to the feeling of a pounding heartbeat. Often the pounding heartbeat will be faster than normal; this is called tachycardia. Heart flutter or fibrillation is a situation in which the normal beating of the heart muscle turns into a rapid twitching. With palpitations the sufferer may become aware of the heart's pumping when sitting or lying on the left side. Palpitations may be an important symptom of heart disease, especially if they are frequent and prolonged or associated with chest pain, dizzy spells, fainting or shortness of breath.

Causes

The causes of palpitations are numerous and may include a combination of some of the following factors: stress, excess alcohol or caffeine intake, smoking, amphetamines, a potassium and/or magnesium deficiency, high blood pressure, extreme fright, coronary artery disease, or an overactive thyroid. Certain drugs, such as thyroid pills or appetite suppressants, can also increase cardiac contractions. Anaemia can also cause the heart to beat faster to supply the necessary oxygen to the tissues.

Before treatment with natural therapies is commenced a medical examination must be taken to determine the cause and extent of the problem.

Nutritional treatment

Nutritional supplements that may be beneficial in the treatment of palpitations are included in the following table (see pages 162–63). See pages xii–xiii for information on how to use these supplements.

Herbal treatment

The herbs that are useful in the treatment of palpitations are listed below. For information on how to use these herbs see pages xiii–xv.

CARDIAC TONICS
- Hawthorn berries
- Lily of the Valley
- Motherwort

NERVINES AND SEDATIVES
- Lady's Slipper
- Lime Blossom
- Skullcap
- Valerian

ANTI-SPASMODIC HERBS
The bitter, anti-spasmodic herb Rue increases peripheral circulation, lowers elevated blood pressure, eases palpitations and anxiety problems. Take 1–4 ml of tincture three times daily or a cup of Rue tea three times daily.

HERBAL TEA
A beneficial combination of herbs that may help relieve palpitations is:

- Hawthorn Berries;
- Mistletoe;
- Motherwort;
- Valerian.

Take as a tea three times daily.

Homeopathic treatment

Treatment that may be prescribed by a homeopath for palpitations varies according to the symptoms. For information on how to use the following homeopathic remedies see page xv.

- Use Aconite when the palpitations occur suddenly as a result of fright, shock or being chilled, or from intense anger.

- Use Argentum nitricum when the palpitations are associated with panic, restlessness or nervous excitement.
- Use Arsenicum album for palpitations in a person who is restless, anxious and frightened of being alone.
- Use Calcarea carbonica for palpitations in a person who is sensitive, melancholic and weeps easily.
- Use Cactus when the palpitations are extremely strong, made worse by lying on left side and may be accompanied by dizziness and shortness of breath.

Nutritional supplements for palpitations

SUPPLEMENT	DOSAGE	COMMENT
Potassium orotate	100 mg daily	Necessary for electrolyte balance. Deficiency may cause irregular heartbeat
Magnesium orotate	750 mg daily at bedtime	Regulates and balances the calcium which is needed for heart muscle function
Folic acid	5 mg daily	Deficiency associated with anaemia and atherosclerosis
L-taurine (an amino acid)	1000 mg daily	Used for cardiac arrhythmias, high blood pressure, valvular heart disease and hyperthyroidism
Coenzyme Q10	100 mg three times daily	Improves heart energetics and increases oxygenation of heart tissue
Vitamin B complex plus	50 mg three times daily	Nourishes the nervous system
Vitamin B1	50 mg daily	Deficiency is associated with tachycardia, stress and hyperthyroidism
Vitamin E	100–200 iu daily and slowly increase to 400 iu daily	Anti-oxidant which also improves blood flows and strengthens the heart muscle
Vitamin A	20,000 iu daily	Anti-oxidant function

Nutritional supplements for palpitations

SUPPLEMENT	DOSAGE	COMMENT
Choline	5–15 g daily	Transports and metabolises fats
Vitamin C with bioflavonoids	1000 mg three times daily	Promotes healing, is an anti-oxidant and is used to treat cardiovascular disease
Essential fatty acids: • Evening Primrose oil • Linseed oil • Sunflower oil • Soy oil • Salmon oil • Cod liver oil • Tofu, seaweed	5–10 g daily or as directed on the label	Helps prevent hardening of the arteries, a deficiency associated with angina, varicose veins and poor circulation
Lecithin granules	One tablespoon before meals	Emulsifies fats to prevent atherosclerosis
Selenium	200 mcg daily	An anti-oxidant. Deficiency of selenium is associated with high blood pressure, angina and heart disease

- Use Lachesis for palpitations in a lively, excitable person with a tendency to overwork.
- Use Moschus when palpitations occur after hysteria, if the patient has a weak pulse and may faint.
- Use Pulsatilla when palpitations are precipitated by a rich and spicy meal.

Aromatherapy treatment

Neroli oil (or Orange Blossom oil) is a specific oil for palpitations, nervous tension, anxiety and shock. It has a very positive and calming effect on both body and mind. Use as a bath or body oil or burn in an oil burner.

Other essential oils which may be helpful are:

- Frankincense;
- Hyssop;
- Marjoram;
- Rose.

For information on how to use these oils see page xvi.

Dietary and lifestyle recommendations

- Avoid tea, coffee and alcohol. Reduce your intake of white sugar and flour as these can cause the release of adrenalin which will increase your heart rate. Also avoid chocolate, colas, red meat, fats, soft drinks, spicy foods and fried foods.
- Reduce or consider giving up cigarettes.
- When feeling stressed, anxious or panicky have a cold shower to slow down your heartbeat.
- Do some regular, moderate exercise such as walking.
- Learn a stress management technique like yoga, tai chi, breathing exercises, relaxation or meditation technique.

VARICOSE VEINS

Description

Veins are the blood vessels that carry the blood from the outside of the body (legs, arms, feet) back to the heart. The veins in our legs have tiny valves that prevent blood from returning to the lower parts of our legs, drawn down towards the earth by gravity. Deeper veins in our legs are surrounded by muscles which support them and assist in returning blood to the heart. Veins closer to the skin are only surrounded by a thin layer of fat which does not provide support for the veins. If the valves in the veins do not work properly, circulation is impaired and blood accumulates in the veins, stretching them.

Symptoms

Symptoms of varicose veins include: heaviness, fatigue and pain in the lower legs, night cramps, restless legs, swollen legs, itchy legs and visibly swollen and widened veins on the legs.

Causes

Factors which are associated with varicose veins include: constipation, being overweight, heavy lifting, sitting or standing in one place for long periods of time, crossing of legs while sitting, pregnancy, tight clothing, lack of proper regular exercise and vitamin C deficiency. Varicose veins are also associated with liver disease, heart disease and abdominal tumours.

Nutritional treatment

Nutritional supplements that may be beneficial in the treatment of varicose veins are included in the table on page 166. See pages xii–xiii for information on how to use these supplements.

Herbal treatment

Herbal treatment for varicose veins can be either external or internal. See pages xiii–xv for information on how to use these herbs.

EXTERNAL APPLICATIONS

The following herbs can be applied externally as ointments, lotions or cold compresses. St John's Wort is also recommended for external application as a lotion. A combination of Marigold, Marshmallow and Echinacea makes an effective compress for varicose veins.

- Calendula
- Chamomile
- Golden Seal (do not use if pregnant)
- Horsechestnut
- Marigold
- Marshmallow
- Witch Hazel

INTERNAL APPLICATIONS

The following herbs can be taken internally as teas or tinctures to improve circulation to the legs and benefit varicose veins.

- Bayberry
- Bilberry
- Chilli (hot)
- Ginko Biloba
- Gotu Kola
- Hawthorn berries
- Horsechestnut
- Motherwort
- Prickly Ash
- Skullcap

Homeopathic treatment

Treatment that may be prescribed by a homeopath for varicose veins includes:

- Carbo vegetabilis if the skin is mottled or discoloured or cold to the touch;
- Ferrum metallicum when the legs look pale but become red easily, if the veins are worse during pregnancy or if the legs are swollen;
- Hamamelis if the veins are worse for touch, worse during pregnancy or worse after childbirth or when the legs are swollen or feet sore and bruised;
- Pulsatilla if the veins have a stinging pain or when the sufferer feels cold.

See page xv for information on how to use homeopathics.

Aromatherapy treatment

The following essential oils may provide relief from the symptoms of varicose veins. They can be used as a bath or body oil or as a compress. See page xvi for information on how to use these essential oils.

- Cypress is a specific oil for varicose veins. Use as a bath or body oil or a compress.
- Rose otto improves circulation and can be used as a bath or body oil or as a compress.
- Chamomile is used to calm inflammation, treat burns and bruises, and relax muscles. Use as a bath or body oil or as a compress.
- Lemon improves circulation and can be used as a bath or body oil or as a compress.

Nutritional supplements for varicose veins

SUPPLEMENT	DOSAGE	COMMENT
Vitamin C with bioflavonoids	3 g daily in divided doses	Necessary for the maintenance of healthy blood vessels and promotes circulation of blood
Vitamin E	500 iu daily	Improves circulation of blood
Vitamin A	10,000 iu daily	Protects the blood vessels and assists tissue repair
Vitamin B complex	100 mg three times daily	Necessary for maintenance of strong blood vessels
Zinc	80 mg daily	Necessary for wound healing and tissue repair
Coenzyme Q10	100 mg daily	Promotes blood circulation and tissue oxygenation

Dietary and lifestyle recommendations

- Rest and elevate your legs. Put your feet up when relaxing and elevate the end of your bed with bricks to facilitate blood flow from your legs as you sleep.
- Any exercise that strengthens the legs can help varicose veins; good muscle tone helps to move blood along the veins.
- Avoid standing for long periods and avoid sitting with your legs crossed.
- Increase fibre in the diet to avoid constipation and to keep the bowels clean. It is recommended to drink six to eight glasses of water daily to keep the stools soft. Acidophilus fibre as a supplement can also be helpful.
- Increase your consumption of fish, fresh fruit (in particular blueberries, blackberries, apricots and cherries), legumes and vegetables, garlic, onions, ginger and capsicum, and buckwheat.
- Avoid junk food, alcohol, salt, sugar, ice-cream, fried foods, cheese, peanuts, refined and processed foods and especially tobacco.

CHAPTER FIVE

THE DIGESTIVE SYSTEM

Maintenance of digestion, absorption and the bowels

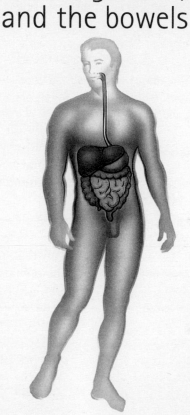

What does it consist of?

The organs of digestion are usually broken into two groups:

1. The gastrointestinal tract which extends from the mouth to the anus.
2. The accessory organs: the teeth, tongue, the salivary glands, liver, gall bladder and pancreas.

What does it do?

The role of the digestive system is the physical and chemical breakdown of food. Food is vitally important for the human body because it provides all the energy which the body needs and the raw materials for the growth and repair of body structures. Energy is required for muscular contraction, for the transmission of nerve impulses and for the metabolic processes of the cells.

After ingestion, food and drink are broken down by the digestive organs into small nutritional molecules which can be absorbed from the intestines and circulated (via the blood and the lymphatic system) around the body. To perform this function the digestive system has a vast network of nervous and hormonal stimulation. Food which cannot be digested and absorbed becomes waste materials (faeces), which is eliminated from the body through the rectum and anus.

What goes wrong with it?

Many common digestive disorders, e.g. peptic ulcers and irritable bowel syndrome, often have a psychological component, as there is a constant interdependence between state of mind and digestive function. Understandably, treatment of digestive disorders may often involve a psychological as well as a physical therapy. Patients who learn to identify emotional problems and stress factors in their lives, and learn ways to cope more effectively, have greater success when they also use other therapies such as herbs, dietary changes and acupuncture.

Nutritional treatment

VITAMIN A
Vitamin A assists the release of gastric juices (pepsin and hydrochloric acid), which are vitally important for protein digestion. Deficiency can lead to gallstones, ulcerative colitis, cirrhosis of the liver, allergies, duodenal and gastric ulcers and Crohn's disease.

VITAMIN B1
Vitamin B1 is required by the stomach to produce hydrochloric acid. Vitamin B1 also assists the body to utilise energy from carbohydrate foods. Deficiency can lead to constipation, abdominal pains, appetite loss and stomach disorders.

VITAMIN B2
Vitamin B2 is also required (with vitamin A) by the stomach for the release of gastric juices, which are necessary for the absorption of proteins, carbohydrates and fats. Deficiency may lead to stomach ulcers, diarrhoea and diabetes.

VITAMIN B3
Vitamin B3 is essential for the proper functioning of the stomach and intestines, and the digestion of carbohydrates, proteins and fats. Deficiency can lead to vomiting, diarrhoea, constipation, bad breath, and inflammation of the mucus membranes in the mouth and gastrointestinal tract.

VITAMIN B5
Vitamin B5 is especially important for the breakdown of fats. Deficiency can lead to anaemia, abdominal pains, ulcers in the digestive tract and hypoglycaemia.

VITAMIN B6
Vitamin B6 plays an important role as a coenzyme in the breakdown and utilisation of carbohydrates, fats and proteins. It is also required for the production of hydrochloric acid and magnesium. Deficiency can lead to ulcers, anaemia, low blood sugar and nausea.

VITAMIN B12

Vitamin B12 is necessary for the metabolism of carbohydrates, proteins and fats. Deficiency may lead to anaemia, weight loss and sore mouth.

VITAMIN C

Vitamin C converts cholesterol into bile acids which are important for good digestion and prevention of kidney stones and gall stones. Deficiency can also lead to gastric ulcers and bleeding gums.

VITAMIN E

Vitamin E is important for the synthesis and use of many amino acids and fats. It regulates the body's use of proteins and fats from the diet. Deficiency can lead to anaemia, colitis, constipation, gallstones, diabetes and coeliac disease.

FOLIC ACID

Folic acid stimulates the appetite and increases the production of hydrochloric acid. Deficiency can lead to anaemia, ulcers, diarrhoea and impaired absorption.

INOSITOL

Inositol promotes the body's ability to produce lecithin, which assists in dissolving fats and in reducing blood cholesterol levels.

SODIUM

Sodium is necessary for the production of hydrochloric acid in the stomach. It functions with potassium to equalise the acid/alkali balance in the blood. A deficiency can lead to anorexia, nausea, weight loss, flatulence and taste impairment.

CHLORINE

Chlorine is necessary for the production of hydrochloric acid and other important gastric juices. Chlorine helps regulate the acid/alkali balance in the blood and assists in the digestion of fats and proteins.

MAGNESIUM

Magnesium assists the digestion of protein and carbohydrates. Deficiency can lead to kidney stones, stomach acidity, diabetes and swollen gums.

POTASSIUM

Potassium assists by balancing the acid/alkaline levels of the body. Deficiency may lead to diabetes, constipation, salt retention, weight loss, colitis and diarrhoea.

Herbal treatment

HERBAL STIMULANTS

Herbal stimulants for the digestive system include bitter herbs, herbs which release the flow of saliva, liver herbs and laxatives.

1. Bitter herbs

Bitter herbs stimulate appetite and stimulate the flow of digestive juices from the pancreas, small intestine and liver. Bitter herbs strengthen the liver and increase the flow of bile. Bitter herbs for digestion include:

- Centaury;
- Chicory;
- Gentian;
- Golden Seal;
- Hops;
- Horehound;
- Mugwort;
- Rue;
- Wormwood.

2. Herbs which enhance the flow of saliva

These help the initial breakdown of carbohydrates in the mouth. They include:

- Cayenne;
- Ginger;
- Licorice;
- Tamarind.

3. Liver herbs

Liver herbs or hepatics strengthen the liver and increase the flow of bile. These include:

- Agrimony;
- Celery;
- Centaury;
- Dandelion root;
- Gentian;
- Golden Seal;
- Horseradish;
- Vervain;
- Wild Yam;
- Wormwood;
- Yarrow;
- Yellow Dock.

4. Herbal laxatives

Herbal laxatives stimulate the bowels to induce bowel movements. These include:

- Aloe;
- Dandelion root;
- Licorice;
- Rhubarb root;
- Senna;
- Yellow Dock.

HERBAL RELAXANTS

Herbal relaxants for the digestive system include: demulcent or soothing herbs, astringents, anti-spasmodic herbs and carminatives.

1. Demulcent herbs

Demulcent herbs are rich in mucilage and can soothe and protect irritated tissues and linings of the intestines. They include:

- Comfrey;
- Hops;
- Irish Moss;
- Marshmallow;
- Oats;
- Slippery Elm.

2. Astringent herbs

Astringent herbs have a binding or tightening action on mucus membranes; this reduces irritation, inflammation and infection. Astringent herbs include:

- Agrimony;
- Comfrey;
- Cranesbill;
- Golden Seal;
- Meadowsweet;
- Sage;
- Witch Hazel.

3. Anti-spasmodic herbs
Anti-spasmodic herbs reduce muscle spasm throughout the body. The anti-spasmodics for the digestive system ease the colic pains that are often associated with digestive upsets. They include:

- Chamomile;
- Cramp Bark;
- Dill;
- Fennel;
- Hops;
- Peppermint;
- Sage;
- Thyme;
- Valerian;
- Wild Yam.

4. Carminative herbs
Carminative herbs are used to cure flatulence by helping the removal of gas from the digestive tract. They include:

- Aniseed;
- Caraway;
- Cardamon;
- Chamomile;
- Dill;
- Fennel;
- Ginger;
- Mustard;
- Parsley;
- Peppermint;
- Sage;
- Thyme;
- Valerian.

ANTI-MICROBIAL HERBS

Anti-microbial herbs help the body to destroy or resist infection from pathogenic organisms. They include:

- Echinacea;
- Garlic;
- Gentian;
- Marigold;
- Myrrh.

Traditional Oriental approach

In traditional Chinese medical philosophy the process of digestion is described in terms of the stomach and spleen (includes the pancreas) organs and meridians. The stomach and spleen are a yin/yang pair: the stomach receives the nourishment of food and drink and 'rots and ripens' it; the spleen and pancreas are responsible for the distribution of nourishment throughout the body. The state of the spleen is one of the most essential factors which determines the quantity of physical energy a person has available to them. The spleen energy is also responsible for lifting and holding the structures of the body in place, therefore hernias, prolapses, poor muscle tone and haemorrhoids are associated with a spleen weakness.

The spleen and stomach organs and meridians are influenced by diet, mental activity and the emotions. The digestion is affected by too much thinking/studying, too much worry, too much sympathy or stress and also by the emotional functioning of the liver (too much anger or frustration).

EMOTIONAL SYMPTOMS OF STOMACH/SPLEEN IMBALANCE

- feeling ungrounded and unearthed
- worry and obsession

- an addictive personality
- needy and selfish behaviour
- apprehension with negative recurring thoughts
- poor concentration
- resisting change

PHYSICAL SYMPTOMS OF STOMACH/SPLEEN IMBALANCE

- dandruff
- brown sacs under eyes
- bloated abdomen
- fluid retention
- tiredness
- excessive urination
- heavy and aching sensations in limbs
- loose stools
- alternating constipation and diarrhoea
- poor memory
- yellowish face and body
- damp hands
- lack of real appetite
- food is tasteless

TRADITIONAL CHINESE MEDICINE RECOMMENDATIONS FOR STRENGTHENING SPLEEN CHI

- Eat mostly cooked food e.g. soups, stews, stirfry, stewed fruits and less raw foods.
- Avoid cold food and liquids from the fridge (allow them to come up to room temperature).
- Chew your food extremely well before you swallow.
- Take your time with meals.
- Eat sweet foods and drinks in moderation.
- Eat a lot of yellow foods and root vegetables (papaya, sweet potato, millet, carrot, pumpkin).

- Use spices like pepper, cardamom, cinnamon, ginger, nutmeg, mace and cloves in your cooking. These spices 'warm' and stimulate the function of the spleen. Ginger tea is excellent for the spleen.
- The bulk of your diet should be composed of complex carbohydrates and vegetables, plenty of fibre and less animal proteins, refined sugars, oils and fats.
- Ginseng is highly recommended as a tonic for the spleen.

Dietary and lifestyle recommendations

FOODS

Foods which strengthen and support the digestive system include:

- acidophilus yoghurt;
- apples;
- asparagus;
- bananas;
- beetroot;
- broccoli;
- cabbage;
- carob;
- celery;
- garlic;
- grapes;
- liquid chlorophyll;
- melons;
- olives;
- onions;
- papaya;
- peaches;
- pears;
- plums;
- spinach;
- sprouts.

JUICES

Juices which strengthen and support the digestive system include:

- carrot;
- papaya;
- parsley;
- potato peel broth;
- whey drinks.

CONSTIPATION

Description and symptoms

Constipation could be described as difficulty in passing stools and incomplete or infrequent passage of stools. Frequency of bowel movements can vary from one individual to another; normal bowel habits can range from two or three times a day to two or three times a week. Generally, regularity and comfort when the bowels are moved are more important factors than frequency.

Constipation if left untreated, can lead to appendicitis, diabetes, mellitus, bad breath, body odour, bloating, depression, cellulite, diverticulitis, fatigue, flatulence, haemorrhoids, headaches, hernia, indigestion, insomnia, meningitis, migraines, obesity, thyroid disease, ulcerative colitis and varicose veins.

Causes

Constipation can be caused by:

- a diet which is low in fibre foods and high in refined foods

- a diet low in fluids, especially water and juices;
- repeatedly ignoring the signals that the bowel needs emptying;
- in the elderly, immobility and weakness of the abdominal muscles;
- structural abnormalities of the bowel;
- bowel diseases (e.g. diverticulitis, irritable bowel disease);
- pregnancy;
- iron supplements, pain killers and antidepressants.

Nutritional treatment

Nutritional supplements that may be beneficial in the treatment of constipation are included in the table on page 175. For information on how to use these supplements see pages xii–xiii.

Herbal treatment

Herbal laxatives stimulate the bowel to promote movements by encouraging greater contractions of the muscle walls of the large intestine. They include:

- Aloe;
- Cascara Sagrada;
- Chamomile;
- Dandelion;
- Fennel;
- Ginger;
- Licorice root;
- Rhubarb;
- Senna pods.

The herbs can be taken as herbal teas. For more information on how to use these herbs see pages xiii–xv.

To prepare Senna pods (stronger than Senna leaf) soak six to twelve pods for six hours in hot ginger tea and drink before going to bed.

Aromatherapy treatment

Use the following essential oils to treat constipation:

- Rose (bath or body oil);
- Rosemary (bath or body oil);
- Fennel (bath or body oil);
- Black Pepper (as a body oil or burn in an oil burner);
- Marjoram (bath or body oil or burn in an oil burner).

For more information on how to use these essential oils see page xvi.

Homeopathic treatment

The homoeopathic repertory for constipation varies according to the symptoms.

- Use Nux vomica when there is a great urge to pass stools but nothing is passed, when there is a constant desire to pass stools and when constipation alternates with diarrhoea. Also use it when the cause of constipation is sedentary habits, pregnancy, overeating or alcohol.
- Use Opium when there is a lack of desire to pass stools.
- Other homeopathic remedies for constipation include Calcarea carbonica, Hepar Sulphuris.

INEFFECTUAL DESIRE TO PASS STOOLS

Use the following homeopathics when there is an ineffectual desire to pass stools:

- Causticum;
- Lycopodium;
- Magnesium carbonate;
- Natrum muriaticum;
- Nux vomica;
- Sepia;
- Silicea.

For more information on how to use homeopathics see page xv.

Dietary and lifestyle recommendations

- Never repress or deny an urge to go the toilet.
- Drink six to eight glasses of water each day to avoid faecal impaction. This is especially important when adding more fibre to the diet. Adding a squeeze of lemon to the water can help.
- Sit on the toilet at the same time every morning even when the urge to pass stools is absent.
- Eat a high-fibre diet which includes fruit, vegetables, legumes and whole grains. Bran and psyllium seeds are the two safest additional sources of extra fibre. Avoid dairy products, fats and spicy foods.
- Stop using chemical laxatives as they eventually weaken the bowel muscles. Prunes or figs are good natural laxatives.

Nutritional supplements for constipation

SUPPLEMENT	DOSAGE	COMMENT
Vitamin B complex	50 mg three times daily before meals	Assists in the digestion of fats, proteins, and carbohydrates
Vitamin B12	100 mcg three times daily	Important for digestion and to prevent anaemia
Vitamin C (buffered form)	10,000 mg daily in divided doses	Regulates cholesterol metabolism and promotes healing
Vitamin E	400 iu daily, before meals	Anti-oxidant which also helps to heal the colon
Folic acid	60 mg daily	Important coenzyme, deficiency can lead to constipation
Essential fatty acids (e.g. linseed oil)	One tablespoon three times daily	Assists in proper stool formation
Digestive enzymes	After meals as directed on label	Assists in breakdown of food
Acidophilus yoghurt	One teaspoon three times daily	Promotes and restores 'friendly' bacteria in intestines
Garlic	Two 500 mg tablets three times daily with meals (or as directed on the label)	Eliminates harmful bacteria from the colon
Fibre (psyllium the husks or bran)	1½ tablespoons three times daily	Bulks the wastes and activates nerve reflexes that signal elimination
Calcium and Magnesium	1500 mg daily 750 mg daily	Regulates muscle tone and muscular contractions

- Exercise for at least 20–30 minutes, three times per week. If appropriate for your level of fitness the aerobic kinds of exercise are recommended: walking, swimming and bicycling.

- If constipation persists seek medical advice.

CROHN'S DISEASE

Description

Crohn's disease is diagnosed when there is a narrowing and thickening of the small or large intestine resulting from a build-up of scar tissue associated with chronic inflammation that may occur anywhere in the digestive tract.

Symptoms

These include bouts of diarrhoea, low grade fever, anorexia, weight loss and flatulence.

Causes

Crohn's disease may be caused by the immune system attacking the body's own tissues, food sensitivity (including lactose intolerance), a genetic predisposition or viral or bacterial infections.

Nutritional treatment

Nutritional supplements that may be beneficial in the treatment of Crohn's disease are included in the following table. For information on how to use these nutritional supplements see pages xii–xiii.

Herbal treatment

Take the following herbs as teas, tablets or tinctures. For more information on how to use these herbs see pages xiii–xv.

- Marshmallow root is a demulcent with soothing and healing properties, used to treat inflammations of the digestive tract.
- Wild Indigo is used to treat gastrointestinal infections.
- Golden Seal is a very useful herb in the treatment of digestive problems. This herb should not be used if you are pregnant.
- Comfrey is a powerful healing herb used to treat Crohn's disease and ulcerative colitis.
- Slippery Elm bark is a soothing demulcent used to treat inflammation of the mucus membrane linings in the digestive tract.

Homeopathic treatment

The homeopathic repertory for Crohn's disease varies according to the symptoms.

- Mercurius corrosivus is used for diarrhoea with severe pain and bloody bowel motions.
- Arsenicum album is used for diarrhoea with exhaustion and fever.
- Podophyllum is used for diarrhoea that alternates with constipation and flatulence.

Nutritional supplements for Crohn's disease

SUPPLEMENT	DOSAGE	COMMENT
Vitamin A	*50,000 iu daily (if pregnant do not exceed 10,000 iu daily)*	*Helps in the repair of the intestinal tract*
Vitamin B12 or Folic acid	*200 mcg daily* *200 mcg daily*	*Helps prevent anaemia and needed for the constant supply of new cells*
Vitamin C	*1000 mg three times daily*	*Improves immunity*
Vitamin D	*400 iu daily*	*Prevents bone disease resulting from malabsorption*
Vitamin E	*500 iu daily*	*Regulates the immune system*
Vitamin K	*As directed on label*	*Important for colon health. inhibiting bile salt Reduces irritation by partially metabolism in the colon*
Garlic	*Two 500 mg capsules three times daily*	*Combats free radicals, aids healing*
Calcium and Magnesium	*2000 mg daily* *1500 mg daily*	*Help prevent colon cancer*
Selenium	*500 mcg daily*	*Anti-oxidant. Important in treating absorption problems*
Zinc	*50 mg daily*	*For healing and boosting immune function*

For information on how to use homeopathics see page xv.

Aromatherapy treatment

The following aromatherapy oils are useful in the treatment of digestive disturbances. Used as massage oils, in a warm bath or as inhalants they can provide relaxation and therapeutic relief. For information on how to use these oils see page xvi.

- Black Pepper
- Chamomile
- Cinnamon
- Eucalyptus
- Juniper
- Lavender
- Marjoram

Dietary and lifestyle recommendations

- It is important that sufferers of Crohn's disease follow a diet which provides them with adequate nutrition, vitamins and minerals. Consult a qualified naturopath or a nutritionist to work out a diet suitable for your individual needs.
- The elimination of lactose-containing foods (milk and milk products) can be of great benefit to sufferers of Crohn's disease.
- Take lactobacillus acidophilus in capsule or tablet form or in yoghurt.
- Avoid smoking as this can worsen the condition.

IT'S IMPORTANT TO SEE YOUR DOCTOR

- For a proper diagnosis of this condition. It is of great importance to eliminate other conditions which produce similar symptoms.

DIARRHOEA

Description

Diarrhoea is the frequent passing of loose watery stools often the result of a weakening or inflammation of the bowel lining caused by a disturbance of the intestinal flora or bacteria.

Chronic diarrhoea occurs when the frequency of bowel movements increases and continues over a longer period of time.

Symptoms

These include frequent loose bowel movements, nausea, vomiting, colicky pains or cramps in the stomach and dehydration.

Causes

The most common cause of acute diarrhoea is through a viral infection such as gastroenteritis (very common in children and easily transmitted). Other notable causes are salmonella bacteria (food poisoning), allergies and stress or anxiety. Symptoms usually disappear in a couple of days.

Possible causes of chronic diarrhoea are diverticulitis, Crohn's disease, ulcerative colitis, irritable bowel syndrome and certain types of malabsorption.

Fluid replacement is essential.

Nutritional treatment

Nutritional supplements that may be beneficial in the treatment of diarrhoea are included in the following table. See pages xii–xiii for information on how to use nutritional supplements.

Herbal treatment

For information on how to use herbal treatments see pages xii–xv. A herbal repertory for the treatment of diarrhoea would include the following herbs:

- Raspberry leaf tea (pour a cup of boiling water onto two teaspoons of dried herbs and let infuse for ten to

Nutritional supplements for diarrhoea

SUPPLEMENT	DOSAGE	COMMENT
Vitamin C	1000–3000 mg daily	Improves the condition of the bowel lining
Vitamin B complex	100 mg three times daily	Necessary for digestion and absorption of nutrients
Charcoal tablets	Four tablets every hour until diarrhoea subsides	Absorbs toxins
Psyllium or oatbran	One tablespoon with meals	For stool formation
Kelp	Five tablets daily	For mineral replacement
Garlic	Two 500 mg capsules three times daily	Kills bacteria and enhances immune system
Acidophilus fibre	One teaspoon in water twice daily	Replaces lost friendly bacteria
Multivitamin and mineral supplement	As directed on label	To help build up immune system
Potassium	As directed on label	To replace potassium lost during diarrhoea

15 minutes. This tea can be taken regularly);
- Slippery Elm bark (taken in powdered form and mixed with a little water or taken in capsule form provides relief from gastric disturbances).

These herbs are also useful in the treatment of diarrhoea:

- Arrowroot;
- Cinnamon;
- Comfrey;
- Meadowsweet;
- Oak bark.

Homeopathic treatment

Homeopathic remedies for diarrhoea vary according to the symptoms.

- Arsenicum album is used to treat diarrhoea related to food poisoning. Use if there is a burning pain after bowel motion or if you have watery, smelly stools.
- Argentum nitricum is used for diarrhoea which is caused by acute anxiety, sometimes accompanied by vomiting. Use if you have green watery stools.

- Sulphur is used for diarrhoea accompanied by flatulence, burning, cramping and a sour smell. It is used to treat children.

Aromatherapy treatment

The following essential oils may provide relief from the symptoms of diarrhoea.

- Chamomile is used for loss of appetite, digestive disturbances, diarrhoea and flatulence. Use as a body oil or compress.
- Cinnamon acts as an antibacterial, an antifungal, and also treats exhaustion. Use in a compress, massage oil or inhalation.
- Fennel is a calmative oil which eases wind, indigestion and colic. It can be used as a body oil or bath oil.
- Lavender is a relaxant oil used for migraines and headaches. It is also an antiseptic. Lavender oil makes an excellent body oil, bath oil or skin compress.

Other essential oils used in the treatment of diarrhoea and other digestive disturbances include:

- Geranium;
- Ginger;
- Nutmeg;
- Peppermint;
- Rosemary;
- Sandalwood.

For more information on how to use these essential oils see page xvi.

Dietary and lifestyle recommendations

- Avoid irritants such as coffee, alcohol, tobacco, spices, laxatives, refined and processed foods, and saturated fats.
- Follow a bland, low-fibre diet while the stools are still loose.
- Do take Acidophilus fibre to replace lost 'friendly' bacteria in the gut.
- Increase your intake of fluids and electrolytes.
- Watermelon juice or Dandelion tea can be taken regularly.

HERNIA

Description

A hernia is a protrusion of part of an organ through a weak area in the barrier muscle which surrounds it. A hiatal hernia is when the stomach protrudes upwards through an opening in the diaphragm muscle into the chest.

Many abdominal hernias are in the groin area and occur most frequently in men.

Inguinal hernia is the protrusion of the hernial sac or bowel into the inguinal opening (the protrusion may extend into the scrotum in males and cause strangulation of the herniated part).

Femoral hernias are more common in women.

Umbilical hernia is uually a mild defect that contains the protrusion of a portion of the abdominal lining through the navel area of the abdominal wall.

Symptoms

The main symptoms of an hiatal hernia occur from stomach acid regurgitating into the oesophagus and throat. Other common symptoms of a hiatal hernia include heartburn, a bitter taste in the mouth, belching, discomfort behind the breastbone as well as a burning sensation in this area. Symptoms are aggravated by lying down after a large meal and exercise which includes bending forward. Acid foods will also aggravate this condition and digestive weakness often accompanies (and contributes to) the problem. Ulcers often accompany a hiatal hernia.

Causes

Hernias are usually the result of an inherited weakness in the abdominal wall. Other possible causes include:

- heavy lifting;
- coughing, chronic bronchitis, smoking and even laughing;
- substantial weight gain;
- poor abdominal muscle tone;
- constipation (see pages 173–75 for more information about the treatment of constipation).

Treatment is aimed towards preventing constipation, supporting the digestive processes and toning up the abdominal muscles.

Nutritional treatment

Nutritional supplements that may be beneficial in the treatment of hernias are included in the table on page 182. For information on how to use nutritional supplements see pages xii–xiii.

Herbal treatment

Herbs that are of benefit in the treatment and prevention of hernias are listed below. For more information on how to use these herbs see pages xiii–xv.

- Comfrey (take as a tea, tablet or tincture)
- Aloe Vera juice (take ¼ cup of Aloe Vera juice twice a day)
- Slippery Elm powder (use one part of the powdered bark mixed with six parts of water; take three times daily)
- Marshmallow (Slippery Elm powder may be mixed with Marshmallow tea to benefit the digestive processes)
- Fenugreek, Red Clover and Golden Seal (make up a herbal infusion using equal parts of each herb then take three cups of the herbal tea daily or 2 ml of each herbal tincture daily). Do not take Golden Seal on a daily basis for more than one week at a time and do not take if you are pregnant. Alternate Golden Seal with the other herbs.

Homeopathic treatment

Homeopathic treatment for hernias is aimed towards treating the symptoms: indigestion, pain, heartburn, and belching.

Nutritional supplements for hernia

SUPPLEMENT	DOSAGE	COMMENT
Vitamin A (use emulsion form)	*30,000 iu daily. (if pregnant do not exceed 10,000 iu daily)*	*Helps regulate stomach acidity and strengthens immune functions*
Vitamin B complex	*As directed on label*	*Facilitates digestion and absorption of carbohydrates, proteins and fats by assisting in enzyme reactions*
Vitamin B12	*100 mcg daily*	*Assists metabolism of fats, protein and carbohydrate and protects gut, mucosal andepithelial cells*
Vitamin C	*500 mg daily*	*Promotes healing and improves immunity*
Zinc	*50 mg daily*	*Involved in many enzyme reactions, immune functions and healing*

FOR INDIGESTION WITH HEARTBURN USE
- Arsenicum
- Calcarea carbonica
- Lycopodium
- Magnesia carbonica
- Nux vomica
- Pulsatilla

FOR INDIGESTION WHICH IS BETTER FOR BELCHING USE
- Argentum nitricum
- Carbo vegetabilis
- Ignatia amara
- Kali carbonicum
- Lycopodium

FOR INDIGESTION WHICH IS WORSE ON BELCHING USE
- China officinalis

FOR INDIGESTION WITH BURNING PAINS IN THE STOMACH USE
- Arsenicum
- Carbo vegetabilis
- Phosphorus
- Sulphur

For a more specific remedy consult your homeopath. For information on how to use homeopathics see page xv.

Aromatherapy treatment

Use the following essential oils as bath or body oils to benefit digestion and relieve constipation. See page xvi for information on how to use these oils.

- Black Pepper
- Fennel (also good for bowel pain and indigestion)
- Ginger
- Marjoram
- Nutmeg
- Peppermint

Use Lemongrass oil as a bath or body oil to tone muscles and benefit digestion.

Dietary and lifestyle recommendations

- Carefully and cautiously exercise to tone up stomach muscles.
- If relevant, lose weight to reduce stress on your stomach muscles.
- Improve your posture when sitting and standing.
- Take extra fibre and digestive enzymes to prevent constipation and straining during bowel movements.
- Avoid large meals; take small meals throughout the day, chew your food well and keep vertical after meals.
- Do not eat within three hours of bedtime.
- Avoid spicy foods, fried foods, chocolate and alcohol as these foods relax the sphincter and can cause heartburn.

HEPATITIS

Description

Hepatitis refers to inflammation of the liver and it can be caused by viruses, drugs and chemicals including alcohol. The inflammation causes the liver to become swollen and tender, and it becomes unable to function properly resulting in a buildup of toxic substances in the body. Clinically, three main types of hepatitis are recognised although more new types are still being identified.

Symptoms and causes

HEPATITIS A

Hepatitis A (infectious hepatitis) is caused by the hepatitis A virus and is caught by eating food that has been handled by someone else who has the disease, through person to person contact, or through contact with contaminated clothing, toys, cutlery, or bed linen. It is generally a relatively mild disease of children and young adults, characterised by anorexia, malaise, nausea, diarrhoea, fever and chills. The usual course of the disease is a worsening of symptoms to a peak when jaundice (yellow colour of skin) is most pronounced. It is most contagious between two to three weeks before and one week after jaundice appears.

A bout of hepatitis A confers immunity to the virus. Most people recover in four to six weeks and it does not cause lasting liver damage, although the liver should be nurtured afterwards.

HEPATITIS B

Hepatitis B (serum hepatitis) is caused by the hepatitis B virus and is spread primarily by sexual or intimate contact with the body fluids of a person who is a carrier of the disease or who has the disease. It can also be caught by sharing contaminated syringes and transfusion equipment. Blood, semen, saliva and tears can spread the virus. People who harbour the active hepatitis B virus are at risk of developing cirrhosis of the liver, liver failure or even liver cancer. General symptoms of hepatitis B are similar to those of hepatitis A.

HEPATITIS C

Hepatitis C (non-A, non-B hepatitis) is caused by a virus that can be passed from one person to another through blood contamination and has often been spread through blood transfusions. It is believed to account for more post-transfusion hepatitis than hepatitis B. Sexual transmission of the disease is uncommon. About a quarter of patients who develop hepatitis C develop chronic liver damage, sometimes only after many years. Hepatitis C sufferers may or may not have acute episodes of symptoms which can include: abdominal discomfort, abdominal fullness, nausea, feverish symptoms, weakness, irritability and muscular pain.

Treatment of hepatitis using alterative therapies is directed towards alleviating the acute symptoms, strengthening the liver and improving its function, improving the function of the immune system, inhibiting viral reproduction and stimulating regeneration of the damaged liver cells. Hepatitis is a disease which can greatly benefit from using alterative therapies.

Nutritional treatment

Nutritional supplements that may be beneficial in the treatment of hepatitis are included in the following table. See pages xii–xiii for information on how to use these supplements.

Herbal treatment

A herbal repertory for treating hepatitis would include the following herbs. For information on how to use these herbs see pages xiii–xv.

Nutritional supplements for hepatitis

SUPPLEMENT	DOSAGE	COMMENT
Vitamin B12	100 mcg twice daily	May shorten recovery time from acute hepatitis
plus Choline	1 g three times daily	For detoxification, synthesis of lecithin and metabolism of fats
plus Inositol	1000 mg daily	Improves liver function
Folic acid	1000 mcg daily	Works with vitamin B12 to shorten recovery time from acute flareups
Vitamin C	2000–5000 mg daily	Improves viral hepatitis and hastens in divided doses recovery

Nutritional supplements for hepatitis

SUPPLEMENT	DOSAGE	COMMENT
Vitamin E	400 iu daily	Strengthens immune system and acts as an anti-oxidant
L-methionine	1 g three times daily	Has a detoxification function, benefits the liver and mobilises fats. Prevents accumulation of fats in the liver
L-cysteine	500 mg twice daily (take with vitamin C and vitamin B6)	Detoxification function
Essential fatty acids • Evening Primrose oil • Cod Liver oil • Linseed oil • Salmon oil	One tablespoon three times daily	Lowers blood fats and heals the liver
Catechin	1 g daily	Anti-oxidant which protects the liver and strengthens the immune system
Coenzyme Q10	50 mg daily	Boosts the immune system and oxygenates the tissue cells
Lecithin granules	One tablespoon three times daily before meals	Mobilises fats and protects the liver
Liver extracts (liver hydrolysate)	500 mg three times daily	Promotes liver regeneration
Calcium	1000 mg daily	Important for blood clotting
Magnesium	1000 mg daily	Assists the function of calcium

- Chinese herbs have also been found to be very helpful, consult your Chinese herbalist.
- Dandelion cleanses the liver and the bloodstream; and benefits the functional capacity of the liver. Take two cups of the herbal tea per day.
- Milk Thistle contains silymarin which protects the liver by inhibiting the factors that are responsible for liver damage. Silymarin benefits cirrhosis, chronic hepatitis, fatty liver and gall bladder inflammation.

- Artichoke has an active ingredient, cynarin, which protects and regenerates the liver. It also helps decongest the liver by clearing bile.
- Burdock root purifies the blood. Take as a tea or tincture.
- Spearmint tea, Ginger and Raspberry Leaf tea all help relieve nausea.
- Licorice has an antiviral activity which benefits viral hepatitis.
- Green tea promotes fat breakdown, aids digestion and benefits the liver. Green tea can be taken with meals.

TEAS OR TINCTURES

These herbs can be taken as teas or tinctures:

- Gardenia;
- Red Clover;
- Skullcap;
- St John's Wort;
- Wormwood;
- Yellow Dock.

Homeopathic treatment

Hepatitis is a serious disease which requires skill and experience to treat effectively, so it is best to consult a qualified homeopath for a treatment program designed specifically for your needs. A homeopathic repertory for treating hepatitis would include the following homeopathics:

- Use Ipecac for vomiting with persistent nausea;
- Use Podophyllum to stimulate the liver and cleanse the bowels where there is congestion;
- Use Bryonia when there is pain and tenderness in the liver region and symptoms come on after exposure to cold;
- Use Mercurius solubilis when the patient is smelly (i.e. bad breath and/or smelly discharges like urine, mucus, stools) and there is a tender liver;
- Use Phosphorus when there is a strong thirst for cold or iced drinks and an empty feeling in the abdomen;
- Use Lachesis when the liver feels swollen and tender and there is a distended abdomen;
- Use Hydrastis for a swollen, tender liver with yellowish discharge from the nose and throat.

For more information about homeopathics see page xv.

Aromatherapy treatment

The following essential oils support the liver. See page xvi for more information on how to use them.

- Juniper can be used as a body or bath oil.
- Lavender can be used as a body or bath oil.
- Lemon can be used as a body or bath oil.
- Rose can be used as a body or bath oil.
- Rosemary can be used as a bath or body oil or burnt in an oil burner.
- Myrrh can be used as a body oil or burnt in an oil burner (avoid during pregnancy).

- Geranium can be used as a bath or body oil or burnt in an oil burner for jaundice.

Dietary and lifestyle recommendations

- Your diet should be reasonably high in complex carbohydrate (60 percent), low in fat (25 percent of calories) and moderate in protein (15 percent of calories). The diet should be low in saturated fats, simple carbohydrates (sugar, white flour, fruit juice, honey, etc.), low in oxidised fatty acids (fried oils) and animal fat.
- Eat five or six small meals per day.
- If you have little or no appetite then vegetable juices and broths are important. Barley broth in particular provides fluid and nourishment. Drink 'green drinks' (green bean juice, cucumber juice, dandelion, greens, wheatgrass, alfalfa sprouts, celery, cabbage), carrot juice and beetroot juice.
- Avoid alcohol, chemicals and food additives, highly processed foods, coffee, raw fish, shell fish and margarine. Take condiments, sauces and spices in moderation.
- Drink plenty of filtered water and get plenty of rest.
- One teaspoon of apple cider vinegar should be taken in water with every meal to improve gastric digestion.

IRRITABLE BOWEL SYNDROME

Description

Irritable bowel – or spastic colon syndrome as it is sometimes known – is characterised by abdominal pain, often accompanied by alternating episodes of diarrhoea or constipation. There is often overproduction of mucus in the colon and the patient may be suffering varying degrees of anxiety or depression. Irritable bowel syndrome (IBS) is the most common digestive disorder reported to physicians. Although there are no signs of diseases of the bowel with this disorder it is important to have a proper diagnosis as the symptoms of IBS are similar to those of Crohn's disease, diverticulitis and lactose intolerance. It is important for sufferers of IBS to look at making changes to their diet, getting regular exercise and replacing lost nutrients.

Symptoms

These include:

- abdominal pain;
- anorexia;
- bloating;
- constipation;

Nutritional supplements for irritable bowel syndrome		
SUPPLEMENT	DOSAGE	COMMENT
Vitamin B complex	50–100 mg three times daily	Needed for proper absorption of food
Acidophilus	As directed on label	To replace lost friendly bacteria in the bowel
Kyolic garlic	As directed on label	Aids in digestion
Fibre, such as: • Oatbran • Flaxseeds • Psyllium seeds	As directed on label	For cleansing and healing
Calcium and Magnesium	2000 mg daily 1000 mg daily	Aids the central nervous system and helps prevent colon cancer

- diarrhoea;
- flatulence;
- nausea;
- mucus in the stools.

Causes

The causes are not entirely clear, however lifestyle factors such as stress and diet are the most common contributors.

An overuse of antibiotics and laxatives which disturb the natural flora of the bowel may also be factors.

Nutritional treatment

Nutritional supplements that may be beneficial in the treatment of irritable bowel syndrome are included in the above table. See pages xii–xiii for information on how to use these supplements.

Herbal treatment

Nervines are used for relaxing the nervous system. These can be beneficial in treating IBS as the condition often results from stress and anxiety.

Use the following nervine herbs as teas or tinctures.

- Chamomile
- Hops
- Skullcap
- Valerian
- Wild Yam

See pages xiii–xv for information on how to use these herbs.

Homeopathic treatment

Treatment that may be prescribed by a homeopath for irritable bowel syndrome includes:

- Colocynthis for colic, griping pains and diarrhoea;
- Nux vomica for constipation alternating with diarrhoea, and griping pains;
- Argentum nitricum if you are anxious or fearful and have indigestion, diarrhoea and flatulence;
- Calcarea carbonica if you are anxious or fearful and have constipation and diarrhoea.

See page xv for information on how to use homeopathics. For a more specific treatment see your homeopath.

Aromatherapy treatment

The following essential oils have therapeutic properties to aid in the symptomatic relief of digestive and stress related illnesses. Used either as massage oils, bath oils or as inhalants (see page xvi for information on how to use essential oils).

- Chamomile is a gentle and relaxing oil that will ease tension.
- Bergamot is used for anxiety, depression and to aid digestion.
- Ginger is used for any digestive problems, flatulence, diarrhoea and headache.
- Peppermint is used to treat digestive disorders, colic, vomiting and diarrhoea.

Dietary and lifestyle recommendations

- Increase fibre in your diet by eating plenty of green vegetables, salads, fruits and wholemeal breads.

- Avoid all processed foods, caffeine, tobacco and alcohol as they will aggravate the problem.
- Reduce stress and anxiety. We can often gain insights into our health problems by re-evaluation of our relationships, work and lifestyle choices. Relaxation, yoga and meditation have a lot to offer here.
- To relieve gas or bloating use charcoal tablets (available in health food stores).
- Early recognition of the disorder, good nutrition, vitamin and mineral supplementation and a positive attitude help minimise complications.

MOUTH ULCERS

Description and symptoms

Mouth ulcers are an extremely common condition and affect a large number of the population.

They are single or clustered, shallow, painful white lesions surrounded by red borders. These lesions are found anywhere inside the mouth including the cheeks, tongue, gums and the inside of the lips.

Causes

Mouth ulcers are often associated with stress, low immunity, dietary excess involving the use of refined sugars, zinc deficiency or ill-fitting dentures.

Nutritional treatment

Nutritional supplements that may be beneficial in the treatment of mouth ulcers are included in the following table. See pages xii–xiii for information on how to use nutritional supplements.

Herbal treatment

The three main herbs used to treat mouth ulcers are listed below. For information on how to use these herbs see pages xiii–xv.

- Echinacea is an anti-microbial used as a mouthwash to treat oral disorders such as mouth ulcers and gingivitis.
- Cleavers is a lymphatic tonic to treat a wide variety of ailments including ulcers.
- Myrrh is an anti-microbial, essential in the treatment of infections in the mouth including mouth ulcers, gingivitis and pyorrhoea.

Homeopathic treatment

Treatment that may be prescribed by a homeopath for mouth ulcers includes:

- Nitricum acidum for painful mouth ulcers on the edge of the tongue.
- Mercurius for mouth ulcers on the gums and the tongue that sting and throb.

For information on how to use homeopathics see page xv.

Aromatherapy treatment

The following essential oils may provide relief from the symptoms of mouth ulcers:

- Cypress (use an inhalant or massage oil);

Nutritional supplements for mouth ulcers		
SUPPLEMENT	DOSAGE	COMMENT
Vitamin A	750 mg daily	Essential for healthy mouth and gums
Vitamin B complex	50 mg three times daily	To aid digestion and heal mouth tissue
Vitamin C	4000 mg daily	Promotes healing
Vitamin E	250 iu daily	Needed to protect the body against infection
Potassium and magnesium	750 mg daily (combined dosage)	For toning the nervous system

- Geranium (use as a bath oil, body oil, inhalant or compress);
- Myrrh (may be used as an antiseptic gargle);
- Tea Tree (a few drops diluted in a glass of water may be used as a mouth wash).

See page xvi for information on how to use essential oils.

Dietary and lifestyle recommendations

- Avoid refined, sugary foods and hot, spicy foods.
- Drink plenty of filtered water.
- Try yoga or meditation for stress relief.
- Eat a well-balanced diet with emphasis on fresh fruit and vegetables.
- Avoid fluoride toothpastes as they can irritate mouth ulcers. Try ones with Myrrh or Tea Tree added. These are available in the health food sections of supermarkets or health food stores.
- Avoid citrus fruit as it may irritate mouth ulcers.
- Take homoeopathic remedies or herbal treatments as they provide quick relief.

OBESITY

Description and symptoms

Obesity can be simply defined as a body condition in which a person is 20 percent or more over the maximum desired weight for their height and build. But perhaps more important than the height to weight ratio is the individual's percentage of fat. For healthy women, fat should not account for more than 30 percent of body weight; for healthy men, fat should not account for more than 25 percent of body weight. Male-patterned obesity, typically seen in the obese male, is when fat is deposited primarily in the upper body (the abdomen and trunk). Female-patterned obesity, typically seen in the obese female, is when fat is deposited primarily in the lower body (the hips and thighs). Obesity puts an undue stress on the body, particularly the back, legs and internal organs. Obesity increases the body's susceptibility to infection and creates a greater risk of developing the following conditions: heart disease, high blood pressure, kidney problems, diabetes, gallstones, stroke, cancer, liver damage, complications of pregnancy and certain psychological conditions.

Causes

Obesity can be caused by or associated with:

- dietary intake of more calories than are converted into energy;
- metabolic disorders such as glandular malfunctions;
- lack of exercise;
- food allergies;
- insatiable appetite from emotional factors, brain injuries or from food sensitivities;

- diabetes;
- hypoglycaemia;
- genetic influences.

Nutritional treatment

Nutritional treatment can assist weight loss in four ways:

1. the use of nutrients to reduce fluid retention;
2. the use of natural appetite suppressants;
3. the use of lipotropic vitamins which support the liver's ability to break down and metabolise fats;
4. the use of certain amino acids which have been found to stimulate the release of growth hormone which converts stored fats into energy.

Nutritional supplements that may be beneficial in the treatment of obesity are included in the following table (see pages 193–94). For information about how to use these supplements see pages xii–xiii.

Herbal treatment

All of the following herbs may be taken as either teas or tinctures. See pages xiii–xv for information on how to use these herbs.

DIURETICS
Herbal diuretics encourage the elimination of excess fluids and wastes. They also support the whole process of inner cleansing. Herbal diuretics include:

- Agrimony;
- Alfalfa;

- Borage;
- Celery seed;
- Corn Silk;
- Dandelion;
- Horsetail;
- Hyssop;
- Juniper berries;
- Parsley;
- Pumpkin seed;
- Thyme;
- Uva Ursi;
- Yarrow.

STIMULANTS
Herbs which improve the body's metabolic rate by stimulating the adrenal glands and the thyroid gland include:

- Bladderwrack;
- Borage;
- Ginseng;
- Hawthorn berry;
- Licorice root;
- Oats;
- Sarsaparilla;
- Wild Yam;
- Wormwood.

APPETITE SUPPRESSANTS
Herbs which suppress appetite include:

- Damiana;
- Ephedra;
- Guarana;
- Kola nut.

BITTER HERBS
Bitter herbs which stimulate digestion include:

- Barberry;
- Boldo;

- Centaury;
- Chicory;
- Gentian root;
- Hops;
- Rue;
- Wormwood.

DIGESTIVE STIMULANTS

Other herbs which stimulate digestion and metabolism include:

- Cardamon;
- Cayenne;
- Cinnamon;
- Ginger;
- Green tea;
- Mustard seed.

LIVER HERBS

Herbs which support the liver's ability to breakdown and metabolise fats include:

- Agrimony;
- Balm;
- Barberry;
- Celery;
- Centaury;
- Dandelion;
- Gentian;
- Golden Seal (avoid during pregnancy);
- Horseradish;
- Wild Yam;
- Wormwood;

Nutritional supplements for obesity

SUPPLEMENT	DOSAGE	COMMENT
Vitamin B3	50 mg three times daily	Lowers blood cholesterol and lessens sugar cravings
Vitamin B6	50 mg three times daily	Important for fat metabolism
Vitamin B12	50 mg three times daily	Important for fat metabolism
Vitamin C with bioflavonoids	2000–3000 mg daily	Regulates cholesterol metabolism and stimulates glandular function
Amino acids:		
• L-carnitine	500 mg daily	Helps fat metabolism and usage
• L-lysine	500 mg daily	Assists digestion of fats
• L-methionine	500 mg daily	Promotes digestion and metabolism of fats
• L-ornithine	500 mg daily	Promotes digestion and metabolism of fats
• L-fyronsine	500 mg daily	Controls appetite and is a precursor of thyroid hormones

(Take amino acids on an empty stomach with water, vitamin B6 and vitamin C with bioflavonoids.)

Nutritional supplements for obesity

SUPPLEMENT	DOSAGE	COMMENT
Coenzyme Q10	As directed on label	Improves cellular energetics
Essential fatty acids: • Cod liver oil • Linseed oil • Corn oil • Evening Primrose oil • Wheatgerm oil • Salmon oil	1000 mg three times daily	Lowers blood fats and controls appetite
Psyllium husks	One tablespoon half an hour before eating (wash down with water or juice)	Provides fibre, reduces appetite and assists bowel movements
Lecithin granules	One tablespoon three times daily before meals	Increases the solubility of cholesterol by emulsifying fats for their removal from the body. Also assists the cells to burn fats
Pancreatin	250–500 mg daily between meals	A digestive enzyme which can reduce appetite and assist weight loss
Spirulina	As directed on label	Good source of vitamins, minerals and useable protein and carbohydrates which also stabilises blood sugar. Acts as a mild appetite suppressant

- Yarrow;
- Yellow Dock.

Homeopathic treatment

Treatment that may be prescribed by a homeopath for obesity includes:

- Phosphorus or Lycopodium for a person who likes chocolate;
- Nitric acidum for a person who likes fatty foods;
- Phosphorus or Veratrum album for a person who likes ice-cream;
- Argentum nitricum, China officinalis, Lycopodium or Sulphur for a person who likes sugar and sweets;
- Calcarea for an obese person who feels chilly, has head sweats, craves

eggs, hot foods and suffers from indigestion;
- Capsicum for an obese person who has burning sensations in the stomach or intestines;
- Ferrum metallicum for an obese person who is also pale-faced and has cold hands and feet;
- Phytolaceca for an obese person who has bad breath, feels exhausted and may be unable to think clearly.

See page xv for more information on how to use these treatments. Consult your homeopath for more specific remedies.

Aromatherapy treatment

Use the following oils as bath or body oils to assist weight loss through fluid loss, or stimulating the digestive processes.

- Cedarwood
- Fennel
- Grapefruit
- Juniper
- Lavender
- Rosemary

Use the following oils as bath or body oils or burn in an oil burner.

- Cypress
- Geranium
- Lemon
- Patchouli

For information on how to use these essential oils see page xvi.

Dietary and lifestyle recommendations

- Drink more water; a glass of water before meals helps you to eat less. Drink six to eight glasses of liquid per day (i.e. filtered water or herbal tea).
- Make breakfast your biggest meal of the day as you burn calories faster and more completely one hour after waking than any other time of day. Eat less food after 3 pm as it is more likely to be converted to fat.
- Eat more complex and simple carbohydrates such as: wholegrain breads, wholegrain cereals and pastas, brown rice, rice crackers, corn tortillas, tofu, lentils, beans and fish (not fried).
- Eat low-calorie raw vegetables and fresh fruits like cauliflower, celery, cabbage, carrots, cucumber, broccoli, green beans, onions, lettuce, spinach, turnips, apples, grapefruit, strawberries, rockmelon and watermelon.
- Avoid alcohol, cakes, lollies, chocolates, ice-cream, refined sugar, white flour, salt, white rice, fats, oils, fast food, processed food and junk food.
- Regular bowel movements and a clean colon are important aspects of weight control. Take additional fibre in the form of bran, psyllium husks or guar gum to keep your bowels regular. Take guar gum or psyllium husks with a large glass of water half an hour before meals; this will also reduce your appetite.

- Get some form of regular aerobic exercise such as brisk walking, jogging, aqua-aerobics, swimming or bicycling.
- Take up yoga or tai chi for an improved breathing pattern, increased flexibility and stress management benefits.
- Consult a counsellor for emotional support as this could potentially be a major source of your weight problem.

PEPTIC ULCERS

Description

Peptic ulcers develop when there is erosion of the membrane lining of either the oesophagus, stomach, or duodenum from excess stomach acid (hydodcholric acid), pepsin (a digestive enzyme) and other substances that are potentially harmful. Normally a layer of mucus secreted by the musosal cells protects this from happening. Peptic ulcers are benign lesions that can be chronic or acute and can affect ten percent of people at sometime in their lives. Duodenal ulcers occur in the duodenum and gastric ulcers occur in the stomach.

Symptoms

These include:

- nausea;
- rising acid in the throat;
- burning pain and discomfort often occurring on an empty stomach.

Causes

The cause of peptic ulcers has been associated with smoking, stress, alcohol and certain medications. Diet also plays a major role in the development of stomach ulcers.

Nutritional treatment

Nutritional supplements that may be beneficial in the treatment of peptic ulcers are included in the following table. For more information on how to use these supplements see pages xii–xiii.

Herbal treatments

The following herbs promote healing and aid in the treatment of peptic ulcers. For information on how to use these herbs see pages xiii–xv.

- Licorice promotes healing of gastric and duodenal ulcers.
- Meadowsweet acts to soothe and protect the mucus membranes of the digestive tract. It also reduces acidity and eases nausea.
- Marshmallow is a specific herb to treat inflammations of the digestive tract, including peptic ulcers.
- Centaury is used to treat sluggish digestion, loss of appetite, liver weakness and dyspepsia.
- Slippery Elm is used to treat digestive problems including gastric or duodenal ulcers.

Nutritional supplements for peptic ulcers

SUPPLEMENT	DOSAGE	COMMENT
Vitamin A	100,000 iu daily	Improves mucus deficiency
Vitamin B complex	50 mg three times daily	Nerve tonic that is needed for proper digestion
Vitamin C buffered	One teaspoon daily in water	Improves immunity
Vitamin E	400–800 iu daily	Potent anti-oxidant promotes healing
Multivitamin and mineral complex	As directed on label	To provide essential nutrients
Pectin	As directed on label	Creates a protective coating in the intestines
Zinc	50–80 mg daily	Promotes healing
Acidophilus fibre	One dessertspoon daily	Delays gastric emptying in water

HERBAL TEA:

A combination of the following herbs makes an excellent tea for dyspepsia:

- Centaury;
- Marshmallow root;
- Meadowsweet.

Pour one cup of boiling water onto one teaspoon of the dried herbs and leave for five to 10 minutes to infuse. Strain away the herbs and drink half an hour before meals.

Homeopathic treatment

Treatment that may be prescribed by a homeopath for peptic ulcers includes:

- Nux vomica for digestive disturbances that follow over-indulgence of food, alcohol, coffee and tobacco.
- Bryonia alba for heartburn, pain and diarrhoea.
- Phosphorus for digestive problems caused by overeating.

See page xv for information on how to use these treatments. For chronic deep-seated conditions such as peptic ulcers it is important to consult your homeopath for a more specific treatment.

Aromatherapy treatment

- Chamomile: a very effective oil for relaxation, nervous tension and stress; use as a bath or body oil.
- Clary Sage: a relaxing tonic for tension, stress and ulcers; use as a bath or body oil.

- Geranium: an excellent oil for digestive upsets; use as a bath or body oil.
- Lavender: use as a body oil, bath oil or compress for digestive problems.
- Myrrh: a highly aromatic oil which has a camphor-like scent and is highly prized for its digestive healing qualities; use as an inhalant or massage oil. Myrrh should be avoided during pregnancy.

See page xvi for information on how to use these essential oils.

Dietary and lifestyle recommendations

- Avoid tea, coffee, sugar, tobacco and alcohol.
- Avoid stomach irritants such as hot and spicy foods.
- Avoid frequent milk ingestion.
- Do not use aspirin.
- Eat bananas as they contain active healing properties.
- Cabbage is also recommended as it contains a substance called vitamin U, which has the potential to heal ulcers.

INDIGESTION and HEARTBURN

Description

Indigestion or dyspepsia is a general term for any pain or discomfort in the upper abdomen or chest. The pain or discomfort is usually caused by incomplete digestion or by gastric reflux. Heartburn often accompanies indigestion and is experienced as a burning pain behind the centre of the chest. The pain may sometimes spread from the top of the stomach right up to the back of the mouth.

Symptoms

Symptoms of indigestion include:

- fullness or bloatedness of the abdomen;
- heartburn (caused by gastric reflux);
- nausea;
- belching, flatulence and rumbling noises in the intestines;
- vomiting;
- hiccups;
- abdominal cramping.

Causes

Occasionally, indigestion can be a sign of gallstones, malabsorption, peptic ulcers, candida albicans, or disorders of the liver, gallbladder or pancreas.

Causative factors associated with indigestion may include:

- emotional stress, excess worry, anger, anxiety and fear;
- overeating or eating too quickly or eating with the mouth open (causes swallowing of air whilst eating);
- an unhealthy diet or a diet which includes too much: alcohol, chocolate, citrus juices, tomato products, salad dressings, coffee, tea, sugar and refined carbohydrates, spicy or oily foods;
- smoking;
- over use of aspirin;
- insufficient digestive enzymes or hydrochloric acid in the stomach;
- the overuse of peppermint or spearmint.

Heartburn is caused by regurgitation of hydrochloric acid from stomach up into the oesophagus where it creates inflammation and pain.

IT'S IMPORTANT TO SEE YOUR DOCTOR IF:
- You are over 40 and develop indigestion suddenly, if your bowel movements are affected and/or you have frequent pain and weight loss.

Nutritional treatment

Nutritional supplements that may be beneficial in the treatment of indigestion are included in the following table (see page 200). See pages xii–xiii for information on how to use these supplements.

Herbal treatment

Herbal medicines used to treat indigestion and heartburn are listed below. For information on how to use these herbs see pages xiii–xv.

BITTER HERBS
Bitter herbs tone and strengthen the digestive process. These include:

- Centaury;
- Gentian;
- Golden Seal (avoid during pregnancy);
- Rue;
- Wormwood;
- Yarrow.

ASTRINGENT HERBS
Astringent herbs can ease inflammation of the digestive passageways. Meadowsweet is an excellent astringent herb for indigestion.

CARMINATIVE HERBS
Carminative herbs are rich in volatile oils to stimulate the gut walls and facilitate bowel movements. They include:

- Aniseed;
- Balm;
- Caraway;
- Chamomile;
- Ginger;
- Lavender.

DEMULCENT HERBS
Demulcent herbs are rich in mucilage to soothe and protect inflamed passageways. They include:

Nutritional supplements for indigestion and heartburn

SUPPLEMENT	DOSAGE	COMMENT
Vitamin A	10,000 iu daily	Promotes the secretion of gastric acid and enzymes
Vitamin B complex plus	100 mg with meals	Helps maintain healthy muscle tone in the gastrointestinal tract
Vitamin B1 plus	100 mg daily	Thiamine is required by the stomach to produce hydrochloric acid
Vitamin B6	100 mg daily	Vitamin B6 is required for the production of vital gastric juices
Vitamin B12	500 mcg twice daily	Required for the metabolism of fats, proteins and carbohydrates
L-methionine	Take as directed on label with water or juice after meals	Promotes digestion and the metabolism of fats
Digestive enzymes	Take as directed on label with meals	Assists in the breakdown of food
Acidophilus fibre	As directed on label	Provides fibre and friendly intestinal bacteria
Garlic	As directed on label	Assists digestion and cleans the bowel
Lecithin granules	100 mg three times daily	Increases the solubility of cholesterol

- Comfrey;
- Marshmallow;
- Slippery Elm bark.

INDIGESTION

For indigestion use:

- Agrimony;
- Barberry bark;
- Chamomile;
- Chilli;
- Dandelion;
- Fennel;
- Fenugreek;
- Gentian;
- Ginger;
- Golden Seal (avoid during pregnancy).

NERVOUS INDIGESTION

For nervous indigestion use:

- Chamomile;
- Hops;

- Lemon Balm;
- Vervain.

HEARTBURN

For heartburn use:

- Alfalfa;
- Aloe Vera juice;
- Catnip;
- Chamomile;
- Marshmallow;
- Meadowsweet;
- Slippery Elm powder.

Homeopathic treatment

Treatment that may be prescribed by a homeopath for indigestion and heartburn varies according to the symptoms.

- For indigestion caused by excess intake of alcohol take Nux vomica. Nux vomica is also used for heartburn and indigestion caused by overeating or mental strain.
- For indigestion and a stomach which is full of wind after eating take Carbo vegetabilis. Carbo vegetabilis is also taken for indigestion with cramping pain in the stomach and/or flatulence and/or a bloated stomach.
- For indigestion aggravated by spicy, fatty or rich foods take Pulsatilla.
- For indigestion caused by, or associated with nervousness take Kali phosphoricum.
- For indigestion with nausea and vomiting take Kali bichromium.
- For heartburn use Lycopodium.

See page xv for information on how to use these treatments.

Aromatherapy treatment

An aromatherapy treatment for indigestion would include the following oils:

- Basil (use as a bath or body oil or burn in an incense burner);
- Clary Sage (use as a bath or body oil);
- Clove (burn a few drops in an oil burner);
- Chamomile (use as a bath or body oil);
- Fennel (use as a bath or body oil);
- Ginger (use as a bath or body oil);
- Lavender (use as a bath or body oil);
- Peppermint (use as a bath or body oil or burn in an incense burner).

Fennel oil is a specific aromatherapy oil for indigestion and Peppermint oil is a specific oil for nausea. For heartburn massage the chest and breastbone with warm olive oil mixed with ten percent lemon oil.

For more information on how to use these essential oils see page xvi.

Dietary and lifestyle recommendations

- Eat five or six small meals per day, do not overeat. The last meal should be eaten three to four hours before going to bed. Chew your food thoroughly, take your time eating and don't eat when you are stressed, angry, anxious or overtired. Avoid lying down after meals and elevate the head of your bed slightly.

- Increase your fibre intake by including in your diet: fresh fruits, vegetables, wholegrains and cereals.
- Include fresh pawpaw and pineapple in your diet as these are excellent sources of the digestive enzymes papain and bromelain. Drink fresh pawpaw or pineapple juice to aid digestion and chew a few of the paw paw seeds.
- Take a few sprigs of fresh parsley or one teaspoon of apple cider vinegar (or lemon juice) before meals.
- Avoid lentils, beans, peanuts, soybeans, caffeine, dairy products, spicy/rich/fatty foods, fizzy drinks, chocolate, citrus juices, tomatoes, sugar, junk foods and processed foods, alcohol and nicotine.
- Do not drink liquids while eating (other than those mentioned here) as they dilute the gastric juices.
- Take fresh potato juice mixed with water three times per day.
- Barley broth is very soothing for heartburn, so too is fresh cabbage juice.
- If heartburn is your problem don't use running as a form of exercise as it can bring gastric acids up in the oesophagus.

IT'S IMPORTANT TO SEE YOUR DOCTOR IF YOUR HEARTBURN IS ACCOMPANIED BY:

- Pain when swallowing;
- Vomiting;
- Shortness of breath;
- Black or blood-stained stools;
- Dizziness or light-headedness;
- Chest pain which begins to travel down your left arm.

COELIAC DISEASE

Description and causes

Coeliac disease is an intestinal malabsorption disorder caused by an intolerance to gluten. Gluten is the protein found in wheat, rye, barley and oats.

For sufferers of coeliac disease ingestion of gluten induces destruction of villi (intestinal lining) and inhibits enzyme secretion accompanied by a variable amount of malabsorption. The condition however can be controlled by excluding cereals and grains except rice and corn from the diet.

Symptoms

Symptoms include:

- weight loss;
- diarrhoea;
- bloating;
- vitamin and mineral deficiencies;
- abdominal distension.

Anaemia can also result from this disorder.

Nutritional treatment

Nutritional supplements that may be beneficial in the treatment of coeliac disease are included in the following

Nutritional supplements for coeliac disease		
SUPPLEMENT	DOSAGE	COMMENT
Vitamin A	15,000 iu daily	Essential for the utilisation of all vitamins and minerals. Aids protein digestion
Vitamin B complex	50 mg (use a wheat and yeast free product)	Important for proper digestion and to correct anaemia problems
Vitamin C	2000–5000 mg throughout day	Helps boost immune response
Vitamin E	400 iu daily	An important anti-oxidant to help heal and balance the body
Magnesium with Calcium	750 mg daily 750 mg daily	Essential in balancing the body's PH levels
Zinc lozenges	Take one 15 mg lozenge five times daily	Helps boost immune system and promotes healing

table. See pages xii–xiii for information on how to use these supplements.

Herbal treatment

The following herbs are recommended to help aid and assist the digestive system and are useful for treating coeliac disease.

- Slippery Elm is used to treat inflammation of the mucus-membrane lining of the digestive system.
- Angelica's calmative qualities ease intestinal colic and flatulence.
- Centaury is an aromatic, mild nervine and gastric stimulant.
- Marshmallow is used for the treatment of inflammation of the digestive tract.

- Take Slippery Elm as a powder mixed with warm water. The other herbs can be taken as teas or tinctures. See pages xiii–xv for information on how to use these herbs.

Aromatherapy treatment

The following essential oils may provide relief from the symptoms of coeliac disease.

- Chamomile is a soothing oil used to treat diarrhoea and flatulence. Use as a bath oil, body oil or as an inhalant.
- Melissa is used to treat nervous tension, stress, diarrhoea and headache. Use as a bath oil or body oil.

- Ginger is used to treat digestive problems, including diarrhoea and flatulence. Use as a massage oil.
- Peppermint is a wonderful aromatic oil used in the treatment of digestive disorders, colic, flatulence, headaches, depression, vomiting and diarrhoea. Use as a bath, body oil or as an inhalant.

For information on how to use these essential oils see page xvi.

Dietary and lifestyle recommendations

- Avoid all foods containing gluten. These include wheat, rye, barley and oats.
- Drink plenty of filtered water and natural juices.
- Substitutes for gluten flour are arrowroot, corn, potato, rice and soybean flour.
- To help avoid coeliac disease breastfeed infants to six months of age and then introduce rice and millet rather than wheat.
- Increase your vitamin and mineral intake as coeliac sufferers are usually extremely deficient.

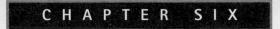
THE REPRODUCTIVE SYSTEM

Maintenance of the reproductive systems

What does it consist of?

Reproduction is the process by which new individuals of a species are produced and the genetic information is passed on from generation to generation. The primary function of the reproductive system, therefore, is to replicate the human being and continue the species.

The organs of the male reproductive system are the testes – a system of long coiled tubes and ducts – and the penis. The testes are a pair of rounded glands, situated in the scrotum, which produce sperm and male sex hormones. The scrotum is a pouch, composed of loose skin, which is divided into two sacs, each containing a single testis.

The organs of the female reproductive system are the ovaries, the fallopian tubes, the uterus (womb), and the vagina, which connects the uterus to the external genitalia. The external genitalia are made up of the clitoris, the labia and the pubic mound and hair.

What does it do?

MALE REPRODUCTIVE ORGANS

From each testis, sperm pass into a long coiled tube where they mature and are stored until they are either ejaculated or reabsorbed into the body. Before ejaculation, sperm are propelled along a long duct called the vas deferens. Fluid secreted by the two seminal vesicles and the prostate gland is added to the sperm to produce semen. Semen provides sperm with a transportation medium and nutrients. The average volume of semen in ejaculation is 2.5–5 ml, with 50–150 million sperm per ml. This large number of sperm is necessary because only a small fraction ever reach the ovum. When the number of sperm falls below 20 million per ml this is termed a 'low sperm count' and the male is likely to be infertile.

FEMALE REPRODUCTIVE ORGANS

From puberty onwards the paired ovaries manufacture the sex hormones (progesterone and oestrogen) which prepare the lining of the uterus for a fertilised egg. The ovaries also store and release the female sex cells, the ova. When a female baby is born each ovary contains all the eggs (about 400,000) that she will ever have. Each month an ovum is released and travels down one of the two fallopian tubes to the uterus. The uterus, situated between the urinary bladder and the rectum, is the size and shape of an inverted pear. The uterus is the site of menstruation, the place where a fertilised ovum embeds itself, and where the foetus develops during pregnancy. If the ovum is not fertilised by the sperm then the egg and the lining of the uterus are shed during menstruation. The lower part of the uterus is called the cervix which protrudes into the vagina and allows sperm, menstrual blood or a body to pass through.

What goes wrong with it?

For men, the most common disorders of the reproductive system are: prostate disorders, impotence, testicular cancer, low sperm count and sexually transmitted diseases.

For women, the most common disorders of the reproductive system are: candida albicans, endometriosis, infertility, cervical cancer and menstrual disorders.

Nutritional treatment

Nutritional supplements that benefit the reproductive system are listed below.

VITAMIN A

Vitamin A protects the mucus membranes of the vagina and uterus and thereby reduces their susceptibility to infection. It is essential for mothers in pregnancy (do not take over 10,000 iu daily if pregnant) and during milk production and breastfeeding. Vitamin

A prevents the formation of cells that could develop into cancerous cells.

VITAMIN B2
Vitamin B2 is essential during lactation and breastfeeding. Deficiency can lead to vaginal itching, eczema of the genitals and some forms of cancer.

VITAMIN B6
Vitamin B6 has been used successfully to treat male sexual disorders. Vitamin B6 alleviates some of the symptoms of premenstrual syndrome (PMS) and as a natural diuretic prevents fluid retention during pregnancy as well as morning sickness. If vitamin B6 deficiency continues through late pregnancy it may result in stillbirths or post delivery infant mortality. Vitamin B6 is also essential for the synthesis and proper functioning of DNA and RNA, which are the genes that are capable of passing on hereditary characteristics.

VITAMIN C
With age, the sex glands develop a greater need for vitamin C. Vitamin C can assist in treating male infertility and cervical dysplasia which can lead to cancer. Vitamin C is drained by menstruation.

VITAMIN E
Vitamin E improves the male sperm count and also prevents the degeneration of the tissues in the testes. Vitamin E normalises the activity of the ovaries in women, improving period regularity and preventing excessive bleeding, dryness and irritation of the genital passages. Vitamin E deficiency in women can be a factor in causing miscarriages and premature births. Vitamin E also prevents haemorrhaging both in the mother and the newborn baby.

ZINC
Zinc is essential for the health of the prostate gland and also for the manufacture of some male hormones and the growth and development of the genital organs. It may also increase the male sex drive and potency, so deficiency of zinc is linked with retarded sexual activity. Zinc deficiency may also cause prostate problems, sperm degeneration and problems with the testicles. Zinc deficiency can also be involved in miscarriages, restricted foetal growth and birth defects such as mental retardation.

CALCIUM
Daily intake of calcium should be considerably increased for mothers during pregnancy, particularly in the third trimester when embryo growth accelerates. The increase should be maintained throughout breastfeeding.

IODINE
Iodine promotes growth and development of the body. Iodine deficiency in pregnancy may result in retarded physical or mental development. These symptoms are reversible if treatment is started soon after birth with iodine supplementation. Kelp is an excellent source of iodine. Iodine deficiency is common.

PHOSPHORUS

Phosphorus is a vital brain and nerve mineral. It plays an important role in the transfer of hereditary characteristics.

IRON

Women need extra iron especially during menstruation and pregnancy. Deficiency can cause anaemia, tiredness and constipation. Difficulty in menstruation (or its absence) may be associated with deficiency of iron and sodium. An expectant mother needs calcium, sodium, iron and silicon in abundance for her growing foetus.

Herbal treatment

There are many herbs that benefit the reproductive system.

UTERINE TONICS

These have a toning and strengthening action on the whole reproductive system. They can be used where no specific acute symptoms are present and general strengthening is indicated. Uterine tonics include the herbs:

- Bayberry;
- Black Cohosh;
- Blessed Thistle;
- Blue Cohosh;
- Chickweed;
- False Unicorn Root;
- Ginseng;
- Motherwort;
- Raspberry;
- Squaw Vine.

RELAXANTS AND ANTISPASMODICS

These relieve menstrual problems such as cramping, headaches, irritability and tension. They include:

- Chamomile;
- Cramp Bark;
- Lady's Slipper;
- Linden;
- Motherwort;
- Passion Flower;
- Skullcap;
- Valerian;
- Vervain;
- Wild Yam.

ALTERATIVES AND LYMPHATIC TONICS

These help to move excess fluid by stimulating the lymphatic system. They also speed up the recovery from any specific illness of the reproductive system. Alteratives and lymphatic tonics include:

- Blue Flag;
- Burdock;
- Cleavers;
- Echinacea;
- Poke Root;
- Sarsaparilla.

DIURETICS

For fluid retention use diuretics such as:

- Celery;
- Corn Silk;
- Cucumber;
- Dandelion;
- Juniper berries;
- Yarrow.

OESTROGENIC-LIKE HERBS

These are used for menopause and some menstrual problems. They include:

- Alfalfa;
- Aniseed;
- Fennel;
- Hops;
- Licorice;
- Parsley;
- Red Clover;
- Sage;
- Soybean sprouts.

PROGESTERONE PRECURSORS

Herbs which act as progesterone precursors are used for menopause and some menstrual problems. They include:

- Fenugreek;
- Sarsaparilla;
- Wild Yam.

MORNING SICKNESS

Herbs for morning sickness include:

- Ginger;
- Peppermint;
- Raspberry leaf.

Aromatherapy treatment

There are many essential oils that benefit the reproductive system.

- Use Jasmine as a bath or body oil, or burn in an oil burner, for menstrual problems, uterine disorders, childbirth and generally for pain in the whole female reproductive system.

- Use Nutmeg as a bath or body oil, or burn in an oil burner for impotence and frigidity.
- Use Frankincense as a bath or body oil, or burn in an oil burner for supporting pregnancy and for uterine disorders.

MENSTRUAL PROBLEMS

For menstrual problems use the following aromatherapy oils:

- Basil (use as a bath, body or burner oil);
- Chamomile (use as a bath or body oil);
- Clary Sage (use as a bath or body oil);
- Cypress (use as a bath, body or burner oil);
- Geranium (use as a bath, body or burner oil);
- Ginger (use as a bath or body oil);
- Hyssop (use as a bath, body or burner oil);
- Juniper (use as a bath or body oil);
- Melissa (use as a bath, body or burner oil);
- Neroli (use as a bath, body or burner oil);
- Rose (use as a bath, body or burner oil);
- Sage (use as a bath or body oil);
- Thyme (use as a bath or body oil).

APHRODISIACS

Use the following oils as bath or body oils, or burnt in an oil burner:

- Cinnamon;
- Jasmine;
- Nutmeg;

- Patchouli;
- Rose;
- Ylang Ylang.

Dietary and lifestyle recommendations

FOODS

There are many foods that benefit the reproductive system. They include:

- asparagus;
- beans;
- beetroot;
- berries;
- blackberries;
- carrots;
- dates;
- egg yolk;
- figs;
- goat's milk;
- grapes;
- lettuce;

- lecithin;
- parsley;
- peas;
- peaches;
- potatoes;
- prunes;
- pumpkin seeds;
- radishes;
- raisins;
- spinach;
- sesame seeds;
- watercress.

JUICES

Juices that benefit the reproductive system are listed below.

- Parsley, pineapple and prune juices are excellent sources of zinc.
- Apricot, beetroot, pineapple, pear, and prune juices are good sources of iron.
- Pineapple juice, egg yolk and wheat germ is a good general tonic for the reproductive system.
- Carrot juice, coconut milk and wheatgerm is another good general tonic.

CANDIDA ALBICANS

Description

Candida, or thrush as it is commonly known, is a fungal infection that inhabits the vagina, intestines, mouth, oesophagus and throat. Normally this fungus co-exists happily in the body with other yeasts and bacteria, however if the immune system becomes run down the fungi can multiply and cause infection known as candidiasis.

If the fungi develops in the vagina it is called vaginitis and there is usually a thick white discharge accompanied by irritation and inflammation. Candida can be transmitted sexually when a woman has vaginal thrush so it is important that both partners be treated to prevent reinfection.

Candida can also manifest in the oral cavity and appears as small white pimples on the throat, tongue, cheeks and gums.

The condition is very common in newborn babies and can be transferred from mother to baby via breastfeeding. The mother's nipples can also be infected.

Symptoms

Symptoms of vaginitis include thick white discharge, severe itchiness and inflammation.

Symptoms of other fungal infections are: lethargy, depression, recurring infections, low immunity, intermittent diarrhoea and constipation, flatulence, skin eruptions, menstrual problems, digestive disorders and poor concentration.

Causes

Causes can often be related to the use of antibiotics, oral contraceptives, food allergies and environmental pollutants.

Nutritional treatment

Nutritional supplements that may be beneficial in the treatment of candida albicans are included in the following table. See pages xii–xiii for information on how to use these supplements.

Herbal treatment

For information on how to use the following herbs see pages xiii–xv.

VAGINAL INFECTIONS

The following herbs can be used in the treatment of vaginal infections.

- Beth Root
- Calendula
- Cleavers
- Comfrey
- Echinacea

Nutritional supplements for candida albicans		
SUPPLEMENT	DOSAGE	COMMENT
Acidophilus fibre	One dessertspoon in water daily	Improves the bowel and vaginal flora
Vitamin B complex	100 mg three times daily	Nourishes the nerves and regulates the conversion of food to energy. Important for building healthy cells
Vitamin B12	1500 mcg three times daily	Essential for the metabolism of fats, proteins and carbohydrates
Vitamin C	1000 mg three times daily	Increases immunity
Garlic	Two capsules three times daily	Inhibits the infection organism
Calcium and Magnesium	1500 mg daily 750 mg daily	People with candida often are deficient in calcium Magnesium enables proper absorption of calcium
Multivitamin and mineral complex	As directed on label	Essential for proper immune system

- Garlic
- Golden Seal (avoid during pregnancy)
- Oak bark
- Periwinkle
- Poke Root

These herbs can be taken as teas or tinctures or a herbal tea can be made by combining two parts Beth Root, with two parts Echinacea, two parts Periwinkle, and one part Cleavers.

This tea should be taken three times daily. The mixture can also be used as a vaginal douche providing relief from irritation and inflammation.

Another vaginal douche recipe uses equal parts of Calendula, Comfrey and Golden Seal. Add two drops of Echinacea.

CANDIDA

- German Chamomile can be used as an effective herbal treatment for candida. Use as a tea or herbal tincture.
- Ginger, Cinnamon and Rosemary contain powerful candida killing substances. Use as a tea, herbal tincture or as a culinary herb in cooking.

For a more thorough diagnosis and prescription of herbal remedies for treating candida consult your herbalist or natural health practitioner.

Homeopathic treatment

Genital and oral thrush can be treated using the following homeopathic remedies.

- Borax is used to treat vaginal discharge that is white and mucusy, accompanied by a burning feeling. It is also used for thrush of the mouth and tongue (especially in children) and thrush that is worse in breastfeeding.
- Mercurius solubilis is used to treat genital thrush, when there is a burning sensation and a strong odour. Also used to treat oral thrush in babies and children that is accompanied by bad breath and excess saliva.
- Natrum muriaticum is used to treat oral thrush, with a white-coated tongue, sore gums and a dry mouth that is accompanied by thirst.
- Nitricum acidum is used to treat genital thrush, with a strong smelling discharge, itching and burning sensations.

For more information on how to use these treatments see page xv.

Aromatherapy treatment

Essential oils that may be of assistance in the treatment of candida are:

- Ginger (use as a massage oil for the treatment of diarrhoea, menstruation problems and fungal infections);
- Rose (a wonderful aromatic oil used as a bath oil, body oil or in a compress to treat nerves, depression, digestion and menstruation disorders);
- Chamomile (use as a bath oil, body oil or compress. Chamomile can be

effective in treating headache, depression, diarrhoea and flatulence);

- Thyme (used as a bath oil or massage oil, thyme is a great healer of anxiety, fatigue and other symptoms of candida).

See page xvi for more information on how to use essential oils.

Dietary and lifestyle recommendations

- Avoid using antibiotics, steroids and birth control pills unless absolutely necessary as these drugs only contribute to causing and worsening candida.
- Avoid refined sugars, found in processed foods, fruit juices, honey and maple syrup.
- Consult your natural health practitioner and ask for a candida control diet.
- Do increase your intake of yoghurt as it contains lactobacillus acidophilus, a type of bacteria which retards the growth of candida.
- For oral thrush avoid medicated mouth wash as this can destroy healthy bacteria.

GENITAL THRUSH
- Avoid soap and vaginal deodorants.
- Make sure to wash the area frequently in cool water. Try adding one cup of cider vinegar to your bath water.
- Apply live yoghurt to the effected area to ease the itching. (See also herbal douches under herbal treatments, pages 211–12).
- Avoid nylon underwear and tight-fitting jeans.

IT'S IMPORTANT TO SEE YOUR DOCTOR OR A NATUROPATH IF:
- The condition has not improved within a few days.

ENDOMETRIOSIS
Description

Endometriosis is a disorder that occurs when the cells from the endometrium – the lining of the uterus – migrate to other parts of the pelvic cavity via the fallopian tubes. These cells attach to other organs such as the bowel, bladder, fallopian tubes, ovaries and intestines. The cells bleed during menstruation and this can cause great discomfort for the woman.

Endometriosis can block the fallopian tubes and in some cases cause infertility. Diagnosis of the condition is often made by a procedure called a laparoscopy. This involves the insertion of a tiny tube called a laparoscope via a small incision in the navel. Orthodox medical practitioners often prescribe medication to suppress menstruation or surgery to cauterise the endometriosis.

Symptoms

These include pain during menstruation (sometimes heavy bleeding occurs), pain and discomfort during intercourse, diarrhoea and cramps.

Causes

These are a number of theories regarding the causes of endometriosis. The theories are related to hereditary, stress and age, however as yet the cause is unknown.

Nutritional treatment

Nutritional supplements that may be beneficial in the treatment of endometriosis are included in the following table. For information on how to use these supplements see pages xii–xiii.

Herbal treatment

The following herbs can be effective in treating reproductive disorders, painful menstruation, ovarian pain and excessive bleeding.

- Beth Root is an uterine tonic that is used to treat excessive blood loss due to menstruation.
- Cranesbill combines well with Beth Root to treat blood loss.
- Cramp Bark relaxes the uterus, relieves ovarian cramp and period cramp.
- Jamaican Dogwood relieves pain during menstruation and ovarian pain. It combines well with Black Haw.

Nutritional supplements for endometriosis

SUPPLEMENT	DOSAGE	COMMENT
Vitamin B complex plus pantothenic acid	As directed on label 100 mg three times daily	Essential for the healthy function of the reproductive organs
Vitamin C with bioflavonoids	1000 mg three times daily	Important for healthy ovaries
Vitamin E	400 iu daily	Normalises ovary activity and improves menstrual regularity
Vitamin K	200 mg daily	Is effective in reducing excessive blood loss during menstruation
Iron	As directed by physician	Essential for the formation of red blood cells. Needs replenishing after menstruation.
Zinc	50 mg daily	Important for the healthy function of the reproductive organs

- Pasque Flower is an excellent herb used to treat pain and discomfort associated with menstruation.
- Valerian is an antispasmodic herb used to relax and relieve cramping.

For a more specific diagnosis and prescription to treat endometriosis see your natural therapist or herbalist. See pages xiii–xv for information on how to use these herbs.

Homeopathic treatment

Some homeopathic remedies that may be helpful in treating problems associated with endometriosis are:

- Belladonna for heavy, painful periods, with bright red, clotted blood. Also use if pain is worse before and during menstruation;
- Nux vomica is used for heavy, painful cramping periods and lower back pain;
- Calcarea phosphorica is used for dark red blood that is often clotted and painful heavy periods. It is used as an effective tonic when women become anaemic following heavy menstruation.

For more information on using homeopathics see page xv.

Aromatherapy treatment

Aromatherapy can be extremely useful in helping treat menstruation pain and other associated problems. The following oils are recommended for disorders such as endometriosis.

- Basil (use as a bath oil or as an inhalant)
- Chamomile (can be used as a bath oil, body oil or compress)
- Frankincense (use as a massage oil, bath oil or burn incense)
- Geranium (use as a bath oil, body oil, compress or inhalant)
- Rose (use as a bath oil, body oil or compress)

A compress is made by soaking a clean cloth in warm water which has a few drops of essential oil in it. Squeeze the cloth out and place on the specific part of the body that needs treating, then wrap this area with a warm damp towel. Leave the compress on until the cloth cools down and repeat.

For more information on using essential oils see page xvi.

Dietary and lifestyle recommendations

- A well-balanced diet is essential. Eat plenty of fresh fruit and vegetables, wholegrains, nuts and legumes.
- Avoid stress by introducing yoga, meditation or relaxation techniques into your daily routine.
- Do have the condition properly diagnosed by a physician. This may involve a short hospital procedure called a laparoscopy.
- Acupuncture can be very effective in treating this condition.
- Avoid caffeine found in coffee, tea, chocolate and cola drinks. Give up smoking.

- Regular exercise can be of great assistance to women suffering from pain associated with endometriosis. Research has proven that women who do regular exercise suffer less pain before and during menstruation.

IMPOTENCE

Description and symptoms

Impotence is the inability to obtain, or to sustain, an erection suitable for penetration and ejaculation.

There are two kinds of impotence: organic and psychogenic. Organic impotence has a physical cause while psychogenic impotence has a psychological cause.

Previously, it was assumed that impotence was primarily a psychological problem but now many therapists believe that as many as 85 percent of all cases of impotence have a physical basis.

Causes

Organic impotence is due to, or associated with, an underlying physical disorder such as:

- disorders of the heart and blood vessels, e.g. atherosclerosis;
- diabetes (probably the most common physical cause);
- kidney failure and liver disease;
- anaemia;
- traumatic injuries (e.g. pelvic fracture, spinal cord damage)

- excess use of alcohol and/or cigarettes;
- high blood pressure;
- the effects of a surgical operations;
- hormonal disturbances such as diminished levels of testosterone or thyroid hormone dysfunction.

Organic impotence usually develops slowly over a period of time.

Impotence which has an underlying psychological nature is known as psychogenic impotence. Causes include guilt, aggression, emotional stress or feelings of inadequacy. Psychogenic impotence can also be associated with depression, anxiety and the use of such drugs as: antidepressants, antihistamines, antihypertensives, diuretics, narcotics, sedatives and ulcer medications.

Nutritional treatment

Nutritional supplements that may be beneficial in the treatment of impotence are included in the following table. For more information on how to use these supplements see pages xii–xiii.

Herbal treatment

All of the following herbs can be taken as teas or tinctures. See pages xiii–xv for more information on how to use these herbs.

- Damiana is a specific herb, used in many cultures, for treating low libido and impotence. Damiana improves blood flow to the genitals and relaxes the mind while increasing vitality.

- Damiana, Ginseng and Saw Palmetto are especially useful for psychogenic impotence.
- If impotence arises from emotional stress and nervous tension then nerve relaxants are useful, such as Lime Blossom, Oats and Skullcap.
- Wild Yam and Sarsaparilla are natural substances which have testosterone and steroid-like effects to increase desire and vigour in sexual activity. Ginseng is also known to increase sexual desire.
- Other herbs that are useful in treating impotence are: Dong Quai, Burdock and Gotu Kola.

Homeopathic treatment

Treatment that may be prescribed by a homeopath includes:

- Lycopodium for persistent cases of impotence or if you feel the surge of sexual desire but anticipate failure;

- Arnica for organic impotence caused by injury or bruising;
- Agnus castus in the early stages of this problem or if the erection in not firm enough for penetration;
- Argentum nitricum if there is definite anxiety and fear of sexual activity;
- Conium for an erection which does not last even though sexual desire is strong.

See page xv for information on how to use these treatments.

Aromatherapy treatment

The following essential oils are recommended for the treatment of impotence. See page xvi for information on how to use these oils.

- Massage the lower back area (definitely not the genital area) with diluted Black Pepper oil and Ginger oil.
- Use Clary Sage or Ylang Ylang essential oils as bath or body oils. Ylang Ylang can be used as a

---

Nutritional supplements for impotence

SUPPLEMENT	DOSAGE	COMMENT
Vitamin A	15,000 iu daily	Important for adrenal cortex and steroid hormone synthesis. It is also an anti- oxidant.
Vitamin B complex	50 mg three times daily	Necessary for rebuilding a healthy nervous system, especially one that has been depleted by stress
Vitamin B6	50 mg three times daily	Involved in the synthesis of essential fatty acids and hormones

Nutritional supplements for impotence

SUPPLEMENT	DOSAGE	COMMENT
Zinc	75 mg daily	Essential for the health of the prostate gland and for the manufacture of many male hormones
Vitamin E	500–1000 iu daily	Improves circulation and regulates the synthesis of sex hormones
Essential fatty acids (e.g. canola oil)	One teaspoon three times daily	Improves blood circulation
L-tyrosine	500 mg twice daily on an empty stomach (do not take if taking an MAO inhibitor)	Used for treating a low libido. Acts as a precursor of many hormones

medicine by taking five drops of the essence on a little brown sugar after meals.

- Sandalwood can be used as a bath or body oil, or burnt in an oil burner for treating impotence.

Dietary and lifestyle recommendations

- Eat a healthy, well-balanced diet which is low in fat, alcohol and caffeine. A high-fat diet affects the penis as well as the heart. Especially avoid alcohol before sexual activity.
- Lose weight if you need to and get some regular exercise, which will increase your blood circulation. Don't exercise right before sex.

- Consult a counsellor or hypnotherapist for emotional problems which interfere with your sexual potency. Acupuncture can also be very helpful.
- Nuts (almonds, cashews, hazelnuts, brazil nuts and walnuts) and seeds (sunflower, sesame and pumpkin) are excellent sources of zinc and should be included in your diet. Rice, barley, garlic, onions, soybeans, and asparagus are also very good sources of zinc.
- Relaxation, meditation, tai chi or yoga may also be extremely helpful in alleviating the stress and performance anxiety component of impotence.

INFERTILITY and STERILITY

Description and symptoms

The usual medical definition of infertility is failure to became pregnant after a year of regular, unprotected sexual intercourse during the period of ovulation. Infertility may also refer to the inability to carry or retain a fertilised egg within the womb for the full term of pregnancy. The failure of intercourse to result in a full-term pregnancy can be due to the man's inability to fertilise the egg, the woman's inability to conceive and/or retain the fertilised egg or to both causes. About 20 percent of couples have problems involving infertility.

Causes

For men, infertility is most commonly associated with a low sperm count, which may be due to:

* varicocele (a varicose vein of the spermatic cord);
* testicular mumps, or other previous genito-urinary infections;
* excessive alcohol consumption and/or smoking;
* raised temperature around the testes caused by recent acute illness, prolonged fever or even by tight pants and being in constantly heated environments;
* certain prescription drugs, such as co-trimoxazole and testerone;
* exposure to radiation, toxins or excessive heat.

For women, infertility is most commonly associated with:

* failure to ovulate;
* blockage of the fallopian tubes (due to scarring from infections);
* endometriosis;
* uterine fibroids;
* an allergic reaction to the male's sperm;
* hormonal imbalances;
* abnormal development of the uterus;
* pelvic inflammatory disease;
* being underweight;
* chlamydia.

The following natural therapy treatments are intended to assist either or both partners to play their role in achieving a full-term pregnancy. The most common and simplest orthodox treatments are ovulation stimulation and artificial insemination. The recommended natural therapies are suggested to complement (not replace) orthodox treatments, although in mild cases of infertility natural therapies may be sufficient on their own. Acupuncture can be very useful. A correct diagnosis (from your doctor and naturopath) is extremely important before choosing your treatment alternatives.

Nutritional treatment

Nutritional supplements that may be beneficial in the treatment of infertility are included in the following table. See pages xii–xiii for information on how to use nutritional supplements.

Herbal treatment

HERBS FOR MEN
Herbs for men which enhance potency, sperm production and motility include:

- Astragalus;
- Damiana;
- Ginseng;
- Sarsaparilla;
- Saw Palmetto.

Astragalus is a specific herb for stimulating sperm motility.

Nutritional supplements for infertility		
SUPPLEMENT	DOSAGE	COMMENT
Vitamin A	10,000 iu daily	Helps regulate hormonal imbalances and is important in the functioning of reproductive glands. Needed for the female reproductive organs
Vitamin B complex plus Vitamin B6	50 mg three times daily 50 mg three times daily	Important for nervous system and for the functioning of reproductive glands Helps infertility in women and reduces the possibility of birth defects
Vitamin C with bioflavonoids	1 g daily	Essential if carnitine is taken and helps maintain the ovaries as well as improving sperm mobility. Revitalises the sperm
Vitamin E	200 iu daily	Helps regulate the production of cervical mucus and sex hormones. Also may stimulate the production of new sperm
Essential fatty acids • Linseed oil or • Sunflower oil or • Soy oil or • Evening Primrose oil	One teaspoon three times daily	Important for normal glandular functioning of the reproductive system

Nutritional supplements for infertility

SUPPLEMENT	DOSAGE	COMMENT
PABA	50 mg daily	May restore fertility in some women by stimulating the pituitary gland
Zinc orotate	100 mg daily	For both partners as it is essential for potency, sperm production and conception
Selenium	200 mcg daily	Deficiency has been linked with both sterility in men and infertility in women
Chromium	250 mcg daily	Deficiency is associated with a low sperm count
Carnitine	200 mg three times daily	An important amino acid found in the testicles
L-arginine plus	8 g daily for a month (not for sufferers of herpes or schizophrenia)	Improves sperm count and mobility. Protects the function of sex glands and hormones
L-cysteine plus	250 mg daily	
L-methionine	500 mg daily	

HERBS FOR WOMEN

Herbs for the female reproductive system include:

- Blue Cohosh;
- Damiana;
- Dong Quai;
- False Unicorn Root;
- Ginseng;
- Gotu Kola;
- Licorice Root;
- Raspberry leaf;
- Squaw Vine;
- Wild Yam Root.

UTERINE TONICS

Herbs which act as uterine tonics include:

- Blue Cohosh;
- Cramp Bark;
- False Unicorn Root.

FEMALE INFERTILITY

Herbs which benefit infertility in women include:

- Raspberry leaf;
- Red Clover;
- Sarsaparilla;
- Sweet Violet.

MISCARRIAGE

Herbs which help prevent miscarriage include:

- Alfalfa;
- Blue Cohosh;

- Cramp Bark;
- False Unicorn Root;
- Raspberry leaf;
- Sarsaparilla.

These herbs can be taken as teas, tinctures and some are available as tablets. See pages xiii–xv for information on how to use these herbs. Consult your naturopath or herbalist for the most appropriate and effective combination of herbs for you.

Homeopathic treatment

Treatment that may be prescribed by a homeopath for infertility includes:

- Sabina for women who have had miscarriages before 12 weeks of pregnancy;
- Sepia for threatened miscarriage around the fifth to seventh month of pregnancy with chronic heaviness and dragging in the pelvis. Sepia is also used for irregular periods, feeling chilly, weepy, irritable and averse to sex. For men, Sepia is used for dragging sensation in the genitals and no desire for sex;
- Kali carbonicum is used for women who miscarry easily around the third month of pregnancy and suffer from tiredness, persistent backache and low uterus;
- Borax veneta is used for female infertility that is accompanied by a strong smelling discharge;
- Conium maculaturn is used for infertility with scanty periods and painful breasts.

See page xv for information on how to use these treatments.

Aromatherapy treatment

The following essential oils may be beneficial in the treatment of infertility.

IMPOTENCE

For treatment of impotence use:

- Ginger as a massage oil;
- Nutmeg as a bath or body oil;
- Ylang Ylang as a bath or body oil;
- Clary Sage as a bath or body oil.

FRIGIDITY

For frigidity use:

- Ylang Ylang as a bath or body oil;
- Clary Sage as a bath or body oil.

INFERTILITY

For infertility use:

- Ylang Ylang as a bath or body oil;
- Sandalwood as a bath or body oil or burn in an oil burner;
- Clary Sage as a bath or body oil.

See page xvi for information on how to use these essential oils.

Dietary and lifestyle recommendations

- Improve your level of fitness with regular, non-vigorous, exercise. Too much exercise can lower sperm count and lessen ovulation.
- Avoid all alcohol as it reduces the sperm count in men and in women it can prevent implantation of the fertilised egg.

- Avoid tobacco and being around smokers, and reduce caffeine intake.
- Eliminate (or reduce) refined carbohydrates such as sugars, soft drinks, chocolate, white flour and ice-cream. Reduce fried foods, junk foods and processed foods. Eat a variety of whole foods, fresh fruit and vegetables, dried beans, fish and lean meat.
- Take some pumpkin seeds, bee pollen (if not allergic) or royal jelly. Also take a strong multivitamin and mineral combination.
- Hot baths and hot tubs (spas and saunas) should be avoided.
- Reduce stress factors in your lifestyle, rest and learn a stress management technique like therapeutic breathing, yoga, tai chi, autogenic relaxation or meditation.

PREMENSTRUAL SYNDROME

Description

Premenstrual syndrome (PMS) covers a number of different symptoms experienced by women in the ten to 14 day period between ovulation and the beginning of menstruation. These symptoms vary from woman to woman. Some women are affected in a minor way while others experience a number of symptoms which at times can be quite disabling. The symptoms experienced by women suffering PMS are not only physical but can be emotional and behavioural as well. In severe but rare cases some women may become suicidal or extremely violent.

Symptoms

Symptoms of PMS include:

- breast tenderness;
- abdominal pain;
- headache;
- backache;
- anger;
- stress;
- irritability;
- sugar craving;
- mood swings;
- skin eruptions;
- fluid retention.

Causes

The causes of PMS are most often related to hormonal imbalance, due to an excess of oestrogen and low levels of progesterone in the second half of a woman's menstrual cycle.

Nutritional treatment

Nutritional supplements that may be beneficial in the treatment of PMS are included in the table on page 224. See pages xii–xiii for information on how to use these supplements.

Herbal treatment

There are number of herbs that can be used to ease the symptoms of PMS.

- Skullcap relaxes nervous tension, and is especially useful when combined with Valerian.

- Valerian has effective sedative and antispasmodic actions that may be useful in treating cramp and period pain.
- Cramp Bark is an antispasmodic herb that relaxes the uterus to relieve painful menstruation cramps.

HERBAL TEA

To make a herbal tea for PMS combine one teaspoon of Valerian root and one teaspoon of Skullcap (the dried herb). Infuse for ten to 15 minutes in a cup of boiling water. This can be drunk three times a day or when needed.

For more information on how to use these herbs see pages xiii–xv.

Homeopathic treatment

Homeopathy can be used very successfully to treat PMS. See page xv for information on how to use the following treatments.

- Sepia is used to treat tender breasts, fatigue and anger.
- Pulsatilla is used when the sufferer is tearful, moody, depressed, craves comforting, and feels better for fresh air.

Nutritional supplements for premenstrual syndrome		
SUPPLEMENT	DOSAGE	COMMENT
Vitamin B complex	100 mg daily	Essential to reduce nervous tension, stress and anxiety. Helps relieve breast pain
Vitamin B6	100 mg daily	Beneficial in reducing fluid retention. Helps restore oestrogen
Vitamin C	500 mg daily	Boosts immune function
Vitamin E	200 iu daily	To help normalise hormone levels
Magnesium and	400–800 mg daily	Needed to balance the nervous system
Calcium	1500 mg daily	Helps relieve cramp and backache
Multivitamin and mineral complex	As directed on label	Needed for the proper function and balance of the immune system
Kelp	Four tablets daily or as directed on label	Excellent source of essential minerals
Zinc	15 mg daily	Needed to boost the immune system
Iron	As directed on label	Helps alleviate anaemia associated with menstruation
Evening Primrose oil	500 mg twice daily	Can relieve symptoms of PMS

- Natrum muriaticum is used when the sufferer has lower back pain, is depressed, and needs to be alone.
- Nux vomica is used when the sufferer is angry, impatient, anxious, and has an aching lower back and cramps.

Aromatherapy treatment

The essential oils used in aroma-therapy can be of great benefit to women suffering from PMS. Included here are a number of oils used to treat symptoms of depression, nervous tension, anxiety, menstrual pain and discomfort. All are conditions associated with premenstrual syndrome. See page xvi for information on how to use these essential oils.

- Chamomile
- Clary Sage
- Frankincense
- Neroli
- Ylang Ylang

These can all be used as uplifting, soothing, calming, bath oils. Just place a few drops of any of these oils in a hot bath, lie back and relax.

The following oils can all be used in a fragrance or oil burner. Place a few drops of the essential oil in the water and light the candle beneath. These fragrances will balance and harmonise the emotions.

- Bergamot
- Geranium
- Lavender

Dietary and lifestyle recommendations

- Eat a well-balanced diet, with plenty of fresh fruit and vegetables, wholegrains, nuts and legumes.
- Avoid caffeine, tobacco and alcohol as they can accentuate the symptoms of PMS.
- Regular exercise helps to eliminate toxins from the body and balance hormone levels.
- Avoid all saturated fats, refined sugars and processed foods as these can contribute to fluid retention and depression.
- Take nutritional supplements, especially vitamin B complex, calcium and magnesium, vitamin C and Evening Primrose oil. They may hold the key to avoiding the symptoms of premenstrual syndrome.

PROSTATE ENLARGEMENT and PROSTATITIS

Description

The prostate gland is a small sex gland which lies at the base of the male bladder, surrounding the urethra, which carries urine from the bladder through the penis to the outside.

The prostate is approximately the size of a golf ball and its main function is to produce a secretion which makes up part of the semen. This secretion is essential for the nutrition of the sperm as they try to fertilise an egg (ovum) in the woman. The prostate is the most common site of disorders in the male reproductive system. The most common prostate problem is benign prostatic hyperplasia (BPH) or prostate enlargement.

Prostatitis is inflammation of the prostate; it is common in older men but can be present in younger men as well.

Symptoms

Symptoms of prostate enlargement include:

* bladder obstruction with the need to urinate more frequently, need to urinate at night, and incomplete emptying of the bladder;
* pain, burning and difficulty in starting and stopping urine flow;
* the presence of blood in the urine;
* sometimes associated kidney damage and bladder infections.

Symptoms of prostatitis include:

* pain between the scrotum and rectum;
* a discharge from the penis;
* frequent urination accompanied by a burning sensation fever;
* aches and pains in the back, rectum and between the legs.

As prostatitis develops it can lead to increasingly difficult urination, premature ejaculation, blood in the urine and impotency.

Prostatitis can be spread to the man's sexual partner in whom it may cause pelvic inflammatory disease.

Causes

The prostate tends to enlarge in middle or old age due to the excessive growth of the glandular cells it contains. This increased growth is benign (not malignant) and is often associated with a drop in sexual activity. This gradual enlargement of the prostate occurs in slightly more than half of all men over the age of 50, and three-quarters of men of 70 years of age. The condition if left untreated will eventually obstruct the bladder outlet, resulting in urine in the blood.

Orthodox treatment of enlarged prostate includes drug treatment, hormone therapy (which can affect libido and potency) and surgery to remove part or all of the prostate. Alternative therapies (dietary, herbal, and nutritional supplements and homeopathy) have been proved to be useful in treating BPH.

Prostatitis is usually caused by a bacterial infection which moves up the urethra from outside or which spreads from other parts of the body. The infection can be sexually transmitted.

Hormonal changes associated with ageing may also be a cause.

Nutritional treatment

Nutritional supplements that may be beneficial in the treatment of prostate enlargement and prostatis are included in the following table (see page 228). See pages xii–xiii for information on how to use these supplements.

Herbal treatment

Use the following herbs as teas, tinctures or tablets. For more information on how to use these herbs see pages xiii–xv.

HERBAL TONICS
Herbal tonics for the male reproductive system include:

- Damiana;
- Ginseng;
- Saw Palmetto.

Saw Palmetto is a specific herb for enlarged prostate gland, or it can be combined with Horsetail and Hydrangea. Horsetail is also a specific herb for prostatitis and enlarged prostate.

PROSTATITIS
A mixture of the following herbs may be useful for prostatitis. Mix equal parts of these herbs to make a herbal infusion or take equal parts of herbal tinctures.

- Barberry
- Echinacea
- Horsetail
- Hydrangea

Barberry and Echinacea deal with infection while the other herbs are diuretics. Horsetail is an astringent and can be used if small amounts of blood are present in the urine.

URINARY TRACT TONICS AND DIURETICS
The following herbs are urinary tract tonics and diuretics:

- Bearberry;
- Juniper berries;
- Parsley;
- Slippery Elm bark.

Homeopathic treatment

Treatment that may be prescribed by a homeopath for prostatitis and enlarged prostate varies according to the symptoms. See page xv for information on how to use these treatments.

- Use Ferrum picricum for frequent urination at night, a feeling of fullness and pressure in the rectum and maybe retention of urine within the bladder.
- Use Pulsatilla for prostate enlargement with yellow, turbid urine. Also use Pulsatilla for prostatitis if there is pain and urgency when urinating but urine is only passed in drops.

Nutritional supplements for prostate enlargement and prostatitis

SUPPLEMENT	DOSAGE	COMMENT
Vitamin A	10,000 iu daily	Involved in steroid hormone synthesis and strengthens the immune system
Vitamin B complex plus	100 mg daily	Nourishes the nervous system and important for building healthy cells
Vitamin B6	50 mg three times daily	Involved in hormone synthesis and helps to prevent arteriosclerosis
Vitamin C	1000–5000 mg daily	Regulates cholesterol and promotes immune function
Vitamin E	500 iu daily	Improves immune system, regulates synthesis of sex hormones and improves circulation
Zinc gluconate lozenges	50–100 mg daily	Reduces the size of the prostate and is involved in many aspects of hormonal metabolism
Magnesium and Calcium	500 mg daily (combined dosage)	Calms the nervous system and may prevent hardening of the arteries, which aggravates the prostate
Amino acids • Glycine • Alanine • Glutamic acid	 200 mg daily 200 mg daily 200 mg daily	This combination relieves many of the symptoms of prostate enlargement
Essential fatty acids • Linseed oil or • Sunflower oil or • Evening Primrose oil or • Soy oil	One teaspoon three times daily	Normalises the levels of prostatic and seminal lipids
Lecithin	One tablespoon three times daily before meals	Regulates cholesterol levels and has a favourable effect on enlarged prostate
Kelp	1000 mg daily	Supplies a range of minerals to improve prostate function

- Use Thuja for prostatitis with a frequent urgent desire to urinate but the urine stream cannot be controlled, being split and weak. Enlarged prostate may also be present.
- Use Saw Palmetto for prostate enlargement with painful intercourse or difficult, painful urination.
- Use Clematis for prostatitis with intermittent urine flow and burning pain with the initial few drops of urine.
- Use Equisetum for pains on passing urine and heavy sensation in the bladder.
- Use Causticum for any accompanying bladder weakness.

Aromatherapy treatment

Use the following essential oils as bath or body oils for fluid retention:

- Cypress (avoid if you have high blood pressure);
- Clary Sage;
- Fennel;
- Geranium;
- Juniper;
- Orange;
- Rosemary;
- Sage.

Geranium is a specific essential oil for the reproductive and urinary organs and can be used as a bath or body oil, burnt in an oil burner or applied as a compress. Soak a clean cloth in warm water, add ten drops of essential oil, squeeze out and place around the bladder area, then wrap with a warm, damp towel.

Clary Sage and Geranium essential oils can be mixed together with a base of almond oil to massage the whole body.

See page xvi for more information on how to use these oils.

Dietary and lifestyle recommendations

- Avoid coffee, tea, chocolate and soft drinks as these tend to tighten the neck of the bladder and make urination more difficult. Eliminate alcohol (especially beer and wine) and tobacco, spicy foods, chlorinated and fluoridated water.
- Increase your fluid intake to avoid dehydration and to promote urine flow. Cranberry juice (250 ml three times daily) is recommended for enlarged prostate.
- Hydrotherapy in the form of a sitz bath is recommended for enlarged prostate; immerse the pelvic region in a hot bath (40°–45° Celsius) for five to ten minutes. The feet can be immersed in a separate small tub (43°–46° Celsius) for extra benefits.
- Check your cholesterol level.
- For prostate gland enlargement drink vegetable juice made of equal parts of carrot, cucumber and beetroot.
- Include more raw onion in your diet.
- Massage the prostate area (particularly with oils mentioned in the aromatherapy treatment

section, page 229), have more sex (for mild to moderate conditions) and remember to empty your bladder before going to bed.

- Get more regular exercise (not cycling) and take up a stress management technique like relaxation, meditation or yoga.

ZINC RICH FOODS

Eat more zinc-rich foods including:

- almonds;
- asparagus;
- brazil nuts;
- brewer's yeast;
- cashews;
- garlic;
- lettuce;
- millet;
- oats;
- onions;
- pumpkin seeds;
- sesame seeds;
- soybeans;
- sunflower seeds;
- walnuts;
- wheat bran;
- wheat germ.

HIV and AIDS

Description

HIV refers to Human Immunodeficiency Virus. This virus damages the body's immune system so that it is no longer able to fight off infections. The HIV virus invades important immune cells called lymphocytes and causes a breakdown of the immune system. The HIV virus causes AIDS (Acquired Immune Deficiency Syndrome). AIDS is still thought to be (eventually) a fatal disease although much new research is constantly improving orthodox treatments. But the disease may develop very slowly.

Symptoms

Many people who are infected with HIV are not even aware that they have it. About a third of those who are affected suffer some generalised flu-like illness around the time of contracting the disease. After the virus has had time to develop and deplete the immune system, symptoms may include:

- lose of appetite and weight;
- fever, and/or night sweats;
- fatigue;
- diarrhoea, thrush, herpes;
- mouth sores and inflamed gums;
- skin disorders;
- swollen lymph nodes.

If the HIV infections progresses to HIV category four the patient is said to have AIDS and the symptoms then may also include:

- Kaposi's Sarcoma (a skin cancer which produces purple marks on the skin);
- pneumonia and other severe infections;
- nerve and brain disorders (e.g. fits, confusion, memory loss and dementia);

- vision problems and eye infections;
- lymph gland cancer.

Causes

HIV is known as a retrovirus that is spread primarily through sexual or blood-to-blood contact (e.g. needle sharing). It can also be spread by blood transfusions or the use of blood products such as clotting factors; although blood is carefully screened for infection, some infected blood may occasionally pass through. It cannot be spread from any casual contact such as: spa baths, kissing, mosquitoes, tears, towels or clothing.

The natural therapy treatments recommended here are not meant to replace orthodox treatments, they are meant to complement orthodox treatments, strengthen the immune system and alleviate the symptoms of HIV and AIDS. Ultimately the individual must weigh up the pros and cons of each treatment option and decide for themselves.

Nutritional supplements for HIV and AIDS

SUPPLEMENT	DOSAGE	COMMENT
Vitamin A (in the form of beta-carotene)	10,000–50,000 iu daily	Stabilises the body's cells so their immune abilities are strengthened. Helps fight disease by increasing the amount of immune cells
Vitamin B complex vitamins plus	100 mg three times daily	Anti-oxidant and anti-stress which support the nervous system and brain function
Vitamin B6 PGE1	50 mg three times daily	Important for the production of (an immune system regulator)
Vitamin C with bioflavonoids	10,000 mg daily in small doses throughout the day	Deficiency is associated with defective T cells (the immune system against viral infection)
Quercetin	500 mg daily	A bioflavonoid which boosts immunity and helps prevent allergic reactions. Also has antiviral properties
Vitamin E (in emulsified form)	200 iu daily for one week increased to 800 iu daily	Stimulates the immune system
Selenium	200–600 mcg daily	Anti-oxidant and powerful immune system enhancer. Supports the liver

Nutritional supplements for HIV and AIDS

SUPPLEMENT	DOSAGE	COMMENT
Iron	50 mg daily	Strengthens the immune system. Deficiency may lead to fatigue, weakness and depleted brain function
Zinc	50–100 mg daily	Zinc deficiency causes a depression of the cells' immune responses
Amino Acids: • L-arginine • L-ornithine • L-cysteine • L-histidene • L-methionine	For all amino acids take thymus as directed on the label on an empty stomach	Argine and Ornithine stimulate the gland to produce killer T cells and thus strengthen the immune system The other amino acids support the liver, and boost the immune system
Coenzyme Q10	50–100 mg daily	Plays a major role in energy production and strengthens the immune system
Acidophilus	Take as directed on the label	Improves colonic bacteria, fights fungal infections (e.g. candida) and supports the liver function
Shark liver oil and Shark cartilage	Take as directed on the label Take as directed on the label	Helps prevent tumour growth and supports the liver
Essential fatty acids: • Salmon oil or • Cod liver oil or • Sesame oil or • Corn oil or • Wheat Germ oil or • Evening Primrose oil	One tablespoon three times daily or as directed	Stimulate the immune system
Garlic	Take as directed on the label	Helps prevent infection. Acts as a natural form of penicillin. Also strengthens lymphatic and immune systems and improves digestion

Nutritional supplements for HIV/AIDS		
SUPPLEMENT	DOSAGE	COMMENT
Digestive enzymes: • Papain • Bromelain	Take as directed, with meals	Supports digestion
Hydrocloric acid	Take as directed, with meals	Supports digestion
Lecithin	One tablespoon three times daily	For cellular protection and antiviral properties

Nutritional treatment

Nutritional supplements that may be beneficial in the treatment of HIV and AIDS are included in the above table. See pages xii–xiii for information on how to use these supplements.

Herbal treatment

Herbal medicines can be used in the treatment of HIV and AIDS to strengthen and detoxify the liver, stimulate digestive juices, cleanse the blood and combat infections by supporting the immune system.

BITTER HERBS

Bitter herbs stimulate digestive juices and detoxify the liver. They include:

- Mugwort;
- Rue;
- Wormwood;
- Yarrow.

HEPATIC HERBS

Hepatic herbs strengthen the liver function. They include:

- Barberry;
- Dandelion;
- Milk Thistle.

ANTI-MICROBIAL HERBS

Anti-microbial herbs are natural antibiotics which help the body strengthen its own resistance to infections. They include:

- Cayenne;
- Echinacea;
- Garlic;
- Marigold;
- Myrrh;
- Wild Indigo.

ALTERATIVE HERBS

Alterative herbs help to eliminate wastes and cleanse the blood. They include:

- Barberry;
- Dandelion;
- Milk Thistle.

Other herbs that can be used in the treatment of HIV and AIDS are listed on page 234.

- Slippery Elm, Aloe Vera and cabbage juice reduce gastric and intestinal irritation and improve digestion.
- Aloe Vera works like the drug AZT, but without the side effects, and appears to inhibit the growth and spread of HIV.
- St John's Wort (Hypericum) has been shown to inhibit retroviral infections. As such, it may also be helpful in the treatment of HIV.
- Wild Yam also has antiviral qualities and strengthens the immune system.
- Siberian Ginseng increases the body's resistance to disease, improves circulation, boosts energy and is helpful for treating bronchial disorders.

CHINESE HERBS

Astragalus (Huang Qi) is an important and useful Chinese herb for strengthening the immune system. Other Chinese herbal tonics which can help include:

- Schizandra (Wu Wei Zi);
- Atractylodes (Bai Zhu);
- Licorice Root (Gan Cao).

The abovementioned herbs can be taken as herbal teas, tinctures and many are available as tablets. Consult your herbalist or naturopath for specific herbs for your condition. See pages xiii–xvi for more information on how to use these herbs.

For complaints accompanying HIV and AIDS, such as pneumonia (pages 25–28) and indigestion (pages

198–202), refer to herbal treatments within those sections of this book.

Homeopathic treatment

Homeopathic prescriptions for HIV and AIDS are complicated and require specific diagnosis of the individual's constitutional strengths and weaknesses. Consult a qualified homeopath.

Aromatherapy treatment

Aromatherapy essential oils may be used to uplift the emotions and to strengthen the immune system. Refer to other sections of this book for aromatherapy treatments of other associated symptoms such as indigestion (page 201) and insomnia (page 107).

IMMUNE SYSTEM

The following oils can be used as bath or body oils to stimulate the immune system:

- Lemon;
- Myrrh;
- Thyme.

MOOD ENHANCERS

The following oils can be used as bath or body oils to elevate the emotions and the spirit:

- Basil (can also be used in an oil burner);
- Bergamot;
- Clary Sage;
- Lavender;

- Melissa (can also be used in an oil burner);
- Neroli (can also be used in an oil burner);
- Rose.

RESPIRATORY WEAKNESSES

The following oils can be used for respiratory weaknesses:

- Bergamot (as a bath or body oil);
- Cypress (as a bath or body oil, or in an oil burner);
- Myrrh (as a body oil or in an oil burner);
- Pine (as a bath or body oil);
- Thyme (as a bath or body oil).

For information on how to use these essential oils see page xvi.

Dietary and lifestyle recommendations

- Avoid all processed foods, saturated fats, alcohol, tea, coffee and simple sugars. Sugar can interfere with the function of the immune system.
- The diet must contain more than the normal amounts of carbohydrates and protein, and a necessary amount of fat. Eat wholegrains which provide fibre (stimulates immune cells), vitamins and trace minerals. Increase your intake of fresh fruit and vegetables. Use plenty of onions, garlic and ginger to stimulate digestion and immune functions. Warming, nourishing soups and stews with onions, garlic and ginger are ideal.
- Eat high quality protein foods such as fish, eggs, yoghurt, liver, chickpeas, lentils, peanuts, cottage cheese, grains and sesame seeds. Amino acid supplements are also beneficial (see page 232).
- Eat plenty of the following vegetables: broccoli, brussels sprouts, cabbage, cauliflower, carrots, pumpkins and yellow or orange sweet potato.
- Avoid foods that contain yeast or foods potentially contaminated with moulds.
- Make sure you get a moderate exposure to sunshine and as much fresh air and rest as you need.
- The best oils to use in cooking are olive and sesame.

SEXUALLY TRANSMITTED DISEASES

Description and causes

There are a number of sexually transmitted diseases (STDs) which are passed on through sexual contact. These include, gonorrhoea, syphilis, genital herpes, genital warts, hepatitis B, candidiasis, chlamydia, pelvic inflammatory disease, pubic lice and HIV and AIDS. The symptoms of these conditions vary greatly and some have no symptoms at all.

Symptoms

The following are a list of the most common STDs and their symptoms:

ACQUIRED IMMUNE DEFICIENCY SYNDROME (AIDS)

See HIV and AIDS, pages 230–35.

CANDIDA ALBICANS

See pages 210–13.

CHLAMYDIA

Between 70 percent and 80 percent of women have no symptoms, however if symptoms do appear they include genital itching, burning and a thick yellowish discharge. There can also be pain in the abdomen and bleeding between periods.

In men the symptoms are more noticeable and include pain and a watery discharge. If left untreated women can suffer infertility and the condition can also lead to pelvic inflammatory disease.

GENITAL HERPES

Symptoms usually appear four to eight days after exposure to the virus. These include itching and burning in the genital area, flu-like symptoms such as headache and fever and painful sores on and around the genitals that can last up to ten days. See pages 53–7 for more information.

GENITAL WARTS

These are caused by the human papilloma virus (HPV). The warts appear either singly or as a mass. They are commonly found in women on the labia and inside the entrance of the vagina. In men they can be found on the penis and under the foreskin. In women the virus has been associated with cervical cancer. If you have had genital warts it is important to have an annual cervical smear test. See pages 74–7 for more information.

GONORRHOEA

A woman may develop no symptoms but can still transfer the disease sexually. If symptoms appear it is usually about three days after infection. These include a vaginal discharge of pus, and pain at the entrance of the urethra and the vagina. Men develop pain and infected urethral discharge. This condition is serious and if left untreated can lead to sterility.

PELVIC INFLAMMATORY DISEASE (PID)

This condition is often referred to as infection of the fallopian tubes. The symptoms are lower abdominal pain, fever and a vaginal discharge of pus. PID can develop from other STDs such as Chlamydia.

SYPHILIS

This is a very serious venereal disease. Infection enters the body via the membranes lining the vagina, mouth or penis. If not treated this disease progresses over the course of many years. There are three main stages in the development of syphilis. The first is a lump that develops into an ulcer at the original point of entry into the body. This may clear up without treatment. The second stage is a skin rash and enlarged lymph nodes, sore throat and fever. The third stage affects the mucus membranes, skin, bones, heart and arteries as well as the nervous system. Penicillin is used to treat syphilis, however if the disease has progressed to the third stage it can be arrested but not cured.

The following natural therapy treatments are recommended to complement orthodox medical treatment, not replace it. As is the case with all sexually transmitted diseases it is important to consult your doctor and undergo a thorough diagnosis of your condition.

Nutritional treatment

Nutritional supplements that may be beneficial in the treatment of STDs are included in the following table (see page 238). See pages xii–xiii for information on how to use these supplements.

Herbal treatment

Use the following herbs as teas, tablets or tinctures. For information on how to use these herbs see pages xiii–xv.

ANTI-MICROBIAL HERBS
Herbs used to treat venereal infections are anti-microbial. These herbs work to help the body destroy infection.

- Echinacea is a very effective anti-microbial herb used in the treatment of STDs.

- Garlic is a natural antibiotic that helps the body to resist infection.
- Wild Indigo is used to enhance immune response to infection. Can also be used as an external ointment to treat infected ulcerations.

LYMPHATIC HERBS
Lymphatic herbs are also extremely important in the treatment of infections because much of the anti-microbial activity takes place in the lymph glands.

- Cleavers is an excellent tonic for the lymphatic system.
- Poke Root is primarily used in the treatment of infections.

ASTRINGENT HERBS
Astringent herbs are used in the treatment of wound healing and the reduction of inflammation. They can also be used effectively as external ointments.

- Oak bark can be used as a douche for vaginal discharge.
- Periwinkle can be used effectively in the treatment of reproductive problems.
- Beth Root makes an excellent uterine tonic. It may also be helpful in treating vaginal ulceration and infection.

HERBAL TEA
The following herbs should be made into a tea and taken three times daily. This combination can also be used effectively as a douche:

Nutritional supplements for sexually transmitted diseases

SUPPLEMENT	DOSAGE	COMMENT
Vitamin C	1500 mg four times daily	Can inhibit the effect of some STD viruses
Acidophilus	Three capsules daily	To help restore friendly bacteria. Is especially important when antibiotics are prescribed.
Vitamin B complex	50 mg daily	Needed to enhance healing
Vitamin E	600 iu daily	Vitamin E oil can also be applied externally on herpes sores
Multivitamin and mineral complex	As directed on label	Necessary to balance the body's function
Kyolic garlic	2 capsules three times daily	Garlic is a natural antibiotic and it stimulates immune function
L-lysine	500–3,000 mg daily	Increases immune function. Used in the treatment of herpes
Calcium	1500 iu daily	Regulates hormonal secretion. Works more efficiently when used with magnesium
Magnesium	750 mg daily	Assists the function of calcium
Zinc	50 mg daily	Helps promote immunity and healing

- Beth Root (two parts);
- Echinacea (two parts);
- Periwinkle (two parts);
- Cleavers (one part).

Homeopathic treatment

HERPES
Homeopathics used to treat herpes are:

- Borax (to treat small blisters, and an itching and burning sensation);
- Rhus toxicodendron (effective when the blisters are pearl-like, hot and puffy);
- Natrum muriaticum (when the genitals are burning and stinging with cracked skin and a red rash).

VAGINAL DISCHARGE
The following homeopathics are used in the treatment of vaginal discharge associated with local infection.

- Sepia – used to treat yellowish discharge, distended abdomen, sharp pain and itching.
- Calcarea carbonica – used when there is a milky discharge causing itching and the irritation is worse

after urination and before menstruation.

CHLAMYDIA AND GONORRHOEA

The following homeopathics can be used in the treatment of chlamydia and may also be recommended for gonorrhoea, depending on the symptoms.

- Apis – used where there is a stinging pain in the urethra, particularly when urinating.
- Argentum nitricum – used when the urine of both men and women may contain blood and there is profuse discharge from the urethra.

For more specific remedies to treat sexually transmitted diseases consult your homeopath. See page xv for information on how to use these treatments.

Aromatherapy treatment

There are no specific aromatherapy essential oils used to treat STDs. See the introduction to the reproductive system at the beginning of this chapter (page 209) for aromatherapy oils used to strengthen the reproductive organs.

Dietary and lifestyle recommendations

- It is important to use a condom until infection has cleared completely as STDs are highly contagious.
- Seek orthodox medical treatment to positively diagnose condition. Antibiotics or penicillin may be recommended.
- Boost your immune function by regularly eating nutritious foods. These include a balance of cereals, vegetables, fruits and whole grains.
- Stress weakens your immune system. Plenty of fresh air and exercise can help to alleviate stress.
- Wear loose clothing to avoid further irritation of the genital area.

CHAPTER SEVEN

THE HORMONAL SYSTEM
Maintenance of the glands, ducts and hormonal secretions

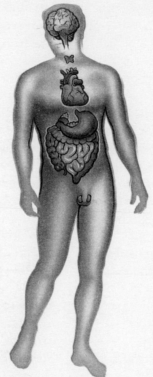

What does it consist of?

The body contains two kinds of glands: exocrine and endocrine. Exocrine glands include sweat glands, oil, mucus and digestive glands.

The endocrine glands, which comprise the hormonal system, include the pituitary (the master gland), the thyroid gland, the parathyroids, the adrenal glands and the pineal gland. Certain organs of the body also contain endocrine tissue. These include the hypothalamus, thymus, pancreas, ovaries, testes, kidneys, stomach, liver, small intestine, skin, heart and placenta.

What does it do?

Endocrine glands secrete their products (called hormones) into the bloodstream. These hormones carry the information that controls the rate at which glands and other organs work. Hormones are the body's internal chemical messengers. Hormones carry out the following functions:

- they regulate the chemical balances (e.g. the blood calcium level) and fluid balances of the body;
- they help regulate metabolic rate and energy levels;
- they regulate contraction of the heart muscle;
- they regulate some functions of the immune system;
- they help maintain the body's functioning in times of infection, stress, trauma, temperature changes, starvation, dehydration and blood loss;
- they play an important role in the smooth, sequential integration of growth and development;
- they play a role in the reproductive process including egg and sperm production, fertilisation, nourishment of the embryo and the foetus, and delivery and nourishment of the baby;
- they regulate the functions of other glands.

PITUITARY GLAND

The pituitary gland is located on the undersurface of the brain and is called the 'master gland' because it releases several hormones that control other endocrine glands. The pituitary gland releases human growth hormone, thyroid stimulating hormone, adrenal stimulating hormone, follicle stimulating hormone (stimulates the ovaries and testes), lutenising hormone (stimulates the production of oestrogen, progesterone and testosterone), prolactin (stimulates mammary glands to produce milk), oxytocin (stimulates uterus and mammary glands) and antidiuretic hormone (decreases urine volume and conserves body water).

THYROID GLAND

The thyroid gland lies in the midline of the front of the neck. The thyroid gland releases the hormones thyroxine (regulates metabolism, growth and development, and activity of the nervous system) and calcitonin (lowers blood levels of calcium and phosphates).

PARATHYROID GLANDS

The parathyroid glands are situated behind the thyroid gland and they produce a hormone which increases calcium in the blood. It acts on the bones to release stored calcium.

PANCREAS

The pancreas secretes hormones directly into the bloodstream. The hormones are glucagon (raises blood glucose levels), insulin (lowers blood glucose levels) and pancreatic hormone (regulates release of pancreatic digestive enzymes).

ADRENAL GLANDS

The adrenal glands are situated one on top of each kidney. The adrenals release several different hormones which affect the body's response to stress, and control the metabolic rate, growth, blood glucose concentration as well as the retention or loss of minerals (e.g. sodium and potassium).

OVARIES AND TESTES

The ovaries and testes produce the sex hormones oestrogen and progesterone (regulates the development and maintenance of female sexual characteristics, the menstrual cycle, maintains pregnancy, stimulates milk production and egg production), relaxin (relaxes pelvis and helps dilate cervix near end of pregnancy) and inhibin (which inhibits the secretion of follicle stimulating hormone from the pituitary gland).

What goes wrong with it?

None of the endocrine glands acts independently of the others. Hormone production is controlled in many cases by a feedback system in which overproduction of a hormone leads to a compensatory decrease in subsequent production until balance is restored. The pituitary gland plays a central role in this feedback system to maintain a state of internal balance (homeostasis). Problems occur when the feedback system breaks down and hormone levels are either too low or too high.

Nutritional treatment

Nutritional supplements that benefit the hormonal system include the following:

VITAMIN B3

Vitamin B3 is necessary for the synthesis of sex hormones and helps to elevate and stabilise blood sugar levels (assisting the hormonal function of the pancreas).

VITAMIN B5

Vitamin B5 stimulates the adrenal glands and increases production of cortisone and other adrenal hormones. Vitamin B5 improves the body's ability to withstand stressful conditions. Deficiency may lead to adrenal exhaustion and low blood sugar level and (if the adrenal function is diminished) may lead to physical and mental depression.

VITAMIN B6

Vitamin B6 helps to produce the hormone adrenalin which is used up under stress. Vitamin B6 deficiency can lead to adrenal exhaustion. It is also necessary for the functioning of the pituitary gland.

VITAMIN C

Vitamin C is essential for the health of the adrenal glands, which are the storehouses of this vitamin. Vitamin C is often termed the stress vitamin. Vitamin C also plays a part in the metabolism of some amino acids that end up as hormones such as thyroxine. Vitamin C promotes a constant flow of many enzyme reactions, which is essential for the pituitary, adrenals, ovaries, heart and brain.

VITAMIN E

Vitamin E is required for the health of the adrenal and pituitary glands and their associated hormone production. The synthetic female hormone oestrogen depletes vitamin E. Vitamin E also helps normalise the functions of the ovaries and testes, by regulating the synthesis of the sex hormones.

MINERALS

Iodine aids in the development and function of the thyroid gland. Iodine is stored in the thyroid gland and is an integral part of thyroxine. Deficiency of iodine may lead to goitre or thyroid enlargement. Iodine-rich foods include kelp, watermelon, spinach, cucumber, asparagus, turnip, peanuts, strawberries, capsicum, eggplant, lettuce, carrot, potato, tomato, beetroot, cabbage, onions, peaches, banana and apples.

Silicon, phosphorus, calcium, chlorine and magnesium are also helpful minerals for the hormonal system.

Herbal treatment

There are many herbs that benefit the hormonal system.

BITTER HERBS

Bitter herbs for the hormonal system include:

- Golden Seal (don't use during pregnancy);
- Mugwort;
- Rue;
- Wormwood;
- Yarrow.

ALTERATIVE HERBS

Alterative herbs (blood cleansers) for the hormonal system include:

- Burdock;
- Cleavers;
- Echinacea;
- Dandelion;
- Sweet Violet leaves;
- Yellow dock.

SPECIFIC HERBS

Specific herbs to support and strengthen the hormonal system include:

- Borage;
- Dong Quai;
- Ginseng;
- Kelp;
- Licorice;
- Wild Yam.

SWOLLEN GLANDS

Specific herbs for swollen glands include:

- Cleavers;
- Echinacea;
- Poke Root.

Dietary and lifestyle recommendations

FOODS

The following foods contain important vitamins, minerals, proteins and oils which support and sustain the hormonal system.

- asparagus
- avocados
- bananas
- beetroot
- berries
- currants
- dates
- garlic
- grapes
- lemons
- olives
- lettuce
- potatoes
- sea vegetables
- kelp
- egg yolks
- wheat germ
- lecithin
- sesame seed butter
- seeds
- nuts
- goat's milk

JUICES

The following juices are beneficial for the hormonal system.

- carrot, beetroot and parsley
- grape
- peach
- pineapple
- strawberry, orange and pineapple

ADRENAL EXHAUSTION or INSUFFICIENCY

Description

The hormones produced by the adrenal glands include adrenalin which causes the stress (or 'fight or flight') response. When the body becomes aware of a threat or a challenge adrenalin is quickly released by the adrenals. Adrenalin makes the heart beat faster, increases the blood sugar level, increases the breathing rate, sends more blood to the brain and the muscles and generally prepares the body for an emergency. Because many of our contemporary stresses do not really demand such a physical response, the release of adrenalin is often excessive and the body has no way of utilising it. If this response happens too frequently it may eventually cause adrenal problems.

If the adrenal cortex is seriously underactive, a rare condition called Addison's disease may develop.

The adrenal glands are also involved in the metabolism of carbohydrates and the regulation of blood sugar. They also produce the sex hormones, androgens (the male hormones) and oestrogens (the female hormones).

Symptoms

Symptoms of adrenal exhaustion include:

- insomnia;
- weakness;
- weight loss;
- loss of appetite;
- vomiting;
- nausea;
- dizziness;
- abdominal pain;
- craving for salt;
- blood sugar disorders;
- headaches;
- memory problems.

Causes

Adrenal exhaustion is the gradual decline of the adrenal glands' function, which may eventually produce a complete functional failure. Adrenal exhaustion may be caused by:

- rapid infection (particularly in the newborn);

- severe stress;
- overwork;
- surgical removal of the adrenals.
- In Chinese medicine, another cause of adrenal exhaustion would be too many ejaculations (for men) which weakens the kidneys and adrenal glands.

Nutritional treatment

Nutritional supplements that may be beneficial in the treatment of adrenal exhaustion or insufficiency are included in the following table.

See pages xii–xiii for information on how to use these herbs.

Nutritional supplements for adrenal exhaustion or insufficiency

SUPPLEMENT	DOSAGE	COMMENT
Vitamin B5	200 mg daily in divided doses	Vitamin B5 is involved in the synthesis of cortisone and is necessary for the function of the adrenal glands
Vitamin B6	150 mg daily in divided doses	Vitamin B6 is involved in the synthesis of noradrenaline and other hormones which are used up in stress. A deficiency may lead to adrenal exhaustion
Vitamin B12	100 mcg daily	Vitamin B12 has been effective in providing relief from fatigue, anaemia and nervous irritability
Vitamin C with bioflavonoids	2000 mg three times daily	Vitamin C is essential for the health of the adrenal glands which store this vitamin. Stress hormones cannot be produced without Vitamin C
Folic acid	3000 mcg daily	Folic acid is needed to prevent anaemia and glandular exhaustion
Potassium	100 mg daily	Stress depletes potassium and it is needed to balance sodium in the body
Copper	3 mg daily	Deficiency may cause weakness and anaemia. Copper works with potassium and zinc

Nutritional supplements for adrenal exhaustion or insufficiency

SUPPLEMENT	DOSAGE	COMMENT
Zinc	100 mg daily	Depleted by stress. Works with copper and potassium
Magnesium	1000 mg daily	Magnesium is required for the conversion of glucose into energy. The adrenal glands regulate the amount of magnesium
L-tyrosine	600 mg daily on an empty stomach	L-tyrosine is a precursor of the adrenal hormones. Deficiency may cause stress exhaustion
Coenzyme Q10	50 mg daily	Oxygenates the cells for energy production

Herbal treatment

CHINESE HERBS

A herbal repertory for the treatment of adrenal exhaustion would include the Chinese herbs:

- Ginseng (Ren Shen);
- Astragalus (Huang Qi);
- Licorice root (Gan Cao).

Ginseng protects against mental and physical fatigue, provides support against stress, and improves adrenal gland function.

These herbs belong to the category of herbs which tonify chi.

WESTERN HERBS

The western herbs Borage and Wild Yam are also used. Borage and Wild Yam are natural precursors of the adrenal hormones and they revitalise the adrenals. They can be taken as teas or herbal tinctures.

See pages xiii–xv for information on how to use these herbs.

Dietary and lifestyle recommendations

- Avoid alcohol, caffeine and nicotine as these substances are toxic to the adrenal glands. Also avoid fatty, oily foods, processed foods, white flour and red meat.
- Green, leafy vegetables are important in the diet. Also include in your diet: garlic, onions, brewer's yeast, brown rice, nuts, olive oil, wheatgerm and whole grains.
- Take steps to resolve stress in your life through relaxation, meditation, counselling, yoga, etc.
- Take regular, moderate exercise, such as walking, to stimulate the adrenal glands and to ease stress.

BREASTFEEDING and LACTATION

Description

During pregnancy the breasts increase in size as the mammary glands develop and prepare themselves for breast-feeding.

Breastmilk provides all the nourishment a newborn baby needs. It also helps to protect against infection. When a baby is placed on the breast immediately after birth it will begin to suckle. This stimulates the release of the hormone oxytocin. Oxytocin is a pituitary hormone that promotes both the flow of milk and uterine contractions.

Breastfeeding is highly recommended to establish early bonding between mother and infant. It provides important antibodies that help prevent gastroenteritis, respiratory infections and meningitis. There is also less likelihood of an allergic reaction in the baby to the mother's breastmilk than to infant formula, and the action of suckling the breast promotes the development of the facial muscles, the jaw and the teeth.

There are a small percentage of women who unfortunately, for a number of different reasons, are unable to breastfeed. For these women and their babies there are some excellent infant formulas available.

Breastfeeding problems

- Engorgement is a common problem that can occur in the early stages of breastfeeding. The breasts become swollen and overfilled with milk, can be extremely tender to touch and the baby may have difficulty attaching to the nipples. Gently massaging the breast under a warm shower to express excess milk usually brings relief.
- Cracked or sore nipples may also be a problem for some women. This problem can be extremely painful and is often related to the baby not attaching properly to the nipple while suckling. It is recommended the baby be fed from the other nipple for a few days to allow healing to take place. There are some excellent homeopathic and natural soothing lotions that can be used to treat this problem.
- Mastitis or breast infection is a condition that occurs when the milk ducts become blocked and inflamed. It may begin with a sore or cracked nipple or it could result from engorgement. The breast becomes red and very tender and the woman may develop fever and flu-like symptoms. It is recommended a physician be consulted immediately if you suspect infection as untreated mastitis can lead to a breast abscess.

Nutritional treatment

Nutritional supplements that may be beneficial for breastfeeding and lactation are included in the following table. See pages xii–xiii for information about how to use these supplements.

Herbal treatment

The following herbal remedies may be useful in the prevention and treatment of breastfeeding problems. For information on how to use these herbal remedies see pages xiii–xv.

- Calendula is especially recommended for external use for a range of skin conditions. Calendula ointment may provide relief for cracked and sore nipples.
- Poke Root has a wide range of uses including providing relief for mastitis. Poke Root can be taken internally or used in a poultice.
- Milk Thistle is a wonderful herb for promoting milk secretion and is perfectly safe for breastfeeding mothers. Milk Thistle can be taken as a tablet or tincture.
- Raspberry tea (made from raspberry leaves) is recommended during and after pregnancy to strengthen and tone the uterus.

Homeopathic treatment

Homeopathic treatment can be of great use when it comes to breastfeeding problems, especially those that centre around painful breasts, sore nipples and problems with milk supply. See

---

Nutritional supplements for breastfeeding and lactation

SUPPLEMENT	DOSAGE	COMMENT
Vitamin B complex	50 mg daily	Needed for milk production
Vitamin C	2000 mg daily	Essential vitamin for bone and teeth growth and strengthening the nervous system. Important in blood cell formation
Vitamin D	400 iu daily	Important for proper absorption of calcium
Multivitamin and mineral complex	As directed on label	Essential for the health and wellbeing of mother and child
Calcium and Magnesium (chelate)	1500 mg daily 500 mg daily	Both of these are essential for bone formation. Requirements are higher during lactation
Iron	As directed by your physician	Pregnancy and lactation increase the mother's demand for iron

page xv for more information on how to use the following treatments.

- Pulsatilla is used when there is too little milk or the milk supply is watery and thin.
- Belladonna is useful when the breasts are inflamed, tender and engorged with an oversupply of milk.
- Bryonia is used when the breasts are hard and extremely tender to touch.
- Sepia is used to treat nipples that are deeply cracked and very sore.
- Sulphur is also used to treat chapped sore nipples.
- Chamomilla is helpful in treating inflamed and sensitive nipples.

Aromatherapy treatment

Aromatherapy essential oils balance and harmonise the emotions. For more information on how to use the following essential oils see page xvi.

- Geranium is used as a bath oil, compress or massage oil. This oil is highly recommended for the female system, especially new mothers.
- Lavender has the ability to restore skin health. Used as a massage oil it can be used as a soothing rub for cracked and sore nipples.
- Neroli is a beautiful perfumed oil that has a deeply relaxing effect on the body and emotions. Use as a body, bath or inhalation oil.

Dietary and lifestyle recommendations

- Breastfeeding mothers need to make sure they get plenty of rest and relaxation. A well-balanced diet is extremely important, with emphasis on fresh fruit, vegetables, whole grains and natural carbohydrates.
- Drink plenty of fluids including fresh fruit and vegetable, juices, water and milk (preferably soymilk).
- Vitamin E will soothe cracked nipples caused by breastfeeding. Rub a small amount of vitamin E oil from a capsule onto the nipple after feeding.
- Avoid soap on your nipples when bathing as this will dry them out and lead to cracking.
- Feeding your baby on demand will help prevent engorgement. Use both breasts when feeding. Begin on one side until baby loses interest, then change to the other. Next time you feed, begin with the side you ended on before.
- Avoid tea, coffee, alcohol and tobacco during pregnancy and lactation as the effects of these drugs are passed directly to the baby.

DIABETES MELLITUS

Description and causes

Diabetes mellitus is a group of disorders that lead to an elevation of glucose in the blood (hyperglycaemia). As hyperglycaemia increases, there is a loss of glucose in the urine. The common hallmarks of diabetes mellitus are excessive urine production, excessive thirst and excessive hunger.

There are two types of diabetes mellitus. The first type (Type I) is called insulin dependent diabetes where regular injections of insulin are required as the body has an absolute deficiency. This type of diabetes usually begins in young people under the age of 20.

Type II diabetes is far more common and usually occurs later in life. Type II is often linked to poor diet and lifestyle factors, and injections of insulin are usually not required. High levels of glucose in the blood can often be controlled by diet, exercise and weight loss. For those who suffer type II diabetes, the condition arises not from a shortage of insulin but because cells become less sensitive to it.

Nutritional supplements for diabetes mellitus

SUPPLEMENT	DOSAGE	COMMENT
Vitamin A	10,000 iu daily	Deficiency common to diabetes. Helps improve sensory nerve function
Vitamin C with bioflavonoids	2000 mg daily	May help reduce insulin doses
Vitamin E	400 iu daily	Helps reduce circulation problems and stabilises blood sugar levels
Garlic	Two 500 mg capsules daily	Stabilises blood sugar levels
Magnesium	750 mg daily	Protects the body against arteriosclerosis
Chromium	Consult with your doctor before using this mineral	Helps lower blood sugar levels
Brewer's yeast	Three tablespoons daily	Natural source of Vitamin B. Helps to normalise blood sugar levels

Nutritional supplements for diabetes mellitus

SUPPLEMENT	DOSAGE	COMMENT
Multivitamin and mineral complex	As directed on label	Essential for the balanced functioning of the body
Zinc	25 mg daily	Diabetics have shown signs of a deficiency of this mineral
Phosphorus	1000 mg daily	Associated with insulin resistance
Potassium	5 g daily	Associated with insulin resistance

Symptoms

The symptoms of both types of diabetes include excessive thirst, excessive urination, weight loss, fatigue, hunger and weakness. Diabetes mellitus is a chronic condition and can cause nerve damage, blindness, kidney failure, hypertension, angina, and circulatory problems. Appropriate medical treatment must be observed otherwise coma and death may result.

Nutritional treatment

Nutritional supplements that may be beneficial in the treatment of diabetes mellitus are included in the above table. See pages xii–xiii for information on how to use these supplements.

Herbal treatment

It is highly recommended that professional advice be sought regarding a specific treatment for diabetes mellitus. The following are herbs that may be suggested in treating this chronic condition. See pages xiii–xv for information on how to use these herbs.

- Bilberry leaf helps to control insulin levels.
- Garlic has many benefits, including preventing infection and reducing blood pressure and blood cholesterol levels.
- Nettle strengthens and supports the whole body. Nettle is also high in iron and vitamin C.
- Ginseng has an antidepressive action. It may be helpful in treating depression associated with weakness and fatigue.

Homeopathic treatment

Homeopathy is very useful in treating some of the symptoms of diabetes mellitus. See page xv for information on how to use the following treatments.

- Antimonium is recommended for treating tender feet associated with corns and bunions.

CATARACTS

- Calcarea carbonica is used to treat dimness of vision, permanently dilated pupils and light sensitivity.
- Silicea is used to treat confused vision, sufferers who are dazzled by light and sharp pain in the eyes.

PYELONEPHRITIS

Pyelonephritis is inflammation of the kidneys.

- Cuprum arsenitum is used to treat garlic smelling urine, abdominal symptoms of colicky pain and diarrhoea.

Aromatherapy treatment

Aromatherapy oils that may be useful to ease depression, fatigue and exhaustion associated with diabetes mellitus are listed below. See page xvi for more information on how to use these oils.

- Geranium is used as a massage oil. It has a therapeutic effect on the circulatory system.
- Lavender is a wonderful healing oil that relaxes and calms the body. Use a few drops in a warm bath or use in a vaporiser. This aromatic oil is very uplifting.

Dietary and lifestyle recommendations

- A diet high in complex carbohydrates and plant fibre including cereal grains, legumes and root vegetables has been proven to be of great benefit to those suffering from diabetes.
- Eat plenty of fresh raw fruit and vegetables as these help reduce the need for insulin.
- Foods that help to normalise blood sugar levels are brewer's yeast, dairy products, eggs, fish, garlic and soybeans.
- An exercise program should be developed in relation to the individual's fitness level. Appropriate exercise has proven benefits of enhanced insulin sensitivity, improved glucose tolerance and, in some cases, a reduction in the need for insulin injections.
- Orthodox treatment should not be neglected. It is extremely important to have the condition properly diagnosed and a course of treatment worked out. This may involve regular insulin injections.
- Natural therapies can play a large role in helping those with diabetes to maintain good health and wellbeing.

HYPERTHYROIDISM

Description

The thyroid gland, in the front of the neck, is responsible for releasing a number of hormones which are collectively called thyroxine. These hormones act as the accelerators for every cell of the body by controlling the body's energy levels.

Hyperthyroidism involves over-production of hormones by the thyroid gland which also influences the pituitary, parathyroid and sex glands. This excess production of thyroid hormones speeds up all body processes, and malabsorption occurs. As a result, many of the body's nutrients are used up at a greater rate. Overactivity of the thyroid gland is called thyrotoxicosis, Grave's disease or hyperthyroidism.

Symptoms

Symptoms of hyperthyroidism include:

- excess sweating;
- weight loss;
- nervousness;
- tiredness;
- irritability;
- increased appetite;
- insomnia;
- mood swings;
- protruding eyeballs;
- palpitations;
- a constant feeling of being hot;
- increased frequency of bowel movements;
- rapid heartbeat;
- less frequent menstruation;
- hair loss;
- goitre.

Causes

The causes of hyperthyroidism include:

- an auto-immune reaction in which antibodies attack the thyroid gland and overstimulate it;
- lumps or tumours that form on the thyroid, disrupting hormone production;
- hereditary factors;
- stress;
- infection or inflammation can cause temporary hyperthyroidism.

Orthodox treatment of hyperthyroidism involves surgically removing most of the thyroid gland or destroying most the cells in the gland by giving the patient radioactive iodine (Iodine 131). If left untreated this condition can lead to heart failure.

Nutritional treatment

Nutritional treatment of hyperthyroidism is aimed at increasing nutrients which are depleted by the condition. Vitamin B complex is important in assisting the body to metabolise extra carbohydrates and proteins. If the patient is losing weight additional protein may be necessary in order to replace lost muscle tissue.

See pages xii–xiii for information on how to use the supplements contained in the table on pages 255–56.

Herbal treatment

Hyperthyroidism is treated with a combination of herbs:

- nervine relaxants;
- digestive bitters;
- specific herbs.

For information on how to use these herbs see pages xiii–xv.

NERVINE RELAXANTS

Nervine relaxants include the herbs:

- Lavender;
- Pasque Flower;
- Skullcap;
- St John's Wort;
- Valerian.

Use these herbs as either teas or tinctures.

BITTER HERBS

Bitter herbs for digestion include:

Nutritional supplements for hyperthyroidism

SUPPLEMENT	DOSAGE	COMMENT
Vitamin A	50,000 iu daily	Resists infection. Deficiency can cause cysts or growths on the glands
Vitamin B complex plus	50 mg three times daily	Assists in the metabolism of additional carbohydrates and protein. Also important for thyroid function
Vitamin B1 plus	100 mg daily	Facilitates blood formation, energy production and stimulates appetite
Vitamin B2 plus	50 mg daily	Depleted by hyperactivity and needed for the normal functioning of all glands
Vitamin B6	100 mg daily	Facilitates hormonal synthesis and regulation. Also important for immune system and antibodies
Vitamin C	2000–5000 mg daily in divided doses	Improves immunity and promotes healing
Vitamin E	500 iu daily	Strengthens immune system, blood flow and acts as an anti-oxidant
Lecithin granules	One tablespoon three times daily before meals	Increases the solubility of cholesterol to digest fats and protects the lining of cells and organs
Essential fatty acids • Linseed oil • Sunflower oil • Evening Primrose oil • Soy oil	one teaspoon per day	Important for glandular functioning and reduces inflammation

Nutritional supplements for hyperthyroidism		
SUPPLEMENT	DOSAGE	COMMENT
Kelp	As directed on label	Regulates both slightly overactive and underactive thyroid gland conditions
Choline	20 g daily	Needed for the transport and metabolism of fats and also for immune response
Brewer's yeast	One–three tablespoons daily	Rich in B vitamins
Folic acid	2000 mcg daily	Deficiency of folic acid affects the hormonal system
Inositol	1000 mg daily	Regulates cell surface functions such as binding of hormones

- Gentian Root;
- Rue;
- Yarrow;
- Wormwood.

SPECIFIC HERBS

A specific herb for hyperthyroidism is Bugleweed (Lycopus virginica). Use it as a tea or tincture.

Take equal parts of the following herbs as teas, or tinctures.

- Bugleweed
- Nettle
- Valerian
- Yarrow

Cabbage, cress and spinach juice are also recommended for hyperthyroidism. Onions are also helpful.

GOITRE

Bladderwrack (seaweed) is an excellent source of iodine and is used to treat goitre. Take in tablet form as a dietary supplement or as an infusion, drunk three times daily.

Homeopathic treatment

Treatment that may be prescribed by a homeopath for hyperthyroidism includes:

- Thyroidinium for hyperthyroidism with goitre;
- Natrum muriaticum when hyperthyroidism is accompanied by palpitations and weight loss;
- Belladonna if the sufferer has a flushed face and staring eyes;
- Lycopus if the heart is fast and pounding with palpitations;
- Iodum for goitre or when the sufferer feels hot, is hyperactive and obsessive about everything.

See page xv for details on how to use these herbs.

Dietary and lifestyle recommendations

- Caffeinated drinks (tea, coffee, colas and chocolate) should be avoided as they increase the metabolic rate even further and expend more calories. Nicotine and alcohol should also be avoided for the same reason.

- A natural wholefood diet is appropriate as digestion speeds up in hyperthyroidism and malabsorption often accompanies it. Onions, seafood and vegetables grown organically (in iodine-rich soils) would be advised.
- Bathing in seawater is recommended for glandular disturbances, especially hypo and hyperthyroidism.

THYROXINE PRODUCTION
The following foods help to reduce thyroxine production, so they should be emphasised in the diet.

- berries
- broccoli
- brussels sprouts
- cabbage
- cauliflower
- peaches
- pears
- soy products
- spinach
- turnips

Eat watercress on a regular basis.

HYPOGLYCAEMIA
Description

Hypoglycaemia is the term given to describe the symptoms that occur due to a significant drop in blood sugar levels. When blood sugar levels drop the body releases the hormones adrenaline, glucagon and cortisol; these hormones compensate by increasing the blood sugar levels.

Nutritional supplements for hypoglycaemia		
SUPPLEMENT	DOSAGE	COMMENT
Acidophilus fibre	One dessertspoon a day with meals	Helps reduce the rise of blood sugar
Vitamin B complex	50–100 mg daily	A lack of these vitamins will significantly effect the breakdown of glucose to form energy
Vitamin B1	30 mg daily	Aids in the production of hydrochloric acid for digestion
Vitamin B3	30 mg daily	Helps in the proper functioning of the digestive system
Vitamin C with bioflavonoids	3000 mg daily	For the healthy function of the adrenals

Nutritional supplements for hypoglycaemia

SUPPLEMENT	DOSAGE	COMMENT
Vitamin E	*400 iu daily*	*Anti-oxidant*
Magnesium chelate	*100 mg daily*	*Important for the metabolism of*
Calcium	*100 mg daily*	*sugar*
Brewer's yeast	*As directed on label*	*Helps stabilise blood sugar levels*
Manganese chelate	*15 mg daily*	*Helps maintain blood sugar levels*
Zinc	*50 mg daily*	*Needed for the release of insulin*

Symptoms

If the blood sugar levels drop rapidly adrenaline will produce the following physical symptoms; sweating, increased heart rate, tremor, hunger and anxiety. If the fall is more gradual the symptoms include headache, depression, dizziness, mood swings, forgetfulness, poor coordination and cravings for cigarettes, drugs, sweets, cakes and coffee.

The only specific way of diagnosing the condition is to undergo a glucose tolerance test (see your physician for details). Also refer to hypoglycaemia on pages 158–60.

Causes

The most common cause of this condition is vitamin and mineral deficiency and poor digestion and absorption of nutrients. Obviously the patient's lifestyle is of considerable importance. Hypoglycaemia can also be associated with diabetes.

Nutritional treatment

Nutritional supplements that may be beneficial in the treatment of hypoglycaemia are included in the above table. See pages xii–xiii for information on how to use these supplements.

Herbal treatment

The following herbs may be helpful in treating hypoglycaemia. Use these herbs as teas, tablets or tinctures.

- Bilberry helps to control insulin levels.
- Oats are useful in treating nervous exhaustion, depression and general weakness. May reduce craving for cigarettes.
- Dandelion is a natural source of calcium that supports the liver and the pancreas.
- Skullcap is used to treat headaches, palpitations and mental fuzziness.

See pages xiii–xv for information on how to use these herbs.

Homeopathic treatment

Homeopathy may be of benefit in treating some of the symptoms that accompany hypoglycaemia.

DEPRESSION
For the treatment of depression try:

- Arsenicum album;
- Calcarea carbonica;
- Chamomilla;
- Ferrum metallicum.

DIZZINESS
Faintness or dizziness can be treated by using:

- Sepia;
- Pulsatilla.

ANXIETY
Anxiety is often a symptom of hypoglycaemia. A few homeopathics that may provide relief are:

- Kali sulphuricum;
- Argentum nitricum;
- Aconite.

SWEET CRAVINGS
For sweet craving use:

- China officinalis;
- Lycopodium;
- Sulphur.

See page xv for more information on how to use these treatments.

Aromatherapy treatment

The following essential oils may be helpful in alleviating some of the symptoms of hypoglycaemia.

DEPRESSION
- Bergamot
- Chamomile
- Lavender
- Ylang Ylang

HEADACHE
The following oils can be used in an oil burner to provide relief from headache:

- Eucalyptus;
- Lemon Grass;
- Peppermint;
- Rose.

See page xvi for more information on how to use these oils.

Dietary and lifestyle recommendations

- Avoid alcohol, caffeine, tobacco, refined and processed foods, salt, sugar and saturated fats as they cause profound changes to blood sugar levels.
- Eat at least six times per day, with an emphasis on complex carbohydrates with moderate protein and fibre.
- Food allergies can often be linked to hypoglycaemia. Testing for allergies may be of benefit to the patient.

HYPOTHYROIDISM

Description

Hypothyroidism is the underproduction of thyroid hormones (thyroxine), resulting in lowered cellular metabolism. Underactivity of the thyroid gland is also called myxoedema. It is more common in females (especially elderly women). Hypothyroidism may be associated with an enlarged thyroid gland (goitre) or the size of the thyroid may be normal.

Symptoms

Symptoms of hypothyroidism include:

- tiredness;
- weakness;
- muscle cramps;
- constipation;
- dry skin;
- headaches;
- nervousness;
- decreased appetite;
- dull and dry hair;
- slurred speech;
- clumsiness;
- numbness and tingling in the hands and feet;
- always feeling cold.

Causes

Causes of hypothyroidism may include:

- Hashimoto's disease, in which the body becomes allergic to thyroid hormone

- iodine deficiency
- genetic factors

Lack of thyroid hormone during foetal life or infancy results in cretinism. Cretins are physically, sexually and mentally underdeveloped. Orthodox treatment of hypothyroidism is by administering oral thyroid hormone.

Nutritional treatment

Nutritional supplements that may be beneficial in the treatment of hypothyroidism are included in the following table (see pages 261–62). See pages xii–xiii for information on how to use these supplements.

Herbal treatment

Herbal treatment of hypothyroidism would include bitter herbs, nerve relaxants and specific thyroid stimulants. The following herbs can be taken as teas, tablets or tinctures. For more information on how to use these herbs see pages xiii–xv.

NERVE RELAXANTS
Nerve relaxants include the herbs:

- Lavender;
- Pasque Flower;
- Skullcap;
- St John's Wort;
- Valerian.

BITTER HERBS
Bitter herbs for hypothyroidism include:
- Gentian Root;
- Rue;

- Wormwood;
- Yarrow.

SPECIFIC HERBS

A specific herb for hypothyroidism is Bladderwrack (Kelp), which is rich in iodine.

Bayberry, Black Cohosh and Golden Seal are also useful in treating hypothyroidism. Do not take Golden Seal internally for more than a week at a time or if you are pregnant.

Homeopathic treatment

For hypothyroidism, Arsenicum album can be taken for up to five days, twice daily whilst a more constitutional treatment is obtained from your homeopath. A homeopathic thyroxine is also available from your homeopath. See page xv for information on how to use homeopathics.

Nutritional supplements for hypothyroidism		
SUPPLEMENT	DOSAGE	COMMENT
Vitamin A	10,000 iu daily	Resists infection and enhances immune function
Vitamin B complex plus Vitamin B6 plus Vitamin B12	100 mg three times daily with meals 50 mg three times daily 15 mg three times daily	The B vitamins are important for energy production, the immune system, digestion and the function of the thyroid gland. Vitamin B6 is important in hormone synthesis
Vitamin C	500 mg three times daily	Vitamin C is important for the adrenal function of producing stress hormones. It also improves immune system
Vitamin E	300–400 iu daily	Improves blood flow and the immune system
L-tyrosine	500 mg twice daily on an empty stomach	Tyrosine is a precursor of thyroid hormones and is specific for treating hypothyroidism
Kelp	As directed on the label	Contains iodine, which is essential in the synthesis of thyroid hormones. This organic form of iodine may be better retained by the body
Brewer's yeast	As directed on the label	Excellent source of B vitamins

Nutritional supplements for hypothyroidism

SUPPLEMENT	DOSAGE	COMMENT
Zinc	50–100 mg daily	Involved in over 80 different enzyme systems. Also important for immune system.
Iron (chelate)	50 mg daily	Take iron if anaemic symptoms are present
Manganese	50 mg daily	Important for the synthesis of thyroxine
Essential fatty acids: One teaspoon daily • Cod liver oil • Sunflower oil • Soy oil • Evening Primrose oil • Wheatgerm oil		Thyroid gland needs essential fatty acids for its hormone synthesis

Aromatherapy treatment

Use the following essential oils to relax the digestive system and to benefit constipation.

- Black Pepper can be used as a body oil or in an oil burner.
- Fennel can be used as a bath or body oil or in an oil burner.
- Marjoram can be used as a bath or body oil, or in an oil burner.
- Orange can be used as a bath or body oil.
- Rose can be used as a bath or body oil.
- Rosemary can be used as a bath or body oil, or in an oil burner.

Use the following essential oils for depression and fatigue.

- Basil can be used as a bath or body oil, or in an oil burner.
- Chamomile can be used as a bath or body oil.
- Clary Sage can be used as a bath or body oil.
- Eucalyptus can be used as a bath or body oil, or in an oil burner.
- Jasmine can be used as a bath or body oil, or in an oil burner.
- Lavender can be used as a bath or body oil.
- Rose can be used as a bath or body oil.
- Sandalwood can be used as a bath or body oil, or in an oil burner.
- Ylang Ylang can be used as a bath or body oil.

For more information on how to use essential oils see page xvi.

Dietary and lifestyle recommendations

IODINE-RICH FOODS

A natural whole-food diet which is rich in vitamins, minerals and fibre is recommended. Foods rich in iodine like iodised salt, seafood, shellfish and seaweed are needed. Other sources of iodine include:

- apples;
- asparagus;
- bananas;
- beetroot;
- blueberries;
- cabbage;
- capsicum;
- carrot;
- cucumber;
- lettuce;
- okra;
- onions;
- peaches;
- peanuts;
- potato;
- spinach;
- strawberries;
- tomato;
- turnip;
- watermelon.

- A moderate form of exercise (such as brisk walking) is beneficial because it stimulates the production of thyroxine.
- Avoid processed and refined foods including white flour and white sugar. Drink only distilled, filtered or tank water to avoid fluoride and chlorine.
- Eat fish or chicken and non-pasteurised, non-homogenised milk and cheeses to keep your protein intake up.

MENOPAUSE
Description

Menopause is not a disease but rather a natural phase that takes place in a woman's life around the age of 50–55 years and usually lasts about five years. It is a time when menstruation ceases and the ovaries slow down production of oestrogen and progesterone. Menopause signifies the end of the woman's childbearing years. For some women this can be a very emotional time and produce a number of psychological symptoms. Other women see this new phase in their lives as a blessing.

Symptoms

There are a range of physical symptoms that occur during this time due to the drop in hormone levels.

- hot flushes
- fatigue
- poor concentration
- night sweats and insomnia
- shortness of breath
- dry skin and hair
- depression
- bladder problems
- painful intercourse
- decreased libido
- vaginal dryness and itching

Nutritional supplements for menopause

SUPPLEMENT	DOSAGE	COMMENT
Vitamin B complex	As directed on label	To improve cellular function and circulation
Calcium (chelate) and	1500 mg daily	Essential for maintaining healthy bones and avoiding osteoporosis
Magnesium	500 mg daily	Helps alleviate anxiety and irritability
Evening Primrose oil	500 mg daily	Important for the production of oestrogen
Vitamin E	400 iu daily	Helpful in reducing hot flushes and other menopausal symptoms
Selenium	100 mcg daily	Helps maintain normal hormone levels
Vitamin C with bioflavonoids	2000 mg daily	Used to treat hot flushes
Multivitamin and mineral complex	One tablet daily	Important for balancing and maintaining normal hormone production
Garlic	Two 500 mg capsules	Helps the body maintain a high level of daily immunity against infection
Brewer's yeast	Six–ten tablets daily	Excellent source of calcium
Zinc	50 mg daily	Helps protect the body against bone degeneration

- heart palpitations
- osteoporosis

Causes

The symptoms that occur during menopause are caused by the decrease in the production of oestrogen and progesterone. The hormone oestrogen is needed for the health of arteries, skin and bone formation. When the ovaries stop producing this hormone the endocrine glands take over and continue to produce a small amount of oestrogen to help maintain the body's natural function.

Nutritional treatment

Nutritional supplements that may be beneficial in the treatment of menopause are included in the above table. See pages xii–xiii for information on how to use these supplements.

Herbal treatment

The following herbs can provide relief from menopausal symptoms.

- Sage helps reduce sweating.
- St John's Wort is very effective in treating tension, anxiety and depression.
- Chaste Tree berry balances hormonal disruptions and works effectively in reducing hot flushes.
- Life Root is used as a uterine tonic to strengthen and aide the body during menopausal disturbances.
- Skullcap is used to treat depression and exhaustion or fatigue.
- Valerian is used for the relief of tension and insomnia.

HERBAL TEA

A combination of equal parts Life Root, St John's Wort and Oats may be helpful in treating menopausal symptoms.

Pour a cup of boiling water onto one–three teaspoons of the dried herbs and let stand for 10–15 minutes. Drink three to four times daily.

For information on how to use herbal treatments see page xiii–xv.

Homeopathic treatment

Homoeopathy is another natural therapy that can be used safely and effectively to treat the symptoms of menopause. For information on how to use the following homeopathics see page xv.

- Ferrum phosphoricum is used to treat hot flushes with a red face.
- Belladonna is used when the hot flushes stop and start suddenly. It is also used where there is redness to the face and head.
- Sepia is used when there is anxiety, irritability and hysteria.
- Sanguinaria is used to treat hot flushes to the face and neck and burning in the ears.
- Kali phosphoricum is used to treat nervousness, anxiety, depression and hot flushes.

Aromatherapy treatment

To ease nervous tension, depression and anxiety associated with menopause try the following aromatherapy essential oils.

- Basil is a soothing, calming and uplifting oil which is best used as a body or bath oil.
- Chamomile is a soothing oil that has healing and calming properties. It is best used in a compress or as a body or a bath oil.
- Clary Sage is a soothing, relaxing and warming oil used to treat depression, anxiety and dry sensitive skin. Use as a bath or a body oil and as a skin care oil.
- Cypress is a strongly aromatic oil that helps balance the female system. Use as a bath or massage oil. (Avoid cypress if you suffer from high blood pressure.)
- Neroli is a wonderful facial and massage oil or inhalation oil. It has a calming influence on the mind and body.

- Rose is used as a bath or body oil. It is a specific for menopause.
- Sage is used as a massage oil to relieve nervous and muscular tension.

See page xvi for more information on how to use these oils.

Dietary and lifestyle recommendations

- Try eliminating all sugar, tea, coffee and cola drinks from your diet as they can often exacerbate the symptoms of menopause.
- Get regular exercise such as walking, swimming, tennis or yoga.
- If sexual intercourse is painful due to lack of vaginal lubrication try using vitamin E oil or Aloe Vera gel.
- The menopausal phase in a woman's life can sometimes last a number of years. For this reason it is highly recommended natural therapies be used to alleviate symptoms as they can be used safely and effectively for long periods. Long-term drug treatment on the other hand may cause a number of unpleasant and dangerous side effects.

CALCIUM-RICH FOODS

It is essential to eat a well-balanced diet with emphasis placed on calcium-rich foods such as:

- almonds;
- brewer's yeast;
- broccoli;
- cheese;
- chickpeas;
- figs;
- hazelnuts;
- kelp;
- lentils;
- olives;
- parsley;
- pistachio nuts;
- sesame seeds;
- soy milk;
- spinach;
- yoghurt.

CHAPTER EIGHT

THE MUSCULO-SKELETAL SYSTEM

Maintenance of the bones, joints, muscles, cartilage, ligaments and tendons

What does it consist of?

The musculo-skeletal system is made up of bones, joints, cartilage, ligaments, tendons and muscles. This system is built around the framework of the skeleton. Skeletal muscle is also called voluntary muscle becasue we can choose to contract or relax it, as opposed to the involuntary cardiac muscle responsible for contracting the heart.

What does it do?

The skeleton provides support and protection for the organs and tissues of the body and provides points of attachment for the skeletal muscles, thus allowing for movement.

Bones store most of the calcium, phosphorus, magnesium and other minerals and salts that the body needs. Within certain parts of bones the red marrow produces red blood cells, white blood cells and platelets. Bones also store energy in the fat cells of yellow bone marrow. The bones are connected to each other by joints which allow movement. The ball and socket joints of the hips and shoulders allow the greatest range of movement.

Muscles make up the bulk of the body and are responsible for about half of the body's weight. Muscles are made up of microscopic cells called muscle fibres. There are two types of muscle tissue:

- involuntary muscles which are not under our conscious mind control, such as the heart and the movements of the intestines during digestion
- voluntary muscles which are under our conscious control, such as the quadriceps in running.

Ligaments bind joints to provide stability, while the muscles can contract and relax to provide movement. All muscles in the trunk and limbs are kept in a partly contracted state, called muscle tone, in order to keep the body upright.

What goes wrong with it?

Injuries to muscles and their tendon attachments are usually the result of overexertion during daily activities or from sudden pulling or twisting movements, such as those occurring during sports. Muscles are more often injured than diseased and in many cases they are capable of self-repair. One of the most common problems of the musculo-skeletal system is damage to the joints by injury or by wear and tear. But the health of our bones, muscles and joints not only depends on the use to which they are put or the overall structure that they are a part of, but also to a large extent on the condition of our internal environment, on the state of our metabolism, on diet, exercise and lifestyle. If our biochemical and metabolic processes are out of balance then wastes and toxins can accumulate in the body and damage the integrity of our musculo-skeletal system.

Nutritional treatment

Nutritional supplements that benefit the musculo-skeletal system include:

VITAMIN A

Vitamin A stimulates the secretion of gastric juices, which are essential for all types of protein digestion. Vitamin A promotes good teeth and bones. Painful joints and bone growth problems may be symptoms of vitamin A deficiency.

VITAMIN B2

Vitamin B2 is stored in the muscles and is used in times of physical exertion. Vitamin B2 also works as an anti-oxidant to track down and destroy abnormal cells in the body.

VITAMIN B6

Vitamin B6 is essential for the conversion of proteins into amino acids, which are the building blocks for muscle tissue. Vitamin B6 deficiency may lead to arthritis.

VITAMIN B12

Vitamin B12 deficiency may cause immature red blood cells or fewer red blood cells which can result in muscular weakness. Vitamin B12 is important in the synthesis of protein.

VITAMIN C
Vitamin C deficiency can cause easy bruising. Vitamin C may provide relief from conditions like arthritis as it helps nourish and lubricate the joints. It is also needed to maintain collagen, which is a protein required for the formation of connective tissue in the skin, ligaments and bones. Vitamin C is important in healing wounds and burns.

VITAMIN E
Vitamin E is necessary for the synthesis and use of many amino acids. It increases the power and activity of muscles, especially the heart. Vitamin E plays an essential role in cellular respiration of all muscles.

BIOTIN
Biotin assists in the maintenance, growth and healing of bones. It also is needed in the breakdown and metabolism of protein. Deficiency of biotin may lead to muscle pain.

CHOLINE
Choline plays an important part in the transmission of nerve impulses.

FOLIC ACID
Folic acid is important for the breakdown and utilisation of protein. It is also required for the absorption of iron and calcium. Folic acid deficiency may lead to arthritis.

CALCIUM
Calcium is necessary for bone and tooth formation. It is important for muscular contraction. Calcium deficiency can lead to muscular cramps, arthritis, bone pain, osteoporosis and backache. Calcium-rich foods are also required for smooth functioning of the heart muscle.

POTASSIUM
Potassium is the foundation mineral of all muscular tissues. It is essential for muscular contraction and for the repair of all the body's muscles. Deficiency may cause muscle weakness, paralysis and rheumatoid arthritis.

MAGNESIUM
Magnesium is involved in muscular contraction and relaxation, protein synthesis and bone growth. Deficiency may lead to muscular twitch, tremors, weakness, lack of coordination and disturbance of the heart rhythm.

IRON
Iron-rich foods improve protein metabolism. Iron is also necessary for the formation of myoglobin, which is an important part of muscle tissue. Iron deficiency may lead to muscle fatigue.

PHOSPHORUS
Phosphorus stimulates muscle contractions, including the regular contractions of the heart. It is important in the utilisation of protein for growth, maintenance and repair of muscle tissue. Deficiency may lead to

muscular weakness, bone pains and joint problems.

Herbal treatment

There are many herbs that benefit the musculo-skeletal system.

ANTI-INFLAMMATORY HERBS

Anti-inflammatory and anti-rheumatic herbs can be used to prevent, relieve or cure rheumatic problems by reducing swelling and pain in the joints. They include:

- Angelica;
- Black Willow;
- Celery seed;
- Devil's Claw;
- Jamaican Dogwood;
- Juniper;
- Poke Root;
- Sarsaparilla;
- St John's Wort;
- Wild Yam;
- Willow Bark;
- Wormwood.

ALTERATIVE HERBS

Alterative herbs cleanse the bloodstream and thus benefit rheumatic and arthritic conditions. They include:

- Black Cohosh;
- Burdock Root;
- Celery seed;
- Guaiacum;
- Sarsaparilla.

DIURETICS

Diuretics can be helpful for arthritic and rheumatic problems by assisting the cleansing action of the kidneys.

They include:

- Boneset;
- Celery seed;
- Juniper berries;
- Yarrow.

ANTISPASMODIC HERBS

Antispasmodic herbs can prevent or ease muscular spasms or cramps. They include:

- Black Haw;
- Cramp Bark;
- Skullcap;
- Valerian;
- Vervain.

RUBEFACIENT HERBS

Rubefacient herbs are commonly used in lotions or liniments to ease pain, stiffness and even inflammation. They include:

- Cayenne;
- Eucalyptus;
- Ginger;
- Mustard;
- Peppermint;
- Wintergreen.

Aromatherapy treatment

There are many essential oils that can be of great benefit to the musculo-skeletal system.

ARTHRITIS

Use the following essential oils for arthritis:

- Camphor (as a body oil or compress);

- Cedarwood (as a bath or body oil);
- Chamomile (as a bath or body oil, or a compress);
- Eucalyptus (as a bath or body oil);
- Juniper (as a bath or body oil, or as a compress);
- Sage (as a bath or body oil, or as a compress).

RHEUMATISM

Use the following essential oils for rheumatism:

- Bay (as a body oil);
- Cajuput (as a bath or body oil);
- Camphor (as a body oil);
- Chamomile (as a body oil);
- Coriander (as a body oil);
- Cypress (as a bath or body oil or as a compress – avoid during pregnancy);
- Eucalyptus (as a bath or body oil);
- Juniper (as a bath or body oil);
- Lavender (as a bath or body oil or as a compress);
- Lime (as a body oil);
- Pine (as a bath or body oil);
- Rosemary (as a bath or body oil);
- Thyme (as a bath or body oil).

BRUISES AND SPRAINS

Use the following essential oils for bruises and sprains:

- Chamomile (as a bath or body oil);
- Eucalyptus (as a body oil);
- Hyssop (as a bath or body oil, or as a compress);
- Marjoram (as a bath or body oil, or as a compress);
- Rosemary (as a bath or body oil).

ACHES AND PAINS

Use the following essential oils for aches and pains:

- Basil (as a bath or body oil);
- Black Pepper (as a body oil);
- Clary Sage (as a bath or body oil).

Dietary and lifestyle recommendations

MUSCULAR SYSTEM

Foods that benefit the muscular system include:

- acidophilus yoghurt;
- apples;
- avocado;
- bananas;
- beans;
- dates;
- legumes;
- lima beans;
- olives;
- parsley;
- peanuts;
- pepitas;
- potatoes;
- raw nuts;
- seeds;
- soybeans;
- sprouts;
- tahini;
- wheatgerm;
- wholegrains.

High-quality protein is needed for building muscles. This can be found in the following foods:

- beef;
- eggs;

- fish;
- soymeal.

Juices that benefit the muscular system include:

- carrot or spinach juice;
- nut milk with liquid chlorophyll;
- potato peeling broth.

Some essential amino acids can only be obtained from foods like:

- beans;
- lentils;
- peas;
- seafood;
- turkey.

SKELETAL SYSTEM

Foods that benefit the skeletal system include:

- acidophilus yoghurt;
- almonds;
- barley;
- celery;
- cheese;
- green vegetables;
- legumes;
- millet;
- parmesan cheese;
- pepitas;
- raw nuts;
- sesame seeds;
- sprouts;
- sunflower seeds;
- tahini;
- tofu;
- unprocessed goat's milk.

Juices that benefit the skeletal system include:

- black cherry juice;
- carrot, beetroot and cucumber juices;
- celery and parsley juice;
- celery, carrot and parsley juice (for joints).

ARTHRITIS
Description

Arthritis is inflammation of one or more joints, characterised by pain, swelling (which may cause deformity of the joint) and stiffness. In the initial stages the symptoms may come and go, and are often more intense in the morning. Types of arthritis include:

- osteoarthritis (the most common form of arthritis)
- rheumatoid arthritis
- gout

Symptoms and causes

OSTEOARTHRITIS

Osteoarthritis involves the breakdown or wearing away of the cartilage, which covers the ends of bones and allows them to move smoothly against each other. It is a degenerative joint disease which is most commonly related to the wear and tear of aging. Other possible causes include: hormonal factors, genetic predisposition, inflammatory joint disease and fracture. It may also result from injury or a defect in the protein that goes to make up cartilage. Osteoarthritis rarely develops before the age of 40 but it seems to affect (sometimes very mildly) most people past the age of 60. Under the age of 45 osteoarthritis is much more common in men; over the age of 45 it is much more common in women.

RHEUMATOID ARTHRITIS

Rheumatoid arthritis is a condition in which the joints become inflamed and painful. Cartilage and connective tissues in and around the joint are damaged or destroyed. The patient feels generally unwell, with weight loss, malaise, fever, fatigue, pain and stiffness in the hands, feet and knees. The body replaces the destroyed tissue with scar tissue which causes the normal spaces within the joints to narrow and the bones to fuse together. While osteoarthritis affects individual joints, rheumatoid arthritis affects all the synovial joints of the body. For detailed information on rheumatoid arthritis see pages 291–93.

GOUT

Gout is a form of inflammatory arthritis caused by an increased concentration of uric acid in the body's fluid. Uric acid crystals are deposited in joints and tendons and can cause inflammation and extreme pain. It occurs most commonly in people who are overweight and/or overindulge regularly in rich foods and alcohol. Gout usually affects the big toe joint though other joints may be affected.

Nutritional supplements for arthritis

SUPPLEMENT	DOSAGE	COMMENT
Vitamin A	10,000 iu daily	Required for the synthesis of normal collagen and maintenance of cartilage. Deficiency may allow joint degeneration
Vitamin B complex plus	100 mg three times daily	Important for nutritional support of the muscles
Vitamin B3 plus	100 mg three times daily (do not take if you suffer from gout or liver disease)	Increases blood flow by dilating capillaries
Vitamin B5 plus	50 mg per day	Stimulates cartilage growth, used therapeutically for osteoarthritis
Vitamin B6	50 mg per day	Involved in the synthesis of essential fatty acid metabolites
Vitamin C	1000–3000 mg daily in divided doses	Deficiency can result in altered collagen synthesis and compromised tissue repair

Nutritional supplements for arthritis

SUPPLEMENT	DOSAGE	COMMENT
Vitamin E	22 iu three times daily	Stimulates cartilage synthesis and inhibits the breakdown of cartilage
Zinc chelate	100 mg daily	May improve joint pain, morning stiffness and overall condition. Needed for bone growth
Calcium chelate and Magnesium	1000 mg daily 500 mg daily	Can reduce the inflammatory response of pain and swelling. Calcium is needed to prevent bone loss
Copper salicylate	2 mg daily	An effective anti-inflammatory agent which may be more powerful than aspirin
Selenium	200 mcg daily	May be deficient in people with osteoporosis
Bromelain	As directed on label, three times daily with meals	A digestive enzyme from the with known anti-inflammatory properties
Essential fatty acids • Evening Primrose oil • Salmon oil	1500 mg twice daily or as directed on label. Take before meals.	Can reduce pain, swelling and joint mobility You may need to take up to three months before you get results
Glycosamine sulphate	1000–3000 mg three times daily	A sublingual form is recommended or injected with doctor's supervision. Has a marked anti-inflammatory effect
Superoxide dismutase (SOD)	As directed on label	Same as glycosamine sulphate

Nutritional treatment

Nutritional supplements that may be beneficial in the treatment of arthritis are included in the above table. See pages xii–xiii for information on how to use these supplements.

Herbal treatment

See pages xiii–xv for information on how to use the following herbs.

ANTI-INFLAMMATORY

Anti-inflammatory herbs help the body to combat inflammation and decrease pain, swelling and joint deformity.

Anti-inflammatory herbs for osteo-arthritis include:

- Black Cohosh;
- Devil's Claw;
- Feverfew (avoid during pregnancy);
- Ginger;
- Meadowsweet;
- Wild Yam;
- Willow Bark;
- Yucca.

These herbs can be taken as tablets, teas or tinctures.

PAIN RELIEF

A herbal formula to relieve pain and assist a good night's sleep includes the herbs:

- Jamaican Dogwood;
- Passion Flower;
- St John's Wort;
- Valerian.

Use in equal proportions, either by making a herbal infusion or by mixing the tinctures.

St John's Wort oil can be rubbed on areas of arthritic pain to provide relief and assist in a good night's sleep.

DIURETICS

Other herbs that can be of use in treating arthritis include the diuretics:

- Buchu;
- Burdock Root;
- Celery seeds;
- Cornsilk;
- Nettle;
- Parsley.

These can be used as teas, tablets or tinctures.

- Alfalfa tea or sprouts contain all the minerals essential for bone formation, and should be taken regularly.
- Hawthorn berries, bilberries and cherries contain cartilage-stabilising flavonoids and should be eaten regularly.

Homeopathic treatment

For information on how to use the following treatments see page xv.

- Take Arnica if the pain is accompanied by stiffness and is as a result of an injury.
- Take Bryonia if there is a severe pain which is worse on movement (and better when absolutely still) and if the joints are swollen and feel hot.
- Take Calcarea phosphorica when joints feel cold or numb, if there is weakness and pain in the hips, if the small joints of the hand are sore and if all the symptoms are worse in cold, damp weather.
- Take Ledum if the pain starts in the feet and moves upwards, if the joints are heard to crack on movement, and if the stiff, painful joints are relieved by cold compresses.
- Take Pulsatilla for joint pain which rapidly moves around the body and which may be accompanied by weeping, the legs feeling heavy, and when the symptoms are improved on exposure to cool, fresh air.
- Take Rhus toxicodendron if there is pain and stiffness that is worse on waking in the morning, aggravated

by the cold and damp, and improved by heat.
- Take Rhododendron for pain and stiffness that is worse before a storm, worse when at rest, and improved by movement, warmth and when the person has had something to eat.

Aromatherapy treatment

The following oils may provide relief from the symptoms of arthritis. For more information on how to use these essential oils see page xvi.

- Juniper removes toxins and can be used as a bath or body oil or as a compress. For arthritis take four drops of juniper oil on a teaspoon of brown sugar after meals. For gout rub affected joint with a mixture of 90 percent olive oil and ten percent juniper oil.
- Rosemary improves circulation of the blood and also removes toxins. It can be used as a bath or body oil.
- Ginger has warming properties for joints which feel painful, stiff and cold. Use as a massage oil.
- Chamomile can be used as a bath or body oil, or as a compress.
- Geranium can be used as a bath or body oil, or as a compress.
- Lavender can be used as a bath or body oil, or as a compress.
- Marjoram can be used as a bath or body oil, or as a compress.

Dietary and lifestyle recommendations

- Meat contains a form of fat that encourages inflammatory agents in the body. Reduce your intake of red meats, dairy foods, salt, tea, coffee, alcohol and processed or refined foods. A vegetarian diet has been beneficial for many arthritic people. Reduce excess weight and take a diet rich in complex carbohydrates and dietary fibre. Many arthritics benefit from taking digestive enzymes (papain and bromelain) or apple cider vinegar with meals.
- Avoid the nightshade group of foods such as tomatoes, potatoes, eggplant, capsicum and chilli peppers. These foods can aggravate the inflammatory response in joints. Reduce the amount of fat and sugar in your diet.
- Eat cold water fish (salmon, tuna, cod, mackerel) at least three times a week.
- Check for possible food allergies.
- Many arthritic patients find copper rings and bracelets helpful for managing pain and stiffness. Copper chelate rub applied to the affected joint may reduce inflammation.
- Get regular moderate exercise, fresh air and sunshine. Walking, easy bicycle riding, aqua aerobics, swimming, etc are essential for reducing pain and reducing joint deterioration.

BENEFICIAL FOODS

Increase your consumption of:

- apples;
- beetroot;
- cabbage;
- carrots;
- celery;
- cucumbers;
- dates;
- ginger;
- hard nuts;
- melons;
- mussels;
- oats;
- onions;
- parsley;
- prunes;
- spinach;
- tripe;
- watercress;
- wholegrain cereals.

JUICES

Raw juice therapy can help relieve the symptoms of arthritis. Take apple juice daily and in the inflammatory period of arthritis (when the symptoms are acute) take all of the following juices on a daily basis.

- 1000 ml celery juice
- 170 ml carrot juice
- 140 ml beetroot juice
- 140 ml cucumber juice

BACKACHE

Description and symptoms

Backache or back pain is a very common malady that affects a large percentage of people at one time or other during their life. Symptoms consist of aches, pain and muscular stiffness in the lower, middle and upper back and neck.

Causes

Backache can arise for a number of different reasons. It may result from an injury such as a fall where a vertebra has been damaged. The pain may be associated with nerve damage due to weight gain or lack of exercise. Lack of tone in the stomach muscles is the postural cause of back pain.

Sciatica, slipped disc and period pain can also cause backache. There is also emotional backache which is the result of constant stress.

The fact that backache often arises for a number of different reasons means there are also a wide variety of treatments available. These include: osteopathy, chiropractic manipulation, the Alexander technique (which teaches the patient to correct their posture), acupuncture, massage and relaxation. For more information about these treatments consult qualified practitioners.

Nutritional treatment

Nutritional supplements that may be beneficial in the treatment of backache

Nutritional supplements for backache

SUPPLEMENT	DOSAGE	COMMENT
Vitamin A	10,000 iu daily	Needed for healing and the formation of connective tissue
Vitamin B12	2000 mg daily	Helps in the absorption of calcium
Vitamin E	400 iu daily	Promotes healing
Multivitamin and mineral complex	As directed on label	Helps strengthen and balance the body
Calcium and	1500 mg daily	Calcium is essential for strong bones
Magnesium	750 mg daily	Magnesium is needed for proper absorption of calcium
Zinc	50 mg daily	Builds immunity

are included in the following table. See pages xii–xiii for information on how to use these supplements.

Herbal treatment

Herbs can be of benefit in relieving the muscular aches and pain that are associated with backache.

- Skullcap is helpful in relieving back pain triggered by menstruation.
- Valerian provides relief from period pain, muscle spasm and tension.
- Wild Yam is commonly prescribed for muscular and joint pain. Wild Yam has anti-inflammatory and anti-cramp properties.
- Willow is used mainly for symptomatic relief of rheumatic conditions, joint and muscle pain.

The above herbs can be taken as teas, tinctures or tablets. For more information on how to use these herbs see pages xiii–xv.

Homeopathic treatment

Homeopathy treatment may be helpful in relieving the discomfort of backache. See page xv for information on how to use the following treatments.

- Ferrum phosphoricum is useful where there is acute pain, inflammation, redness and heat.
- Arnica can be used externally or internally where there is pain due to strain or injury. Also where there is bruising and pain on movement.
- Bryonia is useful in cases of fibrositis or muscular rheumatism in the neck, back and limbs, when the pain is worse on moving and relieved by stillness and pressure.
- Rhus toxicodendron provides relief from stiffness and pain after overuse or exercise.

Aromatherapy treatment

Treat yourself to a regular massage using aromatherapy essential oils and you may find you avoid backaches and pains. The following oils are recommended to lift your spirits and relax and revitalise your body:

- Lavender relaxes and eases aches and pains and can be used as a massage oil, bath oil or in an oil burner.
- Chamomile is a soothing, calming oil. Used as a bath oil or massage oil it will relax muscles as well as being an anti-inflammatory.
- Rosemary is good for rheumatic aches and pains. Use as a massage oil or bath oil.
- Black Pepper is a stimulating oil for muscular aches and poor circulation. Use as a bath or body oil.

For more information on how to use these oils see page xvi.

Dietary and lifestyle recommendations

- Regular exercise such as walking, swimming, cycling or yoga is important in helping build and maintain muscle tone and fitness. Doing exercises that strengthen the abdominal muscles will help to support the back and improve posture.
- Avoid repetitive bending from the waist. Always bend from the knees and use your legs, abdomen and arms to lift objects.

- To relieve back pain soothe those sore muscles in a warm bath or apply a heated compress to the area.
- If the pain is severe or an injury has occurred consult your physician immediately.

BRUISING

Description and symptoms

A bruise occurs when a part of the body is bumped or struck by a blunt object, causing damage to the tissues underneath the skin. Small blood vessels (usually capillaries or veins) rupture causing discoloration of the skin without a break in the overlying skin. The discoloration starts out red then turns a blue/black tinge. The change in colour is accompanied by pain and swelling.

Causes

There are several factors which predispose certain people to bruising easily:

- haemophilia;
- leukaemia;
- anaemia;
- obesity;
- malnutrition;
- vitamin C deficiency;
- heavy smoking;
- during menstruation;
- using anticoagulants, such as aspirin;
- anti-inflammatory drugs.

Nutritional supplements for bruising

SUPPLEMENT	DOSAGE	COMMENT
Vitamin A	20,000 iu twice daily (if pregnant no more than 10,000 iu daily)	For healing and protection of all tissues. Enhances the adhesion between cells
Vitamin B1	100 mg daily	Anti-oxidant
Vitamin B5	100 mg daily	Vitamin B5 deficiency can lead to anaemia. Vitamin B5 strengthens the skin and underlying tissues.
Vitamin B6	100 mg daily	Vitamin B6 deficiency can lead to anaemia. Vitamin B6 is also essential for the production of antibodies.
Vitamin C with bioflavonoids	5000 mg daily	Vitamin C is essential for collagen formation, and it strengthens the walls of blood vessels. It helps to prevent bruising.
Vitamin D	500 iu daily	Assists in blood clotting and protects the skin.
Vitamin E	500 iu daily	Stabilises cell membranes and improves blood flow to body tissues.
Coenzyme Q10	50 mg daily	Important for the construction of body cells.
Calcium and Magnesium	1000 mg of each daily	Calcium facilitates blood clotting. Magnesium helps with the body's absorption of calcium.
Iron	As directed on the label	Iron improves oxygenation of body cells and assists in skin formation. Deficiency can lead to anaemia.
Selenium	500 mcg daily	Anti-oxidant
Zinc	50 mg daily	Zinc is important for wound healing and zinc deficiency can lead to anaemia.

Bruising easily with no apparent cause can be a early sign of cancer. Seek medical attention if this is the case. For more information on bruising see pages 142–45.

Nutritional treatment

Nutritional supplements that may be beneficial in the treatment of bruises are included in the table on page 280. See pages xii–xiii for information on how to use these supplements.

Herbal treatment

For information on how to use the following herbs see pages xiii–xv.

EXTERNAL USE
For external application use the following herbs as ointments, lotions, tinctures or compresses:

* Arnica;
* Marigold;
* Witch Hazel.

You can also make a poultice from crushed Comfrey leaves to apply to the area.

INTERNAL USE
For internal use, to prevent frequent bruising, the following herbs may be beneficial:

* Horse Chestnut and/or Yarrow for their vitamin C content;
* Dandelion and/or Yellow dock for their iron content;
* Alfalfa for its vitamin K content (which is important for blood clotting).

Take these herbs as teas, tablets or tinctures.

Homeopathic treatment

Treatment that may be prescribed by a homeopath for bruising includes the following homeopathics. See page xv for information on how to use these treatments.

* For black eyes take Arnica, Bellis or Ledum.
* For bruises with unbroken skin either apply Arnica tincture externally to the affected area or take Arnica homeopathic drops every three to four hours.
* If the skin is broken and bruising is also apparent apply Hamamelis tincture externally or take Hamamelis homeopathic drops every three to four hours.

Aromatherapy treatment

For the treatment of bruises use the following essential oils as body oils or as compresses.

* Chamomile
* Hyssop
* Lavender
* Sweet Marjoram

To make a compress soak a clean cloth in warm water and add 10–20 drops of essential oil. For information on how to use these oils see page xvi.

Lifestyle and dietary recommendations

* As soon as an injury occurs immediately apply a cold pack

(such as packet of frozen peas or ice cubes wrapped in a cloth) for ten to 20 minutes to minimise the bleeding under the skin. Twenty-four hours later begin to apply hot packs for speedy wound healing.

- Wrap and elevate the bruised limb to help minimise blood flow into the affected area.

BENEFICIAL FOODS

Include the following foods in your diet:

- almonds;
- brazil nuts;
- broccoli;
- buckwheat;
- cashews;
- cheeses;
- citrus fruits;
- eggs;
- green peppers;
- hazelnuts;
- leafy greens are good sources of vitamin K;
- lentils;
- meats;
- sunflower and sesame seeds (for zinc and iron);
- sweet potatoes (for vitamin C);
- walnuts;
- wholegrains.

BURSITIS

Description

Bursitis is inflammation of the bursa which are fluid-filled sacs that lubricate the joints. The bursae are located between the bone and the tendon in areas such as the elbow, hip, knee and shoulder.

Symptoms

Symptoms include pain in the joint, especially when moving; a limited range of motion; an accumulation of fluid and swelling and redness.

Causes

Bursitis is commonly caused by an injury (often a sporting injury) or repeated trauma to the affected area. The problem may also result from an infection or gout.

Nutritional treatment

Nutritional supplements that may be beneficial in the treatment of bursitis are included in the following table. See pages xii–xiii for information on how to use these supplements.

Herbal treatment

Herbs used in the treatment of bursitis include Horsetail, Nettle and Celery. These herbs can be taken as teas, tinctures or tablets. For more information on using these herbs see pages xiii–xv.

- Horsetail has mild antiseptic and astringent qualities and is often recommended for arthritic, urinary and circulatory problems.
- Nettle is very helpful for a range of skin conditions including

rheumatic pain, gout and poor circulation.

- Celery is useful in the treatment of arthritis, rheumatism and gout. To make an infusion pour a cup of boiling water onto one–two teaspoons of freshly crushed celery seeds. Leave to infuse for ten to 15 minutes. Drink three times a day.

Homeopathic treatment

Homeopathy can provide relief and healing to those suffering from bursitis. See page xv for information on how to use the following treatments.

- Ruta graveolens is used to treat tennis elbow, where symptoms include pain in the joint, if the area feels worse when exercising and if

the condition is improved when the sufferer is warm.

- Ferrum phosphoricum is used where there is pain and redness, and when the pain is also increased by movement. It is used in the first stages of inflammation.
- Arnica provides relief for stiffness, bruising and pain after an injury.

Aromatherapy treatment

The following essential oils may be helpful in treating bursitis. For more information on how to use these oils see page xvi.

- Benzoin can be used as a bath oil or massage oil to treat rheumatic and arthritic conditions.
- Eucalyptus can be used as an inhalant, bath oil or rub.

Nutritional supplements for bursitis

SUPPLEMENT	DOSAGE	COMMENT
Vitamin A	10,000 iu daily	A potent anti-oxidant and anti-inflammatory essential for healing wounds
Vitamin C	2000–4000 mg daily	Important in the formation of tendon and bursal tissue
Vitamin E	400 iu daily	An anti-inflammatory
Multivitamin and mineral complex	As directed on label	Essential for the proper balance and function of the body
Calcium and Magnesium	1500 mg daily 750 mg daily	Calcium is needed for connective tissue repair Magnesium aids the proper assimilation of calcium
Zinc	15 mg daily	Essential for the repair of tissue

Eucalyptus oil can be used to treat rheumatic pain and inflammation.

- Juniper can be used as a bath oil or body oil. Juniper may provide relief from arthritic and rheumatic conditions where there is muscle and joint pain and discomfort.

Dietary and lifestyle recommendations

- It is essential to rest the injured area.
- Ice the area as this reduces the inflammation and pain. You may however find relief by alternating ice and heat applications. Try an icepack on the area for 15 minutes, then apply a warm compress for 15 minutes.
- Elevate the injury where possible and firmly wrap the area in an elastic bandage.
- When the pain and inflammation is gone slowly resume your regular activities.

CARPAL TUNNEL SYNDROME

Description

Carpal tunnel syndrome is a very painful condition which affects the wrist area. Strenuous and repetitive use of the wrist or hands can cause a buildup of fluid and tissue, which puts pressure on the median nerve as it passes through a gap under a ligament at the front of the wrist.

Symptoms

These include:

- pins and needles in the fingers;
- pain, numbness and inflammation of the wrist;
- tingling that may radiate into the hand, elbow and sometimes the shoulder.

Causes

The main causes are injuries and overuse of the wrist area. The condition can also be associated with rheumatoid arthritis.

Nutritional treatment

Nutritional supplements that may be beneficial in the treatment of carpal tunnel syndrome are included in the following table. See pages xii–xiii for information on how to use these supplements.

Herbal treatment

Herbs may be of benefit to those affected by carpal tunnel syndrome. Herbs can help to stimulate circulation and bring oxygen and nutrients to the area. They can also be helpful in relieving tension and reducing fluid

Nutritional supplements for carpal tunnel syndrome		
SUPPLEMENT	DOSAGE	COMMENT
Vitamin B complex	100 mg daily	Essential for nerve function
Vitamin B6	50 mg daily	Deficiency of this vitamin is commonly found in patients with carpal tunnel syndrome
Bromelain	250–500 mg between meals	Helps reduce inflammation and pain
Manganese	As directed on label	Improves nerve function

build up. Use the following herbs as teas, tinctures or tablets. See pages xiii–xv for information on how to use these herbs.

- Nettle is helpful in treating rheumatic conditions and improving circulation.
- Skullcap may provide relief to those suffering muscular aches and pains.
- Dandelion is an excellent general tonic. Dandelion can be used very effectively to treat muscular rheumatism and fluid retention.

Homeopathic treatment

Homeopathics used to treat carpal tunnel syndrome and repetitive strain injuries are:

- Bryonia for pain that is made worse by movement but is eased when resting.
- Causticum for tearing pains in the muscles and joints, particularly in the arms and when the symptoms are worse when its dry and cold but improve when warm.

- Rhus toxicodendron for pain that is worsened by initial movement but improves as movement increases. It is also used when the pain becomes worse when muscles tire.

See page xv for information on how to use these treatments.

Aromatherapy treatment

Essential oils can provide relief from muscular pain and inflammation, and also improve circulation. Massage the hands and wrists with the following soothing oils.

- Rosemary is a wonderfully aromatic oil that can be used as a massage rub for aching muscles.
- Sage has a soothing and cooling quality and was once widely used as a remedy for rheumatism. As a massage oil sage can relieve nervous tension and muscle pain (avoid during pregnancy).
- Geranium can be used as massage oil or bath oil. Geranium has anti-inflammatory properties and it relieves aches and pains.

- Relieve pain and improve circulation by soaking your hands and wrists in a warm bath with a few drops of lavender oil.

For more information on how to use these oils see page xvi.

Dietary and lifestyle recommendations

- Carpal tunnel syndrome is most common among those whose jobs or hobbies involve repetitive movement of the wrist. It is therefore important to have regular breaks during activities such as computer work, knitting, jackhammering or building work. Stretch the fingers and loosen and relax the wrist by gently rotating them.
- Make sure your retain good posture and use the arm rests of your chair to rest the elbows when typing.

CRAMPS

Description and symptoms

Cramps are characterised by severe and often sharp pain that occurs when a muscle or a group of muscles contract.

There are two main types of cramps: muscular cramps and menstruation cramps.

The contraction or spasm may result from injury or overuse of the muscle. Cramping usually occurs during the night in the calf muscle or the feet. The best way to relieve a sudden cramp is by massaging and stretching the area. It is important to massage down the muscle, not across it. Gentle stretching will also bring relief.

Causes

A deficiency of calcium and magnesium will cause muscles to contract in different parts of the body. Inadequate potassium levels have also been linked to muscle spasm. Poor circulation and overuse or injury to the muscle may also result in cramping.

Nutritional treatment

Nutritional supplements that may be beneficial in the treatment of cramps are included in the following table. See pages xii–xiii for information on how to use these supplements.

Herbal treatment

The following herbs have been traditionally recommended for cramp and muscle spasm. These herbs can be taken as teas, tablets, or tinctures. See pages xiii–xv for information on how to use these herbs.

- Skullcap is used therapeutically to treat muscle aches and pains, menstruation cramp, palpitations and headaches.
- Valerian is used to treat insomnia, cramps, period pain and anxiety.
- Vervain is used as a digestive tonic to calm frayed nerves and to reduce muscle tension.

- Cramp Bark is used as a muscle relaxant to relieve cramps and muscle spasm. It is also recommended for painful period cramps.

Homeopathic treatment

Homeopathy can be used very effectively to treat muscular and menstruation cramps. For information on how to use these treatments see page xv.

- Magnesium phosphate helps relieve period pain and cramp.
- Calcium phosphate is used to treat cramp in the calf muscles which is worse when walking.
- Chamomilla is used in treating abdominal cramps which tend to be worse when lying down or bending over.

Aromatherapy treatment

The therapeutic use of essential oils to treat muscle spasm and cramp associated with period pain and circulation problems is highly recommended. See page xvi for information on how to use these essential oils.

- Ylang Ylang is used as a bath oil or massage oil. Ylang Ylang can help to improve circulation, relieve anxiety and depression, and deeply relax the body.
- Jasmine is a wonderfully aromatic oil that helps relieve pain associated with the female reproductive system. Use as a body oil, bath oil or in an oil burner.
- Chamomile is a soothing calming oil that relaxes the muscles as well as being an anti-inflammatory. Use as a bath oil or massage oil.

Nutritional supplements for cramps		
SUPPLEMENT	DOSAGE	COMMENT
Vitamin B complex	50 mg three times daily	Vitamin B complex is used for nervous exhaustion. It also improves circulation
Vitamin E	400 iu daily	To improve circulation
Calcium and Magnesium	1500 mg daily 750 mg daily	A lack of these minerals will cause spasming and cramping of the muscles
Potassium	3–8 g daily	Needed for proper absorption of calcium and magnesium
Vitamin C	3000 mg daily	Helps improve circulation
Multivitamin and mineral complex	As directed on label	Helps maintain the body's natural balance

- Black Pepper is a stimulating oil which effectively relieves muscle aches and pains and improves circulation. Use as a massage oil or inhalant.

Dietary and lifestyle recommendations

- Daily exercise is one of the best things you can do to improve circulation and increase muscle tone and flexibility. Yoga and walking are recommended.
- If you have cramps during the day while being active it is important to consult your physician for a thorough diagnosis. This can be a sign of arteriosclerosis.
- Drink plenty of water during the day to help prevent a build up of toxins in the muscles.
- Treat yourself to regular aromatherapy massage to relieve muscular aches and pains.
- Limit your intake of acidic foods such as tomatoes and vinegar as they may inhibit the absorption of calcium by the body.
- Increase your intake of calcium and magnesium (see table for nutritional supplements for cramp, page 287).
- Relax in a hot bath using mineral salts as this increases the flow of blood to the muscles.

OSTEOPOROSIS

Description

Osteoporosis is the acceleration or rapid breakdown of bone mass causing the bones to thin and become brittle. The condition is often associated with post-menopausal women. During menopause the levels of oestrogen in the body declines, this corresponds with a loss of calcium from the bones. When bone mass begins to breakdown the bones become porous and brittle. In the elderly this results in bone fractures.

After the age of about 30 our bodies stop creating bone mass and we become less efficient at absorbing calcium.

Symptoms

Symptoms of osteoporosis are usually not recognised until it is quite advanced. They include rounded shoulders, stooping and a gradual loss of height.

Causes

Conditions that may contribute to osteoporosis are an over-active thyroid, anorexia nervosa, certain malabsorption disorders and an inadequate intake of calcium over a long period of time. There may also be a hereditary predisposition.

Nutritional treatment

Nutritional supplements that may be beneficial in the treatment of osteoporosis are included in the following table. See pages xii–xiii for information on how to use these supplements.

Herbal treatment

Herbs may provide some relief from the pain and discomfort associated with osteoporosis. The following herbs can be taken as teas, tablets or tinctures. See pages xiii–xv for information on how to use these herbs.

- Sarsaparilla is traditionally used to treat skin conditions. It is also very effective as an anti-rheumatic pain reliever.
- Horsetail is highly recommended for arthritic conditions.
- Wild Yam is an anti-cramp and an anti-inflammatory herb. It is commonly prescribed for joint and muscle pain.
- Ginseng can be taken to improve your physical and mental performance. Ginseng tea can be purchased at health food stores.

Nutritional supplements for osteoporosis

SUPPLEMENT	DOSAGE	COMMENT
Vitamin B complex	As directed on label	To improve circulation and cell function
Vitamin B6	50 mg three times daily	Low levels of vitamin B6 may contribute to osteoporosis
Vitamin B12	1000 mcg daily	Helps promote normal bone growth
Vitamin C	1000 mg daily	Important for the formation of connective issue
Vitamin D	400 iu daily	Essential in prevention of osteoporosis when combined with other nutritional supplements
Vitamin E	400 iu daily	Helps the body to assimilate calcium
Calcium and	1500 mg daily	Essential for maintaining strong bones
Magnesium	750 mg daily	Necessary for the absorption of calcium
Kelp	2000 mg daily	A rich source of minerals
Multivitamin and mineral complex	As directed on label	The body needs all vitamins and minerals to maintain optimum health and wellbeing

Homeopathic treatment

The following homeopathics can be used very effectively to treat symptoms associated with osteoporosis. See page xv for information on how to use these treatments.

- Arnica is a general treatment for trauma and bruising often associated with a fall.
- Rutaceae aids in knitting broken bones and providing pain relief for joint pain.
- Calcium phosphate is used to help promote the union of bone when there is a fracture. It is also used effectively to relieve aching bones.

Aromatherapy treatment

Aromatherapy oils used to treat osteoporosis are listed below. For more information on how to use these essential oils see page xvi.

- Hyssop is used as a bath oil, body oil or as a compress. Hyssop can help where there is bruising or trauma.
- Clary Sage is used to treat stress, high blood pressure, and the whole female system. It has a cooling, calming effect on the body. A few drops of Clary Sage can be used in a warm bath or as a massage oil with a base oil of Almond, Grape or Apricot.
- Rosemary is a wonderful aromatic oil used to treat muscular and joint pain. Use it as a body oil, bath oil or in an oil burner.

Dietary and lifestyle recommendations

- Eliminate tea, coffee, cola drinks, alcohol and tobacco from your diet. Cigarette smoking accelerates bone loss, and caffeine can interfere with proper calcium absorption.
- Exercise is important to help maintain mobility, muscle tone and increase bone density. To begin with try gentle exercises such as walking, swimming and yoga.
- Orthodox medical treatment may involve the use of hormone replacement therapy (HRT). This treatment is usually recommended for women entering menopause to avoid the affects of osteoporosis.
- Meditation and relaxation practices may be of great benefit to those suffering anxiety and depression related to osteoporosis.

CALCIUM-RICH FOODS

Introduce calcium supplements and calcium rich foods into your diet. Foods high in calcium are:

- almonds;
- brewer's yeast;
- cheese (natural cheddar);
- eggs;
- figs;
- kelp;
- leeks;
- lentils;
- linseed;
- molasses;
- onions;
- parsley;
- pecan nuts;

- pepitas;
- sesame seeds;
- soybeans.

RHEUMATOID ARTHRITIS

Description

Rheumatoid arthritis is an auto-immune form of arthritis which develops when the body's immune system begins to attack body tissue. This is usually triggered by an antigen in a genetically predisposed person. The joints become inflamed, swollen, stiff and deformed and they can be extremely painful.

With the early stages of rheumatoid arthritis movement can generally improve the symptoms.

Symptoms

The early symptoms of rheumatoid arthritis include fever, anaemia, weight loss, joint pain and fatigue.

If the disease becomes chronic the eyes, lungs, nerves, heart and skin tissues may be affected.

Causes

It is generally accepted that rheumatoid arthritis is an auto-immune disorder. However, what triggers the inflammation responses is largely unknown. Lifestyle factors, poor nutrition, food allergies, micro-organisms and a genetic predisposition are all being investigated as possible causes.

Nutritional treatment

Nutritional supplements that may be beneficial in the treatment of rheumatoid arthritis are included in the table on page 292. See pages xii–xiii for more information on how to use these supplements.

Herbal treatment

The following herbs can be taken as teas, tinctures or tablets to treat rheumatoid arthritis. For information on how to use these herbs see pages xiii–xv.

- Feverfew is used as an anti-inflammatory and pain reliever. Feverfew has a long history in the treatment of fever, migraine and arthritis. (Avoid during pregnancy.)
- Devil's Claw may be helpful in reducing inflammation and pain in the treatment of rheumatoid arthritis.
- Black Cohosh is very helpful in treating pain associated with rheumatoid arthritis.
- Bogbean is used in the treatment of rheumatism, arthritis and rheumatoid arthritis.
- Licorice is used in the treatment of inflammation, allergy, asthma, and conditions that put stress on the adrenal gland.

Nutritional supplements for rheumatoid arthritis

SUPPLEMENT	DOSAGE	COMMENT
Vitamin B complex	100 mg daily	Important for nutritional support of the muscles
Vitamin C	3000 mg daily	Has anti-inflammatory action
Vitamin E	400 iu daily	An important anti-oxidant. Works well combined with selenium
Selenium	200 mcg daily	Selenium levels are low in patients with rheumatoid arthritis. Selenium is an essential anti-oxidant and can protect against arthritis
Manganese	15 mg daily	Important anti-oxidant
Zinc	45 mg daily	Often zinc levels are low in patients with rheumatoid arthritis. Zinc can provide relief from symptoms
Copper salicylate	1 mg daily	Helps to reduce pain and inflammation
L-tryptophan	400 mg four times daily	Increases endorphin activity. Helps reduce pain in chronic or acute conditions of rheumatoid arthritis
Bromelain	250 mg between meals three times daily	A digestive enzyme from the pineapple plant with known anti-inflammatory properties
Multivitamin and mineral complex	As directed on label	Provides nutritional support for the muscles

- Ginseng can be used to treat fatigue, stress and to increase adrenal function.
- Skullcap has an anti-arthritic and anti-inflammatory action.

Homeopathic treatment

Homeopathics can provide relief to those suffering from rheumatoid arthritis. See page xv for information on how to use the following treatments.

- Ferrum phosphoricum is used when the joint is red, swollen and painful.
- Rhus toxicodendron is used where there is pain and stiffness brought about by cold and damp conditions.
- Rhododendron is used where pain is improved by movement or exercise.
- Ruta graveolens is used for pain in the joints, especially the large

joints, and for when the condition improves when warmed.

Aromatherapy treatment

Aromatherapy is highly recommended as a safe and therapeutic treatment for rheumatoid arthritis. See page xvi for information on how to use the following oils.

- A warm bath of Rosemary, Basil and Lavender can relieve pain and promote relaxation.
- Roman Chamomile speeds healing and calms inflammation. Use as a body oil, bath oil or compress.
- Eucalyptus invigorates and stimulates while having an anti-inflammatory action. Use as a bath oil, body oil or as a rub.
- Ginger is very effective in relieving rheumatic aches and pains. Use as a bath oil or massage oil.
- Marjoram can be used as a massage oil for muscular aches and arthritic pain or as a bath oil or compress.

Dietary and lifestyle recommendations

- Exercise is very important in the treatment of rheumatoid arthritis, because unused joints will become stiff. Gentle exercise such as yoga, swimming, tai chi and walking are all recommended.
- Diet can play an important role in the prevention and treatment of this condition. A vegetarian diet may be of benefit to sufferers of rheumatoid arthritis.

- See Arthritis (pages 272–77) for more information regarding dietary recommendations.

SPRAINS and STRAINS

Description and symptoms

A sprain is the partial tearing of a ligament. Ligaments are the tough bands of fibrous tissue attached to the joints. Sprains can be extremely painful and the area is usually bruised and swollen. It is recommended a cold pack be applied immediately to the sprained area and the limb be elevated. By elevating the joint you keep the blood flowing away from the area, which will help reduce the pain and swelling. Strapping the injured joint in an elastic bandage will help prevent further injury and relieves the strain on the damaged ligament.

Causes

Sprains usually result from a fall or stumble which forces the weight of the body onto an area such as the ankle, wrist or knee.

Strains occur when a muscle or tendon is overstretched or torn, usually as a result of physical exertion during a game or sport. Unlike sprains

Nutritional supplements for sprains and strains

SUPPLEMENT	DOSAGE	COMMENT
Vitamin B complex	100 mg daily	Provides stress relief to the body during exercise and increases oxygen supply
Vitamin C	2000 mg daily	Promotes healing and is important for bone formation
Vitamin E	400 iu daily	Biological anti-oxidant. Promotes healing and circulation
Multivitamin and mineral complex	As directed on label	All nutrients are required for promoting healing
Calcium and Magnesium	1500 mg daily / 750 mg daily	Essential for bone growth and muscle contraction
Silica	25 mg daily	Important for bone and muscle formation
Zinc	50 mg daily	Increases immune function essential for growth and wound healing

there is usually no bruising or swelling and the injured muscle may respond better to a heated compress than a cold pack.

Nutritional treatment

Nutritional supplements that may be beneficial in the treatment of sprains and strains are included in the above table. See pages xii–xiii for information on how to use these supplements.

Herbal treatment

The following herbs are recommended for bruises, sprains and strains and should be taken as teas, tablets or tinctures. For more information on how to use these herbs see pages xiii–xv.

- Arnica is one of the best treatments for bruises and sprains. Use externally but do not use where the skin is broken.
- Marigold is an anti-inflammatory herb used specifically for skin inflammation, external bleeding, bruising and sprains.
- Witch Hazel is used in the treatment of inflammation, swelling, bruising and varicose veins.

Combine Arnica and Witch Hazel to make an excellent lotion or rub for bruises, sprains and strains.

Homeopathic treatment

Homeopathics can provide relief and healing to those suffering from sprains and strains. See page xv for information on how to use the following treatments.

- Arnica is an excellent homeopathic remedy taken internally immediately following a sprain injury.
- Ruta graveolens is used for a sprain or strained joint or ligament, where there is pain, bruising and weakness.
- Rhus toxicodendron is used where the muscles or tendons are painful due to over exertion and often when the pain is worse at night in bed but improves when moving.

Aromatherapy treatment

Aromatherapy essential oils can provide relief for sprain and strain injuries. The following essential oils are recommended for use as bath oils or soothing massage oils. For more information on how to use these oils see page xvi.

- Rosemary or Thyme make excellent bath oils when it comes to providing relief from pulled muscles, ligaments or tendons. They help to increase circulation and speed up the healing process.
- Hyssop and Chamomile can be used as external gentle massage oils where there is bruising.
- Nutmeg, used as a body lotion, provides relief from muscular aches and pains.

Dietary and lifestyle recommendations

- It is recommended that after applying initial cold pack treatment to a sprain you then alternate between hot and cold treatments, about every 15 minutes.
- If there is considerable ongoing pain or there is concern a more serious injury has occurred, consult your physician immediately.
- It is important to elevate the injured limb and get plenty of rest following a sprain injury.
- Drink plenty of water and fresh juices.
- Do follow the herbal and homeopathy treatments provided as they will provide relief and speed up the healing process.

SCIATICA

Description and causes

The sciatic nerve is the longest and thickest nerve in the human body. It runs from the lower lumbar vertebrae, sacrum and pelvis down the back of the thigh and calf to the foot. Sciatica is caused by pressure on the sciatic nerve. Pressure on the sciatic nerve and pain can result from: problems with the lumbar vertebrae and discs, problems with the sacroiliac joint, muscle spasm deep in the buttocks (especially the piriformis muscle), trauma or inflammation of the nerve itself, neuritis and even arthritis. In rare cases the pressure may be caused by a tumour.

Symptoms

Symptoms of sciatica include: pain, numbness and tingling of varying degrees of intensity which may radiate from the buttocks down the thigh, calf, into the groin or right down to the foot. There may be an accompanying loss of strength in the muscles affected. Sciatica can be associated with pregnancy and childbirth.

Sciatica is not a serious complaint though it can be extremely painful. If the pain, tingling or numbness persists it could be caused by nerve root compression which requires medical treatment. Acupuncture, osteopathy and deep tissue massage (especially rolfing) can be very helpful in healing sciatic pain, but if pain persists have an X-ray.

Nutritional treatment

Nutritional supplements that may be beneficial in the treatment of sciatica are included in the following table. See pages xii–xiii for information on how to use these supplements.

Herbal treatment

Refer to the herbal treatment for neuralgia and neuritis on pages 113–16. Other herbs which may be helpful in treating sciatica are listed below. These herbs can be taken as teas, tablets or tinctures. See pages xiii–xv for information on how to use these herbs.

- Horsetail is an excellent source of silica, which is essential in wound healing. It can be taken internally as a tea, tablet or tincture for inflammation or applied externally as a lotion or liniment.
- Black Cohosh reduces muscular cramps and spasms and is used for sciatica and neuralgia.
- Jamaican Dogwood is a sedative used for sedating the pain of neuralgia.
- St John's Wort is an anti-inflammatory and can be used internally or externally as a lotion or compress.
- Yellow Dock and Yarrow are also useful in the treatment of sciatica.

Homeopathic treatment

Treatment that may be prescribed by a homeopath for sciatica includes:

- Aconite for pain which arrives quickly after exposure to cold;
- Arsenicum album for sciatica which is improved by walking and warm applications, or for the elderly whose sciatic pain is worse at night;
- Bryonia for sciatica with sensations of pins and needles in the sole of the foot, that is worse for movement or changes in weather;
- Colocynthis for pain that spreads down the leg, that is worse in cold or damp weather;
- Ferrum phosphoricum for general sciatic pain and inflammation;

- Gelsemium if the suspected cause involves the spinal cord and muscles;
- Hypericum for neuralgia to reduce the pain;
- Lycopodium for pain in the right leg that is aggravated by lying on the right side.

For more information on how to use these treatments see page xv.

Nutritional supplements for sciatica		
SUPPLEMENT	DOSAGE	COMMENT
Vitamin B complex plus	*100 mg three times daily*	*B complex is important for repair and to relieve stress in the lower back muscles*
Vitamin B1 plus	*100 mg daily*	*Used to treat stress and neuritis*
Vitamin B12	*100 mg daily*	*Used to treat spinal lesions and nerve repair. Also assists in calcium absorption*
Vitamin D	*400 iu daily*	*Used to treat skeletal abnormalities. Also assists in absorption of calcium*
Vitamin E	*500 iu daily*	*Improves blood flow and is used to benefit neuromuscular disorders*
Essential fatty acids • *Evening Primrose oil* • *Wheatgerm oil* • *Cod Liver oil*	*One tablespoon three times daily*	*Regulates inflammation responses. Also needed for function and repair of muscles*
Calcium and	*1000 mg daily*	*Regulates muscle contraction, and bone formation and repair*
Magnesium	*500 mg daily*	*Works together with calcium in regulating muscular contraction and transmission of nerve signals*
Zinc	*50 mg daily*	*Important for protein synthesis and wound healing*
Phenylalanine	*Take as directed on label*	*Stimulates the production of the body's natural pain killers*

Aromatherapy treatment

The following essential oils may provide relief from the symptoms of sciatica.

- Marjoram can be used as a bath or body oil, or as a compress.
- Juniper can be used as a bath or body oil, or as a compress.
- Sage can be used as a bath or body oil, or as compress (avoid during preganacy).
- Rosemary can be used as a bath or body oil.
- Ginger can be used as a body oil or compress.
- Camphor is a strong essential oil that can be used as a compress.

For more information on using essential oils see page xvi.

Dietary and lifestyle recommendations

- Rest and application of hot and cold compresses is recommended. Grate some ginger into the hot water for the hot compress. Apply the compress to the lower back and buttocks.
- Consult your local yoga teacher for specific stretches and take regular walking exercise.

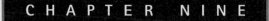
THE LYMPHATIC SYSTEM

Maintenance of the lymphatic organs, lymph nodes, lymphatic fluid and bone marrow

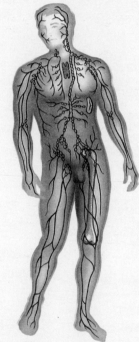

What does it consist of?

The health of the lymphatic system is fundamental to the constant cleansing processes in the body. The lymphatic system is made up of the lymphatic organs (the tonsils, spleen and the thymus gland), the lymph nodes (under the armpits and around the neck, breast, groin and intestines), and the bone marrow where the cells of the lymphatic system are produced. The fluid which passes along the lymphatic vessels is called lymph. Lymph is fluid which seeps out of the blood vessels and is returned to the blood vessels via the lymphatic system.

What does it do?

The functions of the lymphatic system are:

• Draining the fluid which surrounds cells and builds up in body tissue;

- Transporting dietary fats and fat-soluble vitamins through the small intestine.
- Removing any foreign substances such as viruses, bacteria, and any other toxic food substances.

The lymphatic system transports fluids from body tissue, and filters and cleanses the fluid as it returns it to the circulatory system to mix in again with the blood.

The lymphatic system assists the functions of both the immune system and the circulatory system. Movement of lymph fluid through the lymphatic vessels is assisted by muscular contraction as a result of movement, breathing and exercise. Unlike the circulatory system, which has the heartbeat to produce pressure to move the blood, the lymphatic system relies only on movement to push the lymph through the vessels.

What goes wrong with it?

In times of illness or infection the lymph nodes become swollen and inflamed as a result of the invading microbe. Swollen lymph nodes indicate that the body is combating some type of infection. Swollen glands is a term commonly used to describe enlargement of the lymph nodes.

Nutritional treatment

There are many vitamins and minerals which benefit the lymphatic system.

VITAMIN A
Vitamin A is important in resisting infections and slowing the spread of infections. It enhances the body's production of antibodies and immune cells and strengthens the cell walls against infection.

VITAMIN B1
Vitamin B1 is necessary for the improvement of muscle tone in the stomach and intestines, and it also improves food assimilation. Deficiency of vitamin B1 is associated with fluid retention and a weakened immune system.

VITAMIN B2
Vitamin B2 is an anti-oxidant which can detect and destroy abnormal cells in the body and it stands guard against free radicals. It also supports the immune system.

VITAMIN B5
Vitamin B5 is essential for the proper breakdown of fats so they can be transported by the lymphatic system. A deficiency of vitamin B5 can produce a failure to manufacture antibodies to combat infections. A deficiency may also be associated with fluid retention.

VITAMIN B6
Vitamin B6 helps to maintain a balance of the minerals potassium and sodium. This balance is important for the movement of fluids throughout the body. Vitamin B6 is also important in the production of the cells of the immune system.

VITAMIN C

Vitamin C is an anti-oxidant and natural antibiotic, as such it improves the body's immunity. Vitamin C maintains collagen production. Cells in the walls of the lymphatic vessels need collagen to help them expand and contract with the movement of lymph.

BIOTIN

Biotin assists in the breakdown of fatty foods and as such it supports the role of the lymphatic system. Biotin also supports the formation of bone marrow which produces many of the cells of the lymphatic system.

FOLIC ACID

Deficiency of folic acid can result in impaired absorption from the gastrointestinal tract.

Herbal treatment

The function of the lymphatic system is strengthened by the action of anti-microbial, alterative, diuretic and hepatic herbs.

ALTERATIVE HERBS

Alterative herbs are 'blood cleansers' which support the body's ability to eliminate wastes and, therefore, enhance the function of the lymphatic system. Alterative herbs for the lymphatic system include:

- Burdock;
- Cleavers;
- Golden Seal (avoid during pregnancy);
- Poke Root.

ANTI-MICROBIAL HERBS

Anti-microbial herbs support the immune system and the lymphatic system in resisting disease from infective organisms. Anti-microbial herbs which benefit the lymphatic system include:

- Cayenne;
- Echinacea;
- Garlic;
- Marigold.

DIURETIC HERBS

Diuretic herbs assist the lymphatic system in maintaining or restoring fluid balance. They help eliminate fluids in cases of fluid retention. Diuretics which support the lymphatic system include:

- Corn Silk;
- Dandelion leaf;
- Parsley;
- Yarrow.

HEPATIC HERBS

Hepatic herbs support the liver's role in breaking down fats and toxic substances in the body. Hepatic herbs which assist the lymphatic system include:

- Dandelion root;
- Golden Seal (do not take during pregnancy);
- Milk Thistle.

All the above herbs can be taken as teas, tinctures or tablets.

Aromatherapy treatment

FLUID RETENTION

The following aromatherapy oils can be used for fluid retention:

- Cypress;
- Fennel;
- Geranium;
- Juniper;
- Orange;
- Rosemary;
- Sage.

All the above can be used as bath or body oils. They can all (apart from Rosemary) also be used as compresses over parts of the body suffering from fluid retention.

ANTI-VIRAL AND ANTIBACTERIAL

The following aromatherapy oils can be used to help resist or fight viral and bacterial infections.

- Cinnamon can be used as a body oil, a compress or inhaled;
- Eucalyptus can be used as a body oil, a compress or inhaled;
- Oregano can be used as a bath or body oil;
- Tea Tree should be used externally only;
- Thyme can be used as a bath or body oil.

Dietary and lifestyle recommendations

To support the function of the lymphatic system consume plenty of green leafy vegetables, fresh fruit and juices. Also include in the diet berries, apples, celery, okra and watercress.

PURIFICATION

To purify the body include the following in your diet:

- apples;
- apricots;
- beetroot;
- berries;
- broccoli;
- brussels sprouts;
- cabbage;
- carrots;
- cauliflower;
- cucumber;
- lemons;
- lettuce;
- melons;
- onions;
- papaya;
- parsley;
- peaches;
- pears;
- peas;
- pineapple;
- spinach;
- tomatoes.

RESISTING INFECTION

To resist and combat infection include in your diet:

- avocados;
- dates;
- garlic;
- grapes;
- lettuce;
- olives;
- parsley;
- spinach.

Also increase your intake of proteins, fluids and calories.

JUICES

The following juices will all help support the lymphatic system.

- broth made from potato peelings
- apple juice
- grape juice
- carrot juice
- parsley juice
- celery juice

CELLULITE

Description

Cellulite is a condition which affects up to 95 percent of women. It occurs when there is an accumulation of fat, fluid and toxins under the skin causing the surface of the skin to appear dimpled and lumpy. Most women are very aware of this condition and often find it quite distressing. Cellulite usually accumulates around the thighs, bottom and upper arms.

Symptoms

Apart from the cosmetic appearance of cellulite the symptoms are minimal. There may be tenderness of the skin when pinched, pressed or massaged or a feeling of tightness or heaviness in the affected areas.

Causes

Generally it is thought cellulite appears when there is poor circulation and lack of exercise. It is often linked to female hormones as males rarely have cellulite and it may worsen at menopause. A buildup of toxins in the body through poor diet and elimination of waste may also contribute to cellulite.

Nutritional treatment

Nutritional supplements that may be beneficial in the treatment of cellulite are included in the following table (see page 304). See pages xii–xiii for information on how to use these supplements.

See your naturopath for a more comprehensive treatment.

Herbal treatment

Herbs that may be useful to treat cellulite are the lymphatic herbs. The action of these herbs is to help the body eliminate waste products and toxins. All of these herbs can be taken as teas, tablets or tinctures. For more information on how to use these herbs see pages xiii–xv.

- Cleavers is a blood cleanser, lymphatic tonic and diuretic.
- Echinacea helps to cleanse the blood and lymphatic system. It is an antiseptic and an organ tonic.
- Poke Root is very useful in treating lymphatic problems. It aids in cleansing the lymph glands.
- Dandelion cleanses the blood stream and the liver. It is also used as a diuretic.

HERBAL TEA

A herbal tea to aid the lymphatic system is made by combining two parts Echinacea, with one part Cleavers, and one part Poke Root. Seep the herbs in boiling water, strain and drink three times daily.

Nutritional supplements for cellulite

SUPPLEMENT	DOSAGE	COMMENT
Vitamin B complex	100 mg daily	Essential for the health of the nervous system
Vitamin B12	50 mg daily	For proper digestion and absorption of food
Vitamin E	400 iu daily	Helps the body eliminate toxins
Multivitamin and mineral supplement	As directed on label	Essential for the total health and wellbeing of the body

Aromatherapy treatment

Aromatherapy essential oils can play a large part in the treatment of cellulite through massage therapy. See page xvi for information on how to use essential oils.

- Lavender is a versatile healing oil. Lavender can be used as a massage oil in the treatment of cellulite or as an aromatic bath oil.
- Juniper has diuretic qualities and can be used to balance the female system and improve circulation. Use as a massage oil or bath oil.
- Rosemary is a beautiful aromatic oil that invigorates and uplifts the body. Use as a massage oil or bath oil.

Dietary and lifestyle recommendations

- Avoid caffeine, alcohol, tobacco, and a diet high in saturated fats and sugars.
- Maintaining a normal body weight by eating a diet high in fibre and low in saturated fats can be helpful in avoiding cellulite.

- Aerobic exercise for 20–30 minutes three to five times per week can not only help to maintain weight but also reduce cellulite.
- Massage either by hand or using a natural bristle brush or loofah can be beneficial. See the massage recommendations in aromatherapy treatment above.

GLANDULAR FEVER

Description and causes

Glandular fever (mononucleosis) is an infectious illness caused by a virus of the same group as that which causes herpes simplex. The virus is passed from one person to another through all the bodily fluids, but most commonly in the tiny droplets of water vapour that we exhale when breathing. Glandular fever is sometimes called the 'kissing disease' because of its mode of transmission, but also because the group most likely to contract glandular fever is teenagers and young adults aged 12–25 years.

Glandular fever affects the respiratory system; the lymphatic glands in the neck, groin and armpits; the bronchial tubes, the spleen and the liver. Glandular fever can be a very severe illness, sometimes lasting up to three months. After suffering glandular fever tiredness may return a year later and last up to 12 months. Fortunately exposure to the illness creates immunity from contracting it again.

Symptoms

Symptoms of glandular fever include:

- sore throat;
- chills and fever;
- headache;
- bodily aches and pains;
- tiredness;
- swollen glands (at which time the patient is most infectious);
- sometimes a raised, red rash or jaundice;
- the spleen may become enlarged and the liver's function may be affected.

The symptoms of glandular fever are similar to influenza and it is sometimes mistaken for the flu. The symptoms of glandular fever, however, are usually more severe and longer lasting than influenza. The persistent nature of glandular fever can be moderated by using natural therapies.

Nutritional treatment

Nutritional supplements that may be beneficial in the treatment of glandular fever are included in the following table. See pages xii–xiii for information on how to use these supplements.

Nutritional supplements for glandular fever		
SUPPLEMENT	DOSAGE	COMMENT
Vitamin A	10,000–50,000 iu daily (do not take more than 10,000 iu if you are pregnant)	Essential for resisting infection by producing antibodies. Take in an emulsion. Also protects the tissues lining the throat
Vitamin B complex	100 mg three times daily with food	Benefits digestion, increases energy levels and boosts emotional wellbeing
Vitamin C with bioflavonoids	2000 mg three times daily	Improves the body's natural immunity to combat the virus

Nutritional supplements for glandular fever

SUPPLEMENT	DOSAGE	COMMENT
Vitamin E	500 iu daily	Acts as an immune modulator and enhances the production of killer T cells
Acidophilus	As directed on label	Improves the quality and function of the body's friendly bacteria. Supports the digestive system
Digestive enzymes	As directed on label between meals	Benefits digestion and helps maintain energy levels
Garlic	As directed on label with meals	A natural antibiotic which supports the immune system
Kelp	As directed on label	A useful source of minerals
Coenzyme Q10	75 mg daily	An anti-oxidant which improves circulation and strengthens the immune system
Evening Primrose oil	Two capsules three times daily	Regulates the inflammation response
Calcium and Magnesium	1000 mg daily 500 mg daily	Magnesium helps regulate body and temperature and both assist cellular function and repair
Zinc	50 mg three times daily	Supports the immune system
L-lysine	1500 mg daily	Used to treat herpes infections. Supports the immune system

Herbal treatment

For information on how to use the following herbs see pages xiii–xv.

ANTI-MICROBIAL HERBS
Anti-microbial herbs help the body to resist or destroy infections. For glandular fever use:

- Garlic;
- Echinacea;
- Myrrh;
- Wild Indigo.

Myrrh and Wild Indigo are specific anti-microbial herbs for swollen lymphatic glands and are also used to reduce fever. Take all of the anti-microbial herbs as teas, tinctures or tablets.

IMMUNE SYSTEM
To boost the immune system take:

- Astragalus;
- Echinacea;

- Golden Seal (only take internally for one–two weeks and avoid during pregnancy).

Take these herbs as teas, tinctures or tablets.

LIVER

To support the liver take:

- Dandelion;
- Milk Thistle.

These herbs can be taken as teas, tablets or tinctures.

SORE THROAT

For a sore throat and swollen glands in the neck gargle with an infusion made from boiling a handful of cabbage leaves, violet flowers, poppy flowers and elecampane flowers in two litres of water. Gargle the infusion while still warm.

Alternatively, for sore throat take a mixture of two tablespoons of honey with one tablespoon of grated ginger and one tablespoon of lemon juice.

Homeopathic treatment

See page xv for information on how to use the following treatments.

- Ailanthus is used for a throat which is sore and red with swollen neck and maybe also a skin rash, horse voice and headache. Ailanthus is also indicated for weakness and drowsiness.
- Belladonna is used for swollen glands with a fever.

- The tissue salts Kali muriaticum and Ferrum phosphoricum are very useful.
- Aconitum napellus is taken for a constant dry cough which produces a feeling of suffocation. Or when a patient feels anxious and fearful.
- Mercurius solubilis, Phytolacca and Baryta carbonica are also used when glandular symptoms are evident.
- As a preventative measure family members can take glandular fever nosode 30C every 12 hours for two days if exposure to glandular fever has occurred.

Aromatherapy treatment

For information on how to use the following essential oils see page xvi.

FEVER

For fever use the following essential oils as bath or body oils.

- Basil (can also be used in an oil burner);
- Bergamot;
- Black Pepper (can also be used in an oil burner);
- Chamomile;
- Eucalyptus;
- Hyssop (can also be used in an oil burner);
- Lemongrass (can also be used in an oil burner);
- Melissa (can also be used in an oil burner).

SORE THROAT

For a sore throat use the following essential oils as bath or body oils:

- Bergamot;
- Clary Sage;
- Eucalyptus (can also be used in an oil burner);
- Geranium (can also be used in an oil burner);
- Lavender;
- Sage.

Gargle with lukewarm boiled water containing a few drops of Thyme oil.

Dietary and lifestyle recommendations

- Get plenty of rest, keep warm and increase your fluid intake to eight glasses of filtered water daily plus freshly squeezed fruit and vegetable juices (especially apple, grape, carrot, celery or parsley juice).
- Graze don't gorge. Eat four to six small meals daily rather than fewer, larger meals.

INCLUDE IN YOUR DIET
- low fat dairy products
- cod liver oil
- vegetable oil
- wheatgerm
- whole wheat breads
- nuts and seeds
- soybeans
- brown rice
- oatmeal;
- lean meat or a protein supplement
- poultry
- fish
- liver or kidney
- egg yolk

- dark green, yellow or orange fruit and vegetables
- root vegetables

AVOID THE FOLLOWING
- tea and coffee
- processed foods
- fried foods
- soft drinks
- sugar
- alcohol
- nicotine
- white flour products

OEDEMA
Description and symptoms

Oedema is the abnormal accumulation of fluid in body tissues beneath the skin or in the body cavities. The excess fluid causes swelling and bloating which is either spread throughout the whole body or localised in one area. The most common area of swelling is the feet and ankles although it may also affect the hands, breasts, around the eyes, the cheeks or any other area of the body.

Causes

Oedema or fluid retention is often caused by:

- allergies;
- blockage of the lymphatic system;
- deficiencies in the diet;
- sodium retention;
- kidney, bladder, lung, heart or liver dysfunction;

- high blood pressure;
- varicose veins;
- phlebitis;
- long periods of standing in one place;
- premenstrual syndrome (PMS);
- pregnancy;
- reactions to cortisone-based drugs and the contraceptive pill.

The accumulated fluid may cause muscular aches and pains. Oedema of the abdominal region is called ascites.

Nutritional treatment

Nutritional supplements that may be beneficial in the treatment of oedema are included in the following table. See pages xii–xiii for information on how to use these supplements.

Herbal treatment

Diuretic herbs increase blood flow through the kidneys and reduce water reabsorption by the kidneys. Diuretics are inner cleansers which eliminate excess fluids. For oedema use the following diuretic herbs:

- Alfalfa;
- Buchu;
- Burdock;
- Centaury;
- Cornsilk;
- Dandelion;
- Elder flowers;
- Horsetail;
- Kava Kava.

These herbs can be taken as teas, tinctures or tablets. For more information on how to use these herbs see pages xiii–xv.

Carrot juice and celery juice are also diuretics which are high in potassium and are very useful for treating oedema. Take one or two glasses of the fresh juice each day.

Homeopathic treatment

See page xv for information on how to use the following treatments.

- Spartium scoparium has a diuretic action and can be used where there is swelling of the ankles.
- Adonis vernalis is used for pulmonary congestion and swelling of lower limbs.

Nutritional supplements for oedema		
SUPPLEMENT	DOSAGE	COMMENT
Vitamin B complex plus	50 mg three times daily	B vitamins work best when taken together
Vitamin B6	50 mg three times daily	Encourages salt excretion therefore eliminating excess fluids

Nutritional supplements for oedema

SUPPLEMENT	DOSAGE	COMMENT
Vitamin C	2000–3000 mg daily in divided doses	Strengthens blood vessel walls to prevent fluid accumulation and is necessary for proper function of adrenal glands
Vitamin E	500 iu daily	Aids circulation to prevent fluid accumulation
Silica	50 mg daily	Acts as a natural diuretic
Kelp	As directed on the label	A rich source of essential minerals
Garlic	As directed on the label	A powerful cleanser which also stimulates the lymphatic system
Calcium and Magnesium	1000 mg daily 1000 mg daily	Encourages salt excretion and eliminates excess fluid

- Cactus grandiflorus is used for swollen hands and feet (oedema) and can be used for when the hands feel icy cold and when a person has restless legs.

Aromatherapy treatment

For the treatment of oedema the following essential oils can be used as bath or body oils or applied directly to the affected area as a compress. For a compress soak a clean cloth in warm water and add ten drops of the essential oil. See page xvi for more information on how to use these essential oils.

- Cypress
- Geranium
- Juniper
- Orange
- Sage

Rosemary or Fennel can also be used as bath or body oils and Rosemary may also be used in an oil burner.

Dietary and lifestyle recommendations

- Regular exercise is important, especially aquarobics or some other water exercise (about one hour three times a week). Hot baths or saunas twice a week are also recommended.
- Elevate the legs when at rest and avoid tight, restrictive clothing.
- Avoid long periods of stationary standing.
- Don't cross your legs when sitting.
- Drink plenty of water especially the herbal diuretic teas (e.g. parsley).
- Reduce your salt intake. Avoid alcohol, soy sauce, pickled

products, beef, caffeine, white flour, white sugar, chocolate, tobacco, gravies and dairy products.

IT'S IMPORTANT TO SEE YOUR DOCTOR IF:

- You find that pressing on the skin, feet or ankles leaves an indentation. This is a condition called 'pitting oedema', which may be a sign of a more serious condition.

SWOLLEN GLANDS

Description

Swollen glands are characterised by an enlargement of the lymph nodes, usually those located at the sides of the neck and throat. When these glands become swollen it is often a sign they are protecting the body against infection. The term swollen glands may also describe the glands situated in the groin or the armpit.

Symptoms

Symptoms include tenderness and swelling of the glands, localised heat, redness of the area and fever.

Causes

Swollen glands may be associated with the common cold, tonsillitis, mumps, adenoid problems and chicken pox, or other more serious diseases such as leukaemia, measles, tuberculosis, cancer or syphilis.

Nutritional treatment

Nutritional supplements that may be beneficial in the treatment of swollen glands are included in the following table. See pages xii–xiii for information on how to use these supplements.

Herbal treatment

Herbal medicine can aid in the healing and strengthening of the lymphatic system. The following herbs can be taken as teas, tablets or tinctures. See pages xiii–xv for information on how to use these herbs.

- Cleavers is an excellent herb to treat a wide range of problems associated with the lymphatic system. These include tonsillitis and adenoid trouble.
- Echinacea helps to purify the blood and the lymphatic system. It is used to treat a number of infections.
- Garlic has antibacterial properties and is helpful in treating a wide range of conditions including influenza, chronic bronchitis, infections and respiratory catarrh. Up to six garlic capsules or two cloves per day can be taken to help combat infection.

Nutritional supplements for swollen glands

SUPPLEMENT	DOSAGE	COMMENT
Vitamin A	As directed on label	Increases the production of antibodies
Vitamin B complex	100 mg daily	B vitamins work best when taken together
Vitamin B2	Three 50 mg tablets daily	Important for the healthy functioning of the glandular system
Vitamin C	1500 mg daily	Helps fight infection and builds immunity
Vitamin E	400 iu daily	Helps the body eliminate toxins
Multivitamin and mineral complex	As directed on the label	Essential for the balanced function of the body and immune system
Garlic	Up to six 500 mg capsules daily	Used to treat infections and build resistance

Homeopathic treatment

Homeopathy can be very useful in treating conditions where swollen glands are common. See page xv for information on how to use these treatments.

- Baryta carbonica is used in the treatment of swollen glands associated with the common cold and where the throat is inflamed and raw and the tonsils are swollen.
- Belladonna is used where the glands are swollen and sensitive. Belladonna is used to treat inflamed and infected areas of the body, sore throats, earache and sunstroke.
- Calcarea carbonica is used where the symptoms include swollen, painless glands. It is used to treat the common cold, earache, dry night cough and dry sore throats.
- Pulsatilla is used in the treatment of measles with symptoms including swollen glands, cold with cough, weepiness and lack of thirst. Pulsatilla is also used effectively in the treatment of mumps with swollen glands, breast, ovarian and testicle pain and fever.

Aromatherapy treatment

Listed below are essential oils that can be used to treat cold and flu symptoms. These symptoms include sore throat, swollen glands and fever. See page xvi for information on how to use these oils.

- Ginger is used as a bath oil. It can help ward off infections and colds.

- Eucalyptus is a strong anti-microbial oil that can be used as an inhalant, a rub or in a warm bath.
- Lavender is a soothing, relaxing oil, used to treat aches and pains, headaches and a whole range of symptoms. Use as a body oil, bath oil or compress.
- Lemon is a remedy for sore throats. Gargle with two percent oil to warm water.
- A few drops of Black Pepper oil in a warm bath may stop flu symptoms developing.

Dietary and lifestyle recommendations

- Avoid red meat, fatty and fried foods, dairy products, vinegar, alcohol, sugar and tobacco. All artificial food additives should also be avoided.
- In order to aid and support the work done by the lymphatic system it is recommended a day of fasting be undertaken. This should be followed by fresh fruit and vegetable juices for two days.
- In the case of colds and flu see herbal and homeopathic treatment listed on pages 311–12.
- Get plenty of rest and relaxation. Allow the body time to heal.

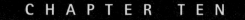

CHAPTER TEN

THE URINARY SYSTEM
Maintenance of the kidneys, urethra and bladder

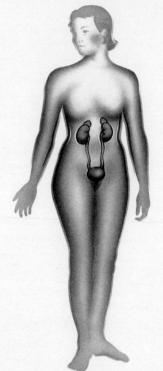

What does it consist of?

The urinary system consists of two kidneys, two ureters, one urinary bladder and a single urethra. The two kidneys are situated at the back of the abdomen and are connected to the bladder by thin tubes call ureters.

What does it do?

The primary function of the urinary systems is to control the composition, volume and pressure of the blood. It does this by filtering the blood, removing and restoring selected amounts of water and solutes.

Urine is excreted from each kidney through its ureter and is stored in the urinary bladder until it is expelled from the body through the urethra. The bladder leads into the urethra but the flow of urine is controlled by a ring of strong muscles (the urethral sphincter and the pelvic floor). The bladder empties when this ring of muscles relaxes and the muscular walls of the bladder contract, thus expelling the urine into the urethra.

Each kidney has around one million microscopic filtering units called nephrons. Each nephron consists of a cup and an attached renal tubule. Nephrons have three basic functions: filtration, secretion and reabsorption. Through the process of filtration some substances are allowed to pass from the blood into the nephron. As the filtered liquid moves through the nephron, wastes and excess substances are secreted into the liquid. Other useful substances (such as glucose and amino acids) are reabsorbed into the blood. As a result of these three functions of the nephrons, urine is formed.

The kidneys also regulate the relative salt balance in the body, excreting excess amounts. The acid/alkali balance of the blood is also the kidney's responsibility. To stay healthy an adult needs to drink between two–four litres of fluid each day to replace water lost in urine, sweat, faeces and exhaled air.

What goes wrong with it?

Common disorders of the urinary system include urinary tract infections, renal failure, cystitis, kidney stones, incontinence and kidney disease.

Nutritional treatment

VITAMIN A
Vitamin A protects the mucus membrane of the vagina and combats infection. Vitamin A also protects the soft tissues of the kidneys and bladder. A deficiency can result in the formation of kidney stones or chronic nephritis.

VITAMIN B6
Vitamin B6 is important for maintaining the mineral balance of sodium and potassium which regulates body fluids. Vitamin B6 has been used successfully in treating certain types of kidney stones. Vitamin B6 is a natural diuretic which assists in the prevention of fluid retention.

VITAMIN C
Vitamin C converts cholesterol into bile acids, which are important for the prevention of kidney stones. Vitamin C also protects the body against invading micro-organisms which cause infection. Vitamin C has been successful in treating inflammation of the urethra, nephritis and kidney stones.

VITAMIN E
A deficiency of Vitamin E can result in nephritis, cystitis and kidney stones. Vitamin E also strengthens the immune system to prevent infection and improves blood circulation.

CHOLINE
Choline helps break down fats and convert cholesterol into bile acids. Choline is used in treating diuresis, nephritis, kidney damage and hemorrhaging of the kidneys.

CALCIUM

Calcium assists the urinary system in maintaining the acid/alkaline balance. Calcium is used in treating nephritis.

POTASSIUM

Potassium also assists in maintaining the acid/alkaline balance in the body. It stimulates the kidneys to eliminate poisonous body waste materials. Deficiency of potassium may be associated with salt retention and kidney damage.

Herbal treatment

Herbal diuretics promote urine flow and generally assist the functioning of the kidney and bladder. Diuretics are part of an ancient repertory of herbs used to eliminate waste products from the body and support the process of internal cleansing. All the herbs mentioned in this section have diuretic properties as well as other actions which benefit the urinary system. They can be taken as teas, tablets or tinctures.

URINARY ANTISEPTICS

Urinary antiseptics are used to treat or prevent infections by strengthening the body's immune system or by directly destroying invading micro-organisms. Urinary antiseptics include:

- Celery seed;
- Couchgrass;
- Echinacea;
- Golden Seal (avoid during pregnancy);
- Juniper;
- Yarrow.

URINARY DEMULCENTS

Urinary demulcents soothe any tissue irritation of the urinary membranes. They also relax painful spasm in the bladder and urinary tract. Urinary demulcents include:

- Corn Silk;
- Couchgrass;
- Marshmallow;
- Parsley;
- Slippery Elm.

URINARY ASTRINGENTS

Urinary astringents are used to stop internal bleeding in the urinary system by helping to tighten and heal damaged tissues. They include:

- Cleavers;
- Couchgrass;
- Golden Seal (avoid during pregnancy);
- Horsetail;
- Tormentil;
- Yarrow.

URINARY ANTILITHICS

Urinary antilithics prevent the formation of stones in the urinary system and can help to break down and eliminate stones which have already formed. They include:

- Corn Silk;
- Hydrangea;
- Stone Root.

Aromatherapy treatment

KIDNEYS

Aromatherapy oils for the kidneys include:

- Black Pepper;
- Cedarwood;
- Cypress (avoid during pregnancy);
- Eucalyptus;
- Fennel;
- Juniper;
- Sandalwood.

These essential oils can all be used as bath or body oils. All of the oils, except Fennel and Juniper, can also be used in an oil burner.

CYSTITIS
Aromatherapy oils for cystitis include:

- Benzoin;
- Bergamot;
- Cedarwood;
- Cypress (avoid druing pregnancy);
- Eucalyptus;
- Juniper;
- Lavender;
- Pine;
- Sandalwood.

These essential oils can be used as bath or body oils. All of the above oils, except for Bergamot and Pine, can also be used in an oil burner.

Dietary and lifestyle recommendations

FOODS
To support the functions of the kidneys and bladder incorporate more of the following foods into your diet:

- alfalfa sprouts;
- apples;
- asparagus;
- beetroot;
- berries;
- carrots;
- celery;
- currants;
- garlic;
- grapes;
- green leafy vegetables;
- kelp;
- leeks;
- lemons;
- lettuce;
- melons;
- parsley;
- potatoes;
- pumpkin;
- spinach;
- watermelon.

JUICES
The following juices will support the function of the urinary system:

- apple;
- asparagus;
- beetroot;
- blackcurrant;
- carrot;
- celery;
- grape;
- parsley;
- pomegranate;
- watermelon.

Alternatively, try the following combinations:

- apple, carrot and celery juice;
- beetroot and grape juice;
- celery and pomegranate juice;
- celery and parsley juice;
- apple and blackcurrant juice.

CYSTITIS

Description and symptoms

Cystitis is a bladder infection that affects women more commonly than men. It is primarily experienced as a burning pain while urinating. There is often an increased need to urinate but only a small amount of urine is excreted causing excruciating, burning pain. Cystitis may be accompanied by lower abdominal pain or, in more severe cases, blood and pus in the urine.

Causes

An acid/alkali imbalance in the bladder encourages the growth of bacteria. This imbalance may result from the diet (over emphasis on refined sugars and carbohydrates) or from poor personal hygiene causing bacteria to be introduced into the urethra from faecal contamination or via women's vaginal secretions. There is also an increased risk of bladder infections during and after pregnancy and following sexual intercourse.

Nutritional treatment

Nutritional supplements that may be beneficial in the treatment of cystitis are included in the following table. See pages xii–xiii for information on how to use these supplements.

Herbal treatment

Herbal medicine can offer valuable remedies to treat bladder infections/cystitis. The following herbs can be taken as teas, tablets or tinctures. See pages xiii–xv for information on how to use these treatments.

- Cranberry juice is widely used to treat cystitis and other bladder infections. Cranberry helps reduce the ability of bacteria to stick to the lining of the bladder or urethra. Cranberry juice is available through supermarkets and health food outlets.
- Cornsilk is a soothing diuretic that is helpful in treating any irritation of the urinary system.
- Garlic is an anti-microbial that helps fight infection including that of the urinary tract.

Nutritional supplements for cystitis

SUPPLEMENT	DOSAGE	COMMENT
Vitamin A	25,000 iu daily	Helps protect the body against infection
Vitamin C with bioflavonoids	500 mg every three hours	Enhances immune function. Has antibacterial effect on urine acidity

Nutritional supplements for cystitis		
SUPPLEMENT	DOSAGE	COMMENT
Multivitamin and mineral complex	As directed on label	Needed to enhance immune system and balance body function
Acidophilus	As directed on label	Helps to restore friendly bacteria and balanced alkalinity and acidity
Garlic	Two capsules three times daily	A natural antibiotic helps fight infection

- Buchu is an excellent herb that is used to treat painful and burning urination associated with cystitis.
- Yarrow can be used as a tea to treat the symptoms of cystitis. Infuse two teaspoons of the fresh herb in a cup of boiling water, let stand for ten to 15 minutes, strain and drink regularly during the day.

Homeopathic treatment

There are a large number of homeopathics and tissue salts that can be used to treat bladder infections and cystitis. Included here are some of the more common ones. If a more specific treatment is required see your homeopathic practitioner.

- Ferrum phosphoricum should be taken at the onset of cystitis when the urge to urinate is strong and frequent and there is pain and burning when passing water.
- Cantharis is used where there is a desire to urinate frequently, where there is a burning pain during and after urination and the bladder never feels empty.
- Causticum is used for a frequent desire to urinate, with pain and burning when urinating, and an urge to urinate but difficulty actually passing water.
- Staphysagria is used for frequent urination with burning pain when not passing water. It is also used for cystitis that follows sexual intercourse.
- Mercurius corrosivus is used for severe cystitis where terrible pain is felt in the rectum and bladder. The urge to urinate is very painful and there may be blood mixed with the urine. It is recommended that if pain is this severe seek medical advice immediately, to avoid kidney infection.

For more information on how to use these treatments see page xv.

Aromatherapy treatment

Aromatherapy can be helpful in relieving symptoms commonly associated with cystitis. See page xvi for more information on how to use essential oils.

- Bergamot can be used as a refreshing body oil or bath oil to treat symptoms of anxiety and depression associated with bladder infection.

- Cypress can be used as an inhalant body oil, bath oil, or compress to help balance kidney energy.
- Eucalyptus is a wonderful aromatic antiseptic oil. Use as a bath oil, body oil inhalant or rub. Eucalyptus can be used to treat cystitis, headache, diarrhoea and depression.
- Juniper has an uplifting effect on the female system. Use as a massage oil or bath oil.
- Lavender is a natural antiseptic that soothes frayed nerves, relieves headaches and depression. Use as a body oil, bath oil or perfume.
- Sandalwood is an exotic oil that has calming, relaxing and soothing qualities. It has antiseptic and diuretic properties. Use as a fragrance, bath oil or body oil.

Dietary and lifestyle recommendations

- Increase fluid intake to at least three litres of filtered or boiled water per day. This will help dilute urine strength and flush out toxins.
- Avoid full strength fruit juice as this can increase the acidity of the urine and cause burning.
- Avoid refined sugars and carbohydrates, tea, coffee and alcohol.
- Eat more fresh fruit, vegetables and complex carbohydrates. Include plenty of garlic and onions.
- Improve personal hygiene by washing genital area regularly and

wiping from front to back after a bowel motion. It is especially helpful for women in avoiding cystitis to wash the genital area and urinate after sexual intercourse.
- Avoid tight-fitting jeans, nylon underpants, perfumed soaps and genital deodorant sprays.

INCONTINENCE
Description

Incontinence is the involuntary passing of urine. It is a very common problem that can take different forms.

Symptoms and causes

Stress incontinence usually occurs as a result of weakness or strain of the pelvic floor muscles. Women who have been through pregnancy and childbirth often suffer from this form of incontinence. In such cases a small amount of urine may escape when a person laughs, coughs or sneezes.

Incontinence or bladder weakness may also manifest in constant urination during the day and throughout the night. This often occurs in the elderly, through loss of control of the bladder sphincters. Other more serious causes of incontinence are: pelvic injuries, damage to the nerves supplying the bladder, kidney disease and bladder infections. Involuntary dribbling after urination in men may be associated with prostate problems. In such cases contact your medical physician.

Nutritional treatment

Nutritional supplements that may be beneficial in the treatment of incontinence are included in the following table. See pages xii–xiii for information on how to use these supplements.

Herbal treatment

Herbal medicine offers valuable remedies to strengthen and heal the urinary system. The following herbs can be taken as teas, tablets or tinctures. See pages xiii–xv for information on how to use these herbs.

- Horsetail is an astringent for the whole urinary system. It has mild diuretic properties, which make it an excellent herb for treating bedwetting problems in children and incontinence problems. It is also used to treat inflammation of the prostate gland.
- Cornsilk is a soothing, non-irritating diuretic with anti-inflammatory properties. It is used to treat urinary tract infections.
- Shepherd's Purse is an astringent with mild antiseptic properties. It is used in the treatment of urinary problems.

Nutritional supplements for incontinence

SUPPLEMENT	DOSAGE	COMMENT
Vitamin A	10,000 iu daily	Helps protect the body against infection. A deficiency can lead to kidney stones or gallstones
Vitamin B complex	50–100 mg twice daily	Helps reduce stress
Vitamin C with bioflavonoids	2000 mg daily	Boosts the immune system and has antibacterial properties
Vitamin E	400 iu daily	Improves the effectiveness of vitamin A. Assists the function of the nervous system
Calcium and	750 mg daily	Calcium aids in preventing bladder problems
Magnesium	1000 mg daily	Magnesium helps reduce stress and works best with calcium
Acidophilus	As directed on the label	Helps restore friendly bacteria to the urinary tract
Garlic	Two capsules three times daily	A natural antibiotic to help fight infection

CORNSILK HERBAL TEA
Infuse the fresh silky part of the common garden corn in a cup of boiling water. Leave for ten to 15 minutes, strain and drink three times daily.

Homeopathic treatment

Homeopathics used in the treatment of incontinence are:

- Ferrum phosphoricum for lack of control over urine function and if a small amount of urine escapes when a person coughs, sneezes or laughs;
- Kali phosphoricum for incontinence due to anxiety, nervousness or weakness;
- Natrum muriaticum for urinating involuntarily when walking or coughing;
- Causticum for incontinence made worse by coughing, sneezing or laughing;
- Nux vomica for dribbling of urine after urination, usually in men.

For more information on how to use these treatments see page xv.

Aromatherapy treatment

Aromatherapy may be useful in treating stress and anxiety often associated with urinary problems. See page xvi for information on how to use the following essential oils.

- Black Pepper is used as a body oil or inhalant. Black Pepper helps stimulate circulation and strengthen kidney function.
- Geranium can be used as a bath oil, body oil, compress or inhalant for urinary problems.
- Sandalwood is a refreshing oil that helps ease nervous tension and anxiety associated with incontinence. Use as a perfume, incense, body oil or bath oil.
- Jasmine is a wonderful aromatic oil that works to ease pain and discomfort in the whole female system. Used to treat anxiety and depression. Use as a perfume, body oil or bath oil.

Dietary and lifestyle recommendations

- Avoid excess fluid intake.
- Avoid stimulants such as coffee, tea and alcohol.
- Exercising the pelvic floor muscles is a simple and effective way to treat incontinence. These muscles support the intestines and bladder, they also increase sexual stimulation during intercourse. By exercising these muscles daily you will avoid further problems relating to stress incontinence. See your natural therapist or yoga teacher for advice on pelvic floor exercises.
- Rosehip tea is an excellent source of vitamin C and is most helpful in treating infections and bladder problems. It can be purchased from any health food outlet.

KIDNEY DISEASE

Description and causes

There are a number of different conditions that can adversely affect kidney function. The most common causes of kidney disease are: infections (pyelonephritis), diabetes, hypertension, gout, lupus, kidney stones, exposure to toxic chemicals or drugs, and obstruction of urinary flow due to injury.

Symptoms

Symptoms of kidney problems include: chills, fever, headaches, nausea, vomiting, decreased appetite, fluid retention, back pain and frequent urination.

It is important if kidney infection or serious kidney problems are suspected you consult your orthodox medical practitioner as certain conditions may lead to kidney failure causing coma and death.

The following natural therapies are recommended to enhance proper kidney function and complement orthodox treatments.

Nutritional treatment

Nutritional supplements that may be beneficial in the treatment of kidney disease are included in the following table. See pages xii–xiii for information on how to use these supplements.

Herbal treatment

Herbal medicine can be used to treat a large range of urinary problems. Herbs aid the body in eliminating waste products and toxins. The following herbs are recommended for treating the urinary system. The following herbs can be taken as teas, tablets or tinctures. See pages xiii–xv for more information on how to use these herbs.

- Buchu helps control bladder and kidney problems, diabetes and fluid retention.
- Dandelion leaves are rich in potassium. They have a diuretic effect and they improve the functioning of the kidneys.
- Yarrow has anti-inflammatory and antiseptic properties. It is recommended for bladder problems, fevers and haemorrhoids.
- Cornsilk is a non-irritating diuretic with soothing anti-fungal and anti-inflammatory properties. It is used to treat urinary tract infection.
- Marshmallow can be used internally or externally. Marshmallow has a healing, soothing action. Used in conjunction with other herbs it is recommended in the treatment of urinary problems.

Homeopathic treatment

Homeopathy can be of benefit in treating the symptoms of kidney infection while waiting to see your medical practitioner. For information on how to use the following treatments see page xv.

- Aconite is used when there is urine retention or pain on urination, where the patient is anxious, feverish, and thirsty and also in cases of sudden onset of the condition.
- Arsenicum is used when the patient is restless and exhausted and when there is burning pain on the passing of urine.

- Cantharis is used when there is pain and discomfort in the kidney area and a constant desire to urinate.

Aromatherapy treatment

Aromatherapy essential oils used in the treatment of kidney problems are:

- Black Pepper;
- Cedarwood;
- Cypress;

Nutritional supplements for kidney disease

SUPPLEMENT	DOSAGE	COMMENT
Vitamin A	Supervised amounts (see your naturopath)	Used to heal the urinary tract and combat infection
Vitamin B6 (pyridoxine) plus	50 mg three times daily	Aids in reducing fluid retention
Choline plus	50 mg daily	
Inositol	100 mg daily	
Vitamin C with bioflavonoids	2000–4000 mg daily	A destroyer of free radicals
Vitamin E	800 iu daily	An important anti-oxidant. Helps strengthen the immune system
Acidophilus	Three tablets daily	Very important if taking antibiotics
Calcium and	1500 mg daily	Assists the urinary system in maintaining the acid/alkaline
Magnesium	750 mg daily	balance
Lecithin	One tablespoon three times daily	Protects the vital organs from the accumulation of fats
Multivitamin and mineral complex	As directed on label	Important for the balance of vitamins and minerals in the body
Potassium	100 mg daily	Helps stimulate kidney function

- Eucalyptus;
- Sandalwood.

These oils can be used as body oils or bath oils. Fennel and Juniper may also be used in an oil burner. For more information on how to use these oils see page xvi.

Dietary and lifestyle recommendations

- It is recommended that a diet high in calories and low in protein be adhered to (see Dietary and Lifestyle Recommendations in the beginning of this chapter, page 318).
- Other natural therapies that may benefit those with this condition include: Chinese herbs, acupuncture and reflexology.
- Yoga and meditation may be of assistance in helping to maintain a stress-free lifestyle. Anxiety, stress and fear can all contribute to a worsening of the condition.
- Avoid toxic chemicals and illicit drugs as they are known to cause kidney problems.

KIDNEY STONES

Description

Kidney stones usually form in the kidney or upper urinary tract. Stones that contain calcium are the most common type of kidney stone. They are made up of calcium oxalate and/or calcium phosphate.

Uric acid stones are usually associated with gout and excess acidity in the urine. Cysteine stones have a hereditary link and they form where there is low pH (low alkaline).

The formation of kidney stones occurs when there is a high concentration of calcium salts and other mineral salts in the urine. This buildup of crystals forms hard deposits of varying size stones or gravel which cause great pain when passing along the urinary tract.

Symptoms

Often there are no visible symptoms until the stone blocks the urinary tract. This blockage results in excruciating pain where the patient may be doubled over in agony. There may also be nausea, vomiting, fever and chills.

Causes

There are a number of causes of kidney stones, the most common of these being dietary. A diet low in fibre and high in refined carbohydrates, fat, salt and animal protein can cause the formation of kidney stones. An excess of vitamin D, calcium and a high alcohol intake also contribute to the conditions. Other causes are antacid abuse, hyperparathyroidism, dehydration and some hereditary conditions.

Nutritional treatment

Nutritional supplements that may be beneficial in the treatment of kidney stones are included in the table on page 328. See pages xii–xiii for information on how to use these supplements.

Herbal treatment

Herbal medicine is highly recommended to treat kidney stones. A good general treatment for this condition is a tea which combines:

- One part Corn Silk;
- One part Gravel Root;
- One part Hydrangea;
- One part Stone Root.

This tea can be taken three times a day to help pass the stone or once a day as a preventative treatment. See pages xiii–xv for more information on how to use these herbs.

Homeopathic treatment

Homeopathy can be of benefit to those suffering the effects of kidney stones. Listed below are a few common homeopathics often recommended for treating this condition. See page xv for information on how to use homeopathics. For a more specific treatment contact a qualified homeopathic practitioner.

- Argentum nitricum is used where there is dull ache in the lower back and bladder, the urine has a burning quality and the patient craves sweets, feels anxious and has gastro-intestinal disturbances.
- Belladonna is used when the patient is red faced and sweaty, is hypersensitive to sudden movement and has colicky abdominal pain.
- Cantharis is used when the patient has excessive thirst and yet has an aversion to food and liquid, there is a cutting and burning pain in kidney area and a continuous desire to urinate.
- Nitric acidum is used specifically where there is pain in the kidneys. It is also used where there is proven raised oxalic acid level, a distinctive urine smell and when the patient feels cold when passing a stone.
- Nux vomica is used for colicky pain extending from the kidneys into the genitals and down the legs. Often the patient feels nauseous and will vomit. Urination requires straining and often there is associated pain in the bladder and urethra.

Aromatherapy treatment

Essential oils may be of benefit to those suffering kidney stones.

Nutritional supplements for kidney stones

SUPPLEMENT	DOSAGE	COMMENT
Vitamin A	25,000 iu daily	Promotes healing of urinary tract following the passing of kidney stones
Vitamin B complex plus	50 mg three times daily	Essential for the wellbeing of the body
Vitamin B6	50 mg twice daily	Taken with magnesium, vitamin B6 can reduce oxalate
Magnesium	500 mg daily	Deficiency can lead to kidney stones
Vitamin C	3000 mg daily	Helps to acidify the urine to prevent kidney stones
Vitamin K (fat soluble Chlorophyll)	As directed on the label	Chlorophyll is an excellent source of naturally occurring vitamin K
Zinc	50 mg daily	Inhibits the formation of crystal buildup

- Bergamot can be used as a bath oil, body oil or compress. Bergamot relieves anxiety and depression.
- Black Pepper is used to stimulate the kidneys. Black Pepper can be added to a bath, used as an inhalant or as a body oil.
- Fennel may assist kidney function. Use as a body oil or bath oil.

For more information on how to use these essential oils see page xvi.

Dietary and lifestyle recommendations

- Avoid antacids as they can cause kidney stones.
- Limit your dairy intake; an over consumption of milk can lead to kidney stones.
- Avoid foods high in oxalates. These include cocoa, tea, rhubarb, spinach, parsley and chocolate.
- Increase your fibre intake if your problem involves calcium stones. Consume more complex carbohydrates and magnesium-rich foods such as bananas, avocados, soybeans, brown rice and rye bread.
- Increase your fluid intake to two–four litres of filtered water daily.
- Although calcium stones are the most common kidney stones it is important to undergo a proper diagnosis and course of treatment. It is therefore recommended you consult a qualified natural health practitioner or your physician.

CHAPTER ELEVEN

ELIMINATION DIETS, EXERCISE, MOVEMENT, RELAXATION AND BREATHING

FASTING

What is it?

Fasting is a wonderful form of self-healing. Animals instinctively know that when they are sick it's best to avoid food and to rest until they feel well again. If you really monitor your appetite when you are sick you will probably find that you have the same natural instincts but they are usually ignored. There are times when the body can use an opportunity to rest the digestive function and to increase the function of the elimination of metabolic wastes and toxins. Fasting can provide such an opportunity for healing and detoxification. It can be used to assist the treatment of a disease or as a preventative measure on more of a regular basis.

Fasting involves, in its purest sense, abstinence from all food and drink, except water. For a first fast, however, water alone can be too severe in that toxins are released too quickly and may cause headaches and discomfort. Juice fasting is safer. By giving the body a rest regularly we can prevent many diseases from manifesting and also reverse (or slow down) the aging process.

A fast may be short (three to five days) or long (five to ten days). Consult your medical practitioner or natural therapist before you commence a five to ten day fast. A three-day fast helps in detoxification and cleansing the blood. A five-day fast begins the process of healing and strengthening the immune system. A ten-day fast is a powerful preventative of many diseases.

Preparing for a fast

A few days of preparation will lessen the shock of fasting. For two days prior to fasting eat only fruit and vegetables. Never begin a fast if you are feeling mentally or emotionally disturbed, anxious or irritated. Make sure you empty your bowels. A herbal laxative may be appropriate to move the bowels.

During the fast

For a juice fast take six glasses of distilled water per day plus two or three glasses of diluted juice (one part water to three parts juice). The best juices to assist detoxification are grape, carrot, celery, apple or grapefruit. For a water fast take eight glasses of distilled water per day.

Cleansing the skin with a natural bristle brush or a loafah is recommended. Moderate exercise, sunlight and plenty of rest will also facilitate the cleansing process. Do not use any deodorants, sprays, detergents, perfumes or synthetic shampoos while fasting.

Breaking a fast

Your first meal, on breaking your fast, should be a small quantity of fresh fruit. Eat slowly, chew well and eat the fruit at room temperature. Your stomach will be relatively small and your digestive juices may have temporarily decreased during fasting. Although you may begin to feel ravenously hungry eat only small meals of fruit or raw vegetable salad with leafy greens, tomato, celery, cucumber and avocado. After two or three days of moderate eating you will be ready to resume a healthy diet of mainly fresh fruit, raw or steamed vegetables, wholegrains, nuts and legumes.

ELIMINATION DIETS

The elimination diet helps an individual to detect food allergies by removing common allergens from the diet and then slowly reintroducing them back into the diet while monitoring allergic responses. Common food and chemical allergens are eliminated from the diet for a period of ten to fourteen days. During this period of restricted diet the individual may eat freely from the list of the following foods:

- apples;
- bananas;
- bream;
- broccoli;
- brussels sprouts;
- buckwheat;
- cabbage;

- celery;
- chicken
- garlic;
- lamb;
- lettuce;
- millet;
- parsley;
- pears;
- potatoes;
- rabbit;
- rice;
- rice crackers;
- sago;
- salt;
- sweet potatoes;
- tapioca;
- tuna;
- turkey;
- veal;
- whiting.

All fruit and vegetables must be washed and peeled before eating; water must be boiled or filtered before use. If the allergic symptoms are food related they should begin to disappear after five to seven days; if the symptoms don't disappear or if they worsen, then the allergen must be among the abovementioned foods. In this case a five day water fast can be used instead of the restricted diet.

After the restricted diet period foods can be reintroduced according to a plan and detailed records should be taken. Reintroduce a single food category for two days. If no allergic symptoms occur then reintroduce the next food category. If allergic symptoms occur record the result, eliminate that food category from the diet and wait for symptoms to subside before reintroducing the next food.

Dairy products should be reintroduced first then wheat and grains (oats, barley and rye, each tested individually) then salicylates (tomatoes, capsicum, zucchini, eggplant and tea are some of the most common) then eggs and egg products, then shellfish, then yeast, then alcohol, then foods containing preservatives and colourings, then cane sugar, then tap water. If the food category tests positive it should be eliminated from the diet for three to four months then tested again.

EXERCISE and MOVEMENT

The human body thrives on movement and good breathing. A sedentary lifestyle (lacking in exercise) is known to be directly related to complaints such as:

- heart disease;
- cancer;
- high blood pressure;
- stroke;
- obesity;
- hardening of the arteries;
- osteoporosis;
- muscular rheumatism;
- lower back pain;
- fibrositis;
- haemorrhoids.

Exercise can help to keep your body looking and feeling younger. It increases energy levels and stimulates the following body functions:

- circulation of blood and oxygen;
- muscle tone;
- immune system in preventing disease;
- breathing;
- digestion and elimination.

Exercise also reduces cholesterol levels, stress and obesity. The effects of exercise on the nervous system are becoming clearly understood; it lifts emotional moods and alleviates depression, anxiety and irritability.

Intensity of exercise

If you haven't exercised for a long time consult your medical doctor or natural therapist before starting. Beginning exercise should be moderate and enjoyable; some moderate forms of exercise are: golf, social tennis, dance, brisk walking, aquaerobics and swimming.

Exercise three times a week for 30 to 40 minutes at moderate intensity (70 to 80 percent of your maximal heart rate). To determine your maximal heart rate simply subtract your age from 220. If you are 45 years old your maximal heart rate is 175 and when exercising moderately your heart rate should be between 122 to 140 beats per minute. To take your pulse while exercising find the pulse in your neck (just to the side of your wind pipe) or in your wrist (on the thumb side). Take your pulse for ten seconds, then multiply by six to get your heart rate in beats per minute.

When you finish your exercise period don't stop abruptly, slow down for two to three minutes before stopping and then stretch the muscles that have been involved in your particular exercise. You may need some guidance from a gym instructor, physiotherapist or exercise trainer. Gradually increase your exercise intensity as your fitness improves.

Some gentle forms of exercise which will help increase your flexibility and range of movement are:

- Qi Gong;
- yoga;
- dance;
- tai chi;
- Feldenkrais technique;
- Pilates exercise technique.

Always seek a qualified instructor for best results.

RELAXATION and BREATHING

In our contemporary society so much value is placed on achievement, success and busyness that many people have become 'human doings' instead of human beings. Our body's nervous systems are over-stimulated by noise, television, radio, music, medical drugs and hyperactive thinking. Stress, anxiety and tension have become a way of life for many people. 'Human doings' are stimulation addicts who are addicted to adrenaline and the 'hype' of the stress response. This constant over-stimulation creates a range of physical, emotional and mental symptoms of disease. Relaxation and breathing techniques can reverse this stressful condition and they can greatly help to restore a feeling of balance and calm. The following books are recommended:

- Ian Gawler, *Peace of Mind*, Hill of Content, Melbourne, 1981
- Paul Wilson, *Instant Calm*, Penguin, Australia, 1995
- Dr Herbert Benson, *The Relaxation Response*, Morrow, New York, 1975
- Ainslie Meares, *Relief Without Drugs*, Angus & Robertson, Sydney, 1995

Relaxation music and guided relaxation processes are available on tape and CD. These can be a wonderful means for achieving a quiet, calm space.

Yoga and tai chi are also immensely effective modalities for combating stress and anxiety. These relaxation therapies particularly benefit the respiratory system, the nervous system and the circulatory system, but the benefits spill over to affect the whole mind–body continuum. These two yogic techniques for opening up the air passageways and clearing the mind are particularly beneficial for the respiratory and nervous systems. The techniques are useful for treating asthma and other respiratory complaints and also stress, anxiety, and other psychological disorders.

(i) Pranayama (alternate nostril breathing)

- Sit comfortably on a chair or cushion. Take three deep, relaxing breaths. Place your right index finger between your eyebrows. Your right middle finger is placed lightly against your left nostril and your right thumb placed lightly against your right nostril. Relax your shoulders.
- Press your right middle finger against your left nostril to close off this nostril. Breathe in through your right nostril and hold the breath for a few seconds.
- Release your right middle finger as your press your right thumb against your right nostril. Breathe out through the left nostril.
- Breathe in through the left nostril and hold the breath. Release your right thumb as you press your middle finger and breathe out through your right nostril.
- Breathe in through your right nostril to commence the cycle again.
- Repeat this cycle of alternate nostril breathing for 20 or more breaths. Do not force the breath; the more gently you breath the easier the rhythm will become. If your nostrils are blocked you may need to use the following technique, Neti, for clearing your nostrils.

(ii) Neti (nasal cleansing)

Neti is an ancient yogic practice for clearing the nasal passageways of excess mucus, bacteria, dirt, etc. It also has a cooling and tranquilising effect on the mind. Neti is a helpful treatment for colds, sinusitis, upper respiratory tract infections, tonsillitis, inflammation of the adenoids and mucus membranes, ear infections, and even myopia. By calming the brain and nervous system it is also useful for treating hysteria, hyperactivity, temper tantrums, migraines and depression.

NETI TECHNIQUE
A special Neti pot is used, which looks like a small teapot. If a Neti pot is not available a small teapot can be used instead. Fill the pot with lukewarm salty water (one teaspoon of salt per litre of water). Open your mouth and breath through your mouth throughout the cleansing process. Slowly tilt your head to the right while simultaneously elevating the Neti pot with the spout in your left nostril. The salty water should flow in through your left nostril and out through your right nostril. Remember to keep breathing through your mouth which remains open. Allow the water to flow freely through the nostrils for about 20 seconds. Remove the spout and clean your nose by blowing fairly vigorously (do not blow too hard). Repeat the process by tilting the head to the left and inserting the Neti pot into the right nostril. Breathe through your mouth. Water should only pass through the nose. If any water enters the throat or mouth it is an indication that the head position is incorrect. Adjust the head until the water only flows through the nose.

If you have any problems consult a qualified yoga teacher. At first a slight burning sensation may be felt when the water passes through the nose. Your mucus membranes are not accustomed to contact with salty water. This possible discomfort will disappear after practising Neti a few times.

DRYING THE NOSE AFTER NETI
Stand up straight with your feet shoulder width apart and your hands clasped behind your back. Bend forward from the waist until your head is inverted. Remain in this position for about 30 seconds while any remaining water drains from your nose. Still in this forward position, blow vigorously through the nose five times, then return to the erect position. Close one nostril by pressing one finger against the side of the nostril then breathe in and out vigorously 30 times. Repeat the same process with the other nostril. Then repeat the same process with both nostrils open.

CONTRA-INDICATIONS
People who suffer from chronic nose bleeding should not do Neti. Also, those who have a structural blockage in the nose may not be able to pass the salty water freely through the nostrils.

FREQUENCY
Daily Neti in the mornings is an excellent preventative measure for opening the air passageways. In cases of acute disease, such as common cold, more frequent cleansing may be necessary.

NETI POT
To obtain a Neti pot in Australia by mail-order ring:

Colin and Janet Drake
Tomewin Pottery
Phone: (07) 5533 0298

CHAPTER TWELVE

Meditation for Health and Healing

The vast majority of illnesses are caused or aggravated by a stress component. The most immediate and insidious aspect of stress is what I call 'excessive thinking'.

Excessive thinking creates defensiveness, contraction and stagnation of the natural energy movement throughout the body. Excessive thinking contributes to ill health and can also prevent a sick body from healing. Understanding the 'thinking mind' and knowing how to let go of excessive thinking is enormously helpful for healing the body.

Our body has a myriad of healing mechanisms which are most effectively mobilised when we are relaxed. When we are stressed, challenged or worried, our body constantly prepares itself for 'fight or flight' – this is the Stress Response. In our contemporary society, many people use the Stress Response as a way of life – it becomes a habit, an identity and a lifestyle.

The Stress Response causes the following physiological responses:

- muscular contraction (we become 'uptight', literally);
- a shorter, faster breathing pattern;
- increased heart rate and blood pressure;
- a decrease in digestion, absorption and assimilation of nutrients;
- release of stress hormones: adrenalin, cortisol etc.

In other words, when we perceive a threat or a challenge (real or imaginary), our body reacts defensively. At these times, our body postpones resting, nurturing, repairing and recovery work as it moves into 'fight or flight' mode for self-protection and control – even if there is no real threat.

To create a healing environment in the body/mind, we need to be able to switch on the Relaxation Response, which has the following qualities:

- muscular relaxation;
- slower, deeper breathing (diaphragmatic breathing);
- a relaxed, open, present state of mind;
- letting go of control, worry and 'holding on';
- the body/mind is able to nurture and heal itself;
- the immune system is activated.

Meditation enables us to choose to step out of the Stress Response and rest in the Relaxation Response for prolonged periods of self-soothing, self-nurturing and healing through doing less. Meditation allows us to get out of our own way and to let healing happen naturally.

The Nature of Thinking and 'Excessive Thinking'

When used consciously and creatively, our thinking mind has enormous positive potential; when used unconsciously and unrestrained, our thinking mind can become destructive and create more problems than it solves. So, let's understand the strengths and limitations of the thinking mind so that we can learn to maximise its potential and avoid the stressful effects of excessive thinking.

The thinking mind is a goal-oriented mechanism. The tools of the thinking mind are memory and imagination. With these tools we are able to create and fulfil goals. We can recall desirable or undesirable experiences from the past and project desirable outcomes for the future. The thinking mind is able to step out of the flow of direct, felt experience (in the body and emotions) and remember the past or speculate about the future.

Thinking involves such functions as:

- judgement;
- evaluation;
- analysis;
- comparison;
- naming and labelling;
- future or past orientation;
- speculation.

These are the normal functions of the thinking mind, but if left unrestrained and unbalanced (by the other parts of our being) then these abilities become limitations, a strength becomes a weakness, i.e. excessive thinking.

Excessive thinking creates and sustains:

- worry, excessive speculation, 'awfulising', the 'what if' syndrome;
- guilt and shame;

- blame and resentment;
- pride, righteousness, stubbornness, intolerance;
- expectations of oneself or others that are too high;
- perfectionism;
- anxiety;
- excessive control of self or others;
- rigidity, i.e. 'taking a position' and holding onto it;
- an argumentative nature, needing to win or be right.

Buddhist philosophy tells us that these forms of excessive thinking are fuelled by the Three Poisons:

- Greed/Desire;
- Fear;
- Ignorance.

Excessive thinking is an attempt at control, which comes out of a lack of relaxation and trust and the inability to be 'in the moment'. By overusing the mechanisms of memory and imagination, we become overly attached to (or insistent on) our ideas of:
- good and bad;
- right and wrong;
- should and shouldn't;
- what I like and dislike;
- what I agree with and disagree with.

With excessive thinking, we take our thinking too seriously; we listen to it too closely and believe in the content of our thinking too much, when after all, it is only memory and imagination. Through excessive thinking, we make

our ego too rigid and we lose the healing abilities of forgiveness, humility, trust, acceptance, compassion and gratitude. We create a defensive, controlling internal environment instead of a healing environment. The regular practice of meditation enables us to take thinking less seriously and, hence, to break habits of being too judgemental, too critical, too analytical and too attached to our ideas of good/bad, right/wrong, agree/disagree, like/dislike. Then we can breathe, relax, let go and heal.

TYPES
of
MEDITATION

The types of meditation, which are most relevant for healing of the body/mind, are:

- Stillness Meditation;
- Creative Meditation using imagery.

Stillness meditation is the more passive of the two types of meditation. It consists of physical relaxation coupled with the practice of taking thoughts less seriously, i.e. learning to let go of the attachment to any particular train of thought. Stillness Meditation requires letting go of involvement with physical sensations, emotions and thoughts, but this does not mean that sensations, emotions or thoughts disappear altogether. This style of meditation creates a deeply relaxed internal environment in which the body is able to do its own work of repairing, re-balancing and healing. Imagery is a more active form of meditation utilising the creative power of the conscious mind by forming images which are conducive for health and healing.

Stillness Meditation

The first requirement for Stillness Meditation is to relax the physical body.

Here I will describe two techniques for physical relaxation:

- the Progressive Muscle Relaxation (PMR);
- the Body Scan.

Beginners should start by practising the Progressive Muscle Relaxation and gaining familiarity and competence with it. Then the Body Scan can be used instead of the PMR if preferred, as it takes less time. Both the PMR and the Body Scan are practised with calmness and thoroughness. The PMR involves taking your attention into each group of muscles in your body; actually squeezing and tensing the muscles then feeling the muscles relax and soften. Feel into the relaxation of that muscle group. If you lose track of your place in the PMR, i.e. if your attention drifts away, keep coming back and continuing with the practice. It is preferable to sit on a cushion or a chair for meditation as lying down easily leads to sleepiness. Meditation is not sleepy, wafty or dreamy – it is a state of relaxed, alert presence.

Sit up straight with your shoulders above your hips, not leaning too far forward or backward. Open your shoulders so that you are not slouched forward. Lower your chin slightly (without tilting your head down) and lift the top of your head to allow the muscles at the back of your neck to be long. Your ears are aligned over the tops of your shoulders. With this aligned posture, you will be able to 'sit like a mountain' – solid but very relaxed. Close your eyes gently, not squeezed tightly, eyelids just touching.

Note: You may wish to record the following PMR script and play it back to yourself at the beginning of your meditation.

PROGRESSIVE MUSCLE
RELAXATION TECHNIQUE

Bring your attention down to your feet. Feel into your feet, feel the pressure on the bottoms of your feet, the contact between the floor and your feet. By curling your toes under, squeeze the muscles of the feet … tighten … now relax and feel the feet soften as the muscles loosen and lengthen.

Now bring your attention to your calves. Feel into your calves. Squeeze the muscles of your calves by pushing your heels into the floor … tighten … now relax and allow the calf muscles to soften and loosen. Feel into the calves, feel the muscles … open and relaxed right through your calves.

Now bring your attention to your thighs, feeling into your thigh muscles. Feel the contact between your thighs and the cushion or chair. Now squeeze the muscles of your thighs by pushing your knees together but resisting the movement of your knees by tightening all the muscles of your thighs … squeeze and tighten … now soften and relax the thighs right through all the muscles … open and relaxed.

Bring you attention to your buttocks, feel the contact between your bottom and the chair/cushion … squeeze your buttocks, feel yourself lifting up slightly … relax and soften the muscles of your buttocks … feel yourself sinking down onto the chair/cushion as your buttocks soften and relax … the whole length of both legs softening and letting go.

Bring your attention to your belly, feel into it … and around the sides of your abdomen, right around to your lower back area … feel into the muscles of your belly and lower back. Now as you inhale, push out the belly and squeeze the muscles of the lower back … pushing and squeezing. Now relax the belly and soften the lower back area … soft belly, just letting go … the lower back area soft and loose.

Bring your attention to your chest and ribcage area, feel into your chest and right around the sides of your ribcage to your middle and upper back. Now as you inhale push out your chest like a barrel and squeeze the muscles of the middle and upper back … push and squeeze … now soften and relax. Feel the chest softening as the breath flows in and out, and your back muscles loosening and lengthening … the whole length of your torso just letting go.

Now sweep your attention down your arms, feeling into the muscles of the upper arms, lower arms, hands and fingers. Curl your fingers to make fists and begin to squeeze the fists … feel the contraction creeping up your arms as the muscles tighten. Now relax the fists and let your fingers uncurl ... feel the forearm and upper arms relax and loosen as the muscles soften ... the whole length of both arms just letting go.

Bring your attention to your shoulders, feel into the shoulder muscles from the base of the neck across to the tips of your shoulders. Now begin to lift your shoulders towards your ears, squeezing the shoulder muscles as you lift. Now let the shoulders drop and feel the muscles lengthening and loosening right through the shoulders.

Bring your attention to your neck. Feel into the neck muscles ... now tilt your head towards your left shoulder ... slowly return your head to the centre. Now tilt your head towards your right shoulder ... slowly return your head to the centre ... tilt your head forward, chin towards your chest. Now return your head to the centre and feel all of the neck muscles softening, loosening and lengthening.

Bring your attention to your jaw muscles, your tongue and lips. Feel into this whole jaw and mouth area ... now bite your teeth together, squeeze the muscles of your jaw and purse your lips ... relax the jaw, soften the tongue and lips ... your lips just softly touching. Now feel into your cheek muscles and all the tiny muscles around your eyes ... squeeze your cheek muscles as you squint your eyes and screw up all the muscles of your face. Now relax your cheeks, soften all the tiny muscles around your eyes with your eyelids just gently touching.

Now bring your attention to your forehead and scalp. Feel across the forehead and into the scalp right over your head ... raise your eyebrows, wrinkle the muscles of your forehead and squeeze.

Now relax and soften, allow the eyebrows to drop, your forehead smooth and the whole scalp relaxed ... your whole body just letting go. Starting from the top of your head, slowly scan your whole body right down to the tips of your toes, just checking that every muscle, every joint is soft and relaxed ... just letting go.

THE SECOND RELAXATION TECHNIQUE

The Body Scan, follows the same sequence as the PMR exercise, feeling into each muscle group, but without the muscular contraction. You simply place you attention into each area in turn, feeling for any sensations in that area such as tightness, tingling, coldness, heat, hardness, softness, etc. and you consciously allow each area to soften and relax, each body part just letting go.

The Body Scan takes less time than the PMR but ensure you do it thoroughly with attentiveness and presence. If you lose your focus, simply come back and continue to soften and let go. Don't worry about any areas that are resistant to letting go and relaxing, do the best you can and then continue on to the next part.

Now that your body is more relaxed and open, you can move further into Stillness Meditation by calming the mind. This does not mean fighting or struggling with thoughts in order to empty your mind. By fighting with thoughts or through any attempt to censor or suppress thoughts, we actually give too much importance or 'weight' to our thoughts. We make the mistake of bringing goal-orientation, judgement, evaluation and comparison into meditation. We cannot tame the 'monkey mind' by trying to catch it, chain it down, shut it up.

All such efforts only create more striving, more struggle and actually generate more thoughts and expectations.

In Stillness Meditation, we neither fight nor feed thoughts; we neither indulge nor deny thoughts. In other words, we don't take thoughts too seriously. Thoughts will come, we don't fight them; but when we find ourselves involved in a thought, we simply choose to let it go, i.e. we don't feed the thought.

The attitude of mind regarding thoughts can be summarised as no thought is a problem and no thought is important.

The importance of this attitude is that it takes energy away from the thinking mind, whereas if we fight or feed our thoughts, we give energy and importance to the thinking mind. Just as a child can be tied to their parents by rebellion or compliance, we become stuck in the thinking mind by reacting to it in any way. This reaction comes out of the thinking mind itself.

The technique of Stillness Meditation is designed to help practise this untroubled attitude towards thoughts.

Once you have relaxed the body, then create a focus for your attention. Each time a thought comes and takes your attention away from the focus of the meditation, you simply choose to let go of the thought and return to the focus. The focus for your attention may be your breathing; a word or mantra repeated in your mind; sensations in the body; a candle flame or a spot on the floor in front of you

When you let go of a thought, it may not disappear altogether. It may chatter away in the background but you re-establish the focus of the meditation as the foreground for your attention. The active aspect of meditation is constantly choosing to let go of any thought (even thoughts about meditation) and to return to the focus of the meditation. This simple act of will gradually builds mastery over the thinking mind … an essential step on the road to freedom and healing of the past. Remember, however, that meditation should be practised with ease, acceptance and compassion, not pushing, fighting or struggling to achieve a goal. Each breath, each instant to be enjoyed and accepted as it is.

Your concentration, when practising meditation, is a light concentration. If you try to concentrate too hard, you slip into a goal-oriented frame of mind, which only generates expectations, more thoughts and stress. Many beginners frustrate themselves by trying too hard and expecting too much, too soon.

Let's talk now about the focus that I recommend for the practice of Stillness Meditation. On completing the PMR or the Body Scan, become aware of the space behind your closed eyelids. This is the natural darkness you see when you close your eyes. The 'space behind your closed eyelids' is a very useful focus for your attention; it acts as a central point or an anchor for your mind. In Yogic philosophy, this area is called 'the Third eye'. You will notice that as thoughts come and take your attention, you lose the awareness of the space behind your closed eyelids.

As you let go of the thought, simply re-establish the focus on this space behind your closed eyelids. A secondary focus for your attention is your natural breathing. As you meditate, whenever a thought dominates your attention, simply choose to bring your attention back to the space behind your closed eyelids and feeling into the flow of your breathing.

Feel the touch of the air on your nostrils, the slight movement of your belly and ribcage as you breathe in and out; listen to the slight sound of your breathing. Allow the space behind your closed eyelids and the flow of your breathing to be the central focus for your attention, even if thoughts continue to chatter in the background. Remember that no thought is important and no thought is a problem.

Keep coming back to the central focus, without trying to analyse why you were distracted and without worrying about the fact that you were distracted. Continue to practise with patience, perseverance and presence.

SO LET'S REVIEW THE STEPS OF STILLNESS MEDITATION

a) Mentally give yourself permission to use the time to relax, heal and to be present. You don't have to fix anything, solve any problems or anticipate anything in the future. This is your time to be present.

b) Use the Progressive Muscle Relaxation or the Body Scan to relax the physical body.

c) Establish the focus of the meditation by becoming aware of the space behind your closed eyelids and feeling into each breath. This creates a sensual, in-the-moment, experiential focus for your attention. This sensual focus on NOW takes your attention away from the conceptual involvement in thoughts.

d) Patiently persevere, keep coming back to the focus of the meditation each time you get caught up in a thought.

e) Every now and again, check your posture and make sure that every part of your body is as open and relaxed as it can be.

f) Enjoy the meditation; it isn't a rigid discipline or something that requires an enormous effort. Stay relaxed, loose and natural.

g) To conclude your meditation, dedicate the meditation. Consciously direct the value (or the virtue) of the meditation towards self-healing, your peace of mind or you may send some thoughts/well wishes to someone else or a group. The traditional Buddhist dedication is 'may all beings find happiness and true peace'.

h) Allow your breathing to become a little deeper, move your hands and feet and, when you are ready, slowly open your eyes.

A full meditation session, as described above, may take 30–40 minutes or even longer, if you choose. Shorter periods of meditation are also beneficial. You can shorten the relaxation time to five minutes and then practice ten–15 minutes of breath awareness whilst looking into the space behind your closed eyelids.

If you find that your mind is very active and the meditation focus as described above isn't strong enough to hold your attention, you can strengthen the focus by repeating silently to yourself the word 'calm' as you inhale, and the word 'relax' as you exhale; keep bringing your mind back to this focus whenever you get caught up in a thought. As the mind calms you can stop repeating 'calm/relax' and use the focus on the third eye coupled with breath awareness.

At first, you may become bored with the Stillness Meditation but with practise and familiarity, you begin to appreciate the moments of stillness, and you realise that the emptiness and letting go create a wonderful space of peace and healing. You become acquainted with your calm, still centre of being ... a place of healing and peace.

Healing Imagery

Meditation and Healing Imagery can assist and complement any other therapies that you might choose to overcome illness and restore balance. Healing Imagery is a technique for creating positive, healing images with the mind and directing healing intentions to any part of the body/mind. Negative thoughts depress the immune system and stifle all the healing mechanisms of the body; whereas consciously created healing images accelerate the processes of repair and recovery from illness.

I use the word 'imagery' in preference to 'visualisation' because an image has more dimensions than just seeing pictures with your mind. An image can also have a feeling component and an auditory component as well as a picture. For example, to create an image of a 'waterfall' you may be able to create the picture of tumbling, cascades of water; you may also be able to sense the exhilarating, refreshing energy that surrounds the waterfall and you may be able to recall the sound of the waterfall. All these components of an image strengthen the image and make it more vivid. Some people find it difficult to create pictures inside their mind, but have less difficulty in creating the feeling component of an image. Even repeating the word 'waterfall' inside your mind creates some part of the image. Don't be despondent if you can't get a strong picture inside your mind – fleeting glimpses and the feeling sense of an image is enough to create the desired effect of imagery.

Imagery may be personal and specific to a certain situation or it may be universal and archetypal. Universal images are cross-cultural and have been used throughout human history. Universal images of healing are water, light and movement; whereas universal images of illness are darkness, hardness and stagnation.

In Chinese Medicine, there is a wise old saying, which goes: 'Qi follows Yi!' (translated: Energy follows Thought) An uplifting thought raises the spirits and stimulates the body's natural healing powers. Here I will describe two powerful healing imagery techniques:

• White Light Imagery;
• Inhaling the Light, Exhaling the Dark.

Imagery is most effective when coupled with Relaxation or used in conjunction with the Stillness meditation. The 'seeds' of imagery go deeper into the subconscious areas of the mind when the mind is relaxed and uncluttered.

WHITE LIGHT IMAGERY

a) Relax the body and calm the mind to some degree using Stillness Meditation.

b) Bring your awareness to the natural flow of your breathing and to the space behind your closed eyes.

c) Allow an image to form of a source of healing, life-affirming energy. You may choose an abstract image like a brilliant light, a more concrete image like the sun or a bright star, or you may choose a spiritual image like Buddha, Jesus, Mohamed or the Virgin Mary, or some saint or Holy person. Imagine that the source of healing energy is in front of you and just above the level of your head.

d) Feel yourself being open and receptive to healing energy. The healing source responds by sending streams of healing white (gold or silver) light towards you, radiating from the very centre of the healing source and extending towards you.

e) Feel or imagine that the white light begins to flow over the top of your head and trickle down, like a liquid nectar, flowing over and through your body. Feel into each body part as you imagine the white light washing through that part of your body, bringing light, cleansing, purifying healing energy into your body.

f) Wherever the white light meets hardness, tension or sickness in your body, imagine the white light softening the hardness, releasing the tension and healing the sickness. Continue to imagine and feel the white light flowing down through your body until it flows smoothly and evenly through every muscle, joint, tissue and cell of your body.

g) Give thanks for the healing white light.

INHALING THE LIGHT, EXHALING THE DARK

a) Relax the body and calm the mind to some degree using Stillness Meditation.

b) Bring your awareness to the natural flow of your breathing and to the space behind your closed eyes.

c) As you inhale, imagine that you are breathing in a white (gold or silver) mist that spreads through your whole body (or you may direct it towards a specific part of your body that needs healing).

d) As you exhale imagine that you are breathing out a black or dark light, releasing toxins and expelling disease from your body. Imagine that dark, heavy energy moving far away from you and being transmuted.

e) Continue this imagery for five–ten minutes.

f) Give thanks for the healing light.

Practice either of these imagery techniques diligently and patiently. Inject the imagery with your own attitude of enthusiasm and positivity. When finishing the imagery return to the Stillness Meditation for at least five minutes before ending the session. It can be very useful to remember the imagery, in an informal way, at any time of the day to strengthen the healing intention and to keep it working throughout the day.

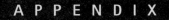

FOOD SOURCES OF COMMON VITAMINS AND MINERALS

The following foods are excellent sources of vitamins or minerals.

Vitamin A

- apricot
- asparagus
- banana
- broccoli
- carrots
- cod liver oil
- dark green leafy vegetables
- eggs
- liver
- papaya
- peach
- mango
- organ meats
- parsley
- pumpkin
- sweet corn
- sweet potato (yellow)
- whole milk dairy products

Vitamin B1

- beets
- blackstrap molasses
- brazil nuts
- brewer's yeast
- brown rice
- cashew nuts
- chicken
- chick peas
- eggs
- fish
- kelp
- kidney beans
- lentils
- peanuts
- peas
- port
- sesame seeds
- soya beans
- sunflower seeds
- turkey
- veal
- walnuts
- wheatgerm
- wholegrains

Vitamin B2

- almonds
- asparagus
- avocado
- brewer's yeast
- broccoli
- brussels sprouts
- chicken

- eggs
- fish
- lentils
- meat
- milk
- millet
- pork
- rice bran
- rye
- sesame seeds
- sprouted seeds
- sunflower seeds
- wheat bran
- wheatgerm
- wholegrains
- yoghurt

Vitamin B3

- almonds
- beets
- brown rice
- carrots
- chicken
- dates
- fish
- leafy greens
- millet
- mung beans
- peanuts
- pinto beans
- potatoes
- pumpkin seeds
- rice bran
- sesame seeds
- sunflower seeds
- tomatoes
- wheat bran
- wheatgerm

Vitamin B5

- almonds
- brewer's yeast
- cashews
- eggs
- kidney
- legumes
- liver
- mushrooms
- peanuts
- pork
- pumpkin seeds
- rice bran
- sesame seeds
- wheat bran
- wheatgerm

Vitamin B6

- bananas
- beans
- brewer's yeast
- broccoli
- brown rice
- carrots
- corn
- hazelnuts
- lentils
- potatoes
- rice bran
- salmon
- sesame seeds
- soybeans
- sunflower seeds
- tuna
- walnuts
- wheat bran
- wheatgerm
- yoghurt

Vitamin B12

- brewer's yeast
- cauliflower
- cheese
- eggs
- herring
- leafy greens
- liver
- mackerel
- milk
- mushrooms
- spirulina
- yoghurt

Biotin

- almonds
- chicken
- eggs
- leafy greens
- liver
- meat
- milk
- peanuts
- rice
- sardines
- soybeans
- walnuts
- wholegrains

Folic acid

- almonds
- bran
- brewer's yeast
- brown rice
- cheese
- chicken
- green leafy vegetables
- legumes

- milk
- mushrooms
- oranges
- root vegetables
- salmon
- soybeans
- sprouted seeds
- tuna
- wholegrains

Vitamin C

- acerola cherries
- asparagus
- avocado
- berries
- blackcurrants
- broccoli
- brussels sprouts
- capsicum
- cauliflower
- citrus fruits
- guava
- kiwi fruit
- lychees
- mangos
- papaya
- parsley
- rosehips
- spinach
- tomatoes

Vitamin E

- almonds
- avocado
- brazil nuts
- brown rice
- cashews
- cold pressed oils
- cornmeal

- eggs
- hazelnuts
- kelp
- leafy vegetables
- liver
- millet
- molasses
- peanuts
- pecans
- sunflower seeds
- sweet potatoes
- walnuts
- wheatgerm

Coenzyme Q10

- beef
- mackerel
- tuna
- salmon
- sardines
- spinach
- tuna
- peanuts

Calcium

- almonds
- asparagus
- bananas
- blackstrap molasses
- brazil nuts
- brewer's yeast
- broccoli
- brussels sprouts
- cabbage
- dairy products
- dandelion greens
- figs
- green leafy vegetables
- hazelnuts
- mackerel

- okra
- olives
- parmesan
- prunes
- ricotta
- salmon
- sardines
- sesame seeds
- shellfish
- soya beans
- spinach
- sunflower seeds
- wheat bran
- yoghurt

Iron

- almonds
- apricots
- avocados
- beets
- brown rice
- cashew nuts
- chick peas
- dates
- kelp
- kidney beans
- lentils
- lima beans
- millet
- mung beans
- parsley
- peaches
- pears
- prunes
- pumpkin seeds
- rice bran
- sesame seeds
- soya beans
- sunflower seeds
- wheat bran

Iodine

- asparagus
- blueberries
- cucumber
- garlic
- kelp
- lima beans
- mushrooms
- okra
- peanuts
- sea salt
- sesame seeds
- soya beans
- spinach
- strawberries
- turnip greens
- watermelon

Magnesium

- apples
- apricots
- avocados
- bananas
- blackstrap molasses
- brown rice
- dairy products
- dates
- fish
- green leafy vegetables
- hazelnuts
- lentils
- lima beans
- millet
- meat
- peaches
- peanuts
- pecan nuts
- pistachio nuts
- sesame seeds
- soya beans
- wheatgerm
- wholegrains

Potassium

- almonds
- apricots
- avocados
- bananas
- blackstrap molasses
- brazil nuts
- brewer's yeast
- brown rice
- chick peas
- dates
- figs
- garlic
- hazelnuts
- lentils
- parsley
- pecan nuts
- pistachio nuts
- potatoes
- raisins
- sesame seeds
- soya beans
- sweet potato (yellow)
- wheatgerm
- wholegrains

Zinc

- almonds
- barley
- brazil nuts
- brewer's yeast
- brown rice
- cashew nuts
- chicken
- eggs
- fish
- hazel nuts

- kelp
- legumes
- lima beans
- liver
- meat
- olives
- oysters
- pecan nuts
- pumpkin seeds
- rye
- sardines
- soya beans
- soy lecithin
- sunflower seeds
- walnuts

BIBLIOGRAPHY

Allardice, Pamela, *Essential Oils*, Ken Fin. Harper Collins, 1994

Balch, James and Phyllis, *Prescriptions for Nutritional Healing*, Avery Publishing Group, New York, 1998

Beckham, Nancy, *The Australian Family Guide to Natural Therapies,* Greenhouse Publications, 1988

Bradford, Nikki, *The Hamlyn Encyclopedia of Complementary Health*, Hamlyn, 1996

Callinan, Paul, *Australian Family Homeopathy*, Penguin, Australia, 1995

Castro, Miranda, *The Complete Homeopathy Handbook*, Macmillan, London, 1990

Hoffman, David, *The New Holistic Herbal,* Element Books Ltd, 1991

Jacka, Judy, *A–Z of Natural Therapies*, Lothian, Melbourne, 1987

Jelinek, Professor George, *Taking Control of Multiple Schlerosis*, Hyland House, Flemington, 2001

Jensen, Dr Bernard, *Foods That Heal*, Avery Publishing Group Inc., 1993

Kirchheimer, Sid, *The Doctor's Book of Home Remedies*, Prevention Magazine Health Books, 1993

Kirschmann, Gayla and John, *Nutrition Almanac*, McGraw-Hill, New York, 1996

Koch, Manfred Urs, *Laugh with Health*, Mastertech Publishing, 1996

Lu, Henry, *Chinese System of Food Cures*, Sterling Publishing Co, 1996

Murray, Michael and Pizzorno, Joseph, *Encyclopedia of Natural Medicine*, Little, Brown and Company, UK, 1998

Osiekck, Henry, *The Physicians Handbook of Clinical Nutrition*, Bioconcepts Publishing, 1990

Shreeve, Dr Caroline, *The Alternative Dictionary of Symptoms and Cures*, Leopard Books, 1995

Tierra, Michael, *Planetary Herbology*, Lotus Press, 1997

Werback, Melvyn, *Nutritional Influences on Illness*, Thorsons Publishers Ltd., 1989

Webb, Peter, *Family Encyclopedia of Homeopathic Remedies*, Book Company, NSW, 1997

Vogel, Dr. H.C.A. – *The Nature Doctor.* Mainstream Publishing, 1991

INDEX